Pharmaceutical Technology I

Pharmaceutical Technology I

Gaurav Agarwal MPharm (BITS-Pilani) PhD
Dean, Faculty of Pharmacy
RP Educational Trust
Karnal, Haryana

Atul Kaushik MPharm (BITS-Pilani) PhD
GM, Watson Pharma
Mumbai

CBSPD

CBS Publishers & Distributors Pvt Ltd

New Delhi • Bengaluru • Chennai • Kochi • Kolkata • Lucknow • Mumbai
Hyderabad • Jharkhand • Nagpur • Patna • Pune • Uttarakhand

Pharmaceutical Technology I

ISBN: 978-81-239-2294-2

First Edition: 2014

Reprint: 2017, 2019, 2022

Published by Satish Kumar Jain and produced by Varun Jain for

CBS Publishers & Distributors Pvt Ltd

4819/XI Prahlad Street, 24 Ansari Road, Daryaganj, New Delhi 110 002, India
Ph: 011-23289259, 23266861, 23266867   Website: www.cbspd.com
Fax: 011-23243014   e-mail: delhi@cbspd.com; cbspubs@airtelmail.in
Corporate Office: 204 FIE, Industrial Area, Patparganj, Delhi 110 092

Ph: 011-4934 4934   Fax: 011-4934 4935   e-mail: publishing@cbspd.com;
publicity@cbspd.com

Branches

• **Bengaluru:** Seema House 2975, 17th Cross, K.R. Road, Banasankari 2nd Stage, Bengaluru 560 070, Karnataka, India
  Ph: +91-80-26771678/79   Fax: +91-80-26771680   e-mail: bangalore@cbspd.com
• **Chennai:** 7, Subbaraya Street, Shenoy Nagar, Chennai 600 030, Tamil Nadu, India
  Ph: +91-44-26680620, 26681266   Fax: +91-44-42032115   e-mail: chennai@cbspd.com
• **Kochi:** 42/1325, 1326, Power House Road, Opp. KSEB, Power House, Ernakulam 682018, Kochi, Kerala, India
  Ph: +91-484-4059061-65   Fax: +91-484-4059065   e-mail: kochi@cbspd.com
• **Kolkata:** 147, Hind Ceramics Compound, 1st Floor, Nilgunj Road, Belghoria, Kolkata-700056, West Bengal, India
  Ph: 033-25633055, 033-25633056   e-mail: kolkata@cbspd.com
• **Lucknow:** Basement, Khushnuma Complex, 7, Meerabai Marg (Behind Jawahar Bhawan), Lucknow 226001 (UP), India
  Ph: 0522-4000032   e-mail: tiwari.lucknow@cbspd.com
• **Mumbai:** PWD Shed, Gala No. 25/26, Ramchandra Bhatt Marg, Next to JJ Hospital, Gate No. 2, Opp. Union Bank of India, Noorbaug, Mumbai 400009 Maharashtra, India
  Ph: +91-22-66661880/89   e-mail: mumbai@cbspd.com

Representatives

• **Hyderabad**   0-9885175004   • **Jharkhand**   0-9811541605   • **Nagpur**   0-9421945513
• **Patna**   0-9334159340   • **Pune**   0-9623451994   • **Uttarakhand** 0-9716462459

Printed at Neekunj Print Process, Haryana, India

to
Shreya, Danya and Vaidish

Foreword

It is our privilege to write a few words about Dr Gaurav Agarwal's and Dr Atul Kaushik's textbook "Pharmaceutical Technology-I". This book is a ready reckoner for B. Pharmacy students.

The efforts have been mainly taken to focus on the primary aspects of students of Pharmacy undergoing degree and diploma courses of various degree/diploma awarding bodies. It seems to be one of the finest efforts of its own kind to offer a wide range of various fundamentals in the field of pharmaceutics from the very traditional to the modern trends of sciences and cutting edge technologies of today. Pharmaceutics, being an interdisciplinary subject, is today covering a wide range of interest both among the students and teaching communities. We compliment authors for simple and explicit presentation. And sure that this book is going to become popular and sought after by pharmacy students. We wish the authors success in their present venture and urge them to continue this good and noble work by publishing more books for the benefit of pharmacy students.

Dr Agarwal and Dr Kaushik are to be congratulated for the tremendous efforts they have taken in compiling this useful work for budding pharmacy technocrats. The present book admirably fills up the various gaps between the pharmacy students and the basic knowledge required for specialized training of the subject. Authors have distilled their vast experience of teaching and research in this compact and concise text for students and teachers of pharmacy.

Presently Dr Gaurav is working with **RPIIT**. RPIIT, an institution of par excellence, has reached unflinching success in its strides for imparting quality education. It is the largest *integrated*, hi-tech, state-of-art facilitated private campus in Northern India located at **Karnal (Haryana).** RPIIT institute is presently offering various technical and professional courses like **B. Tech, B. Arch, B. Pharmacy, MBA, PGDBM** affiliated to Kurukshetra University and Pt B. D. Sharma University of Health Sciences, Haryana (India). The main objective of the institute is to train the student in such a manner that they can consider every problem as a challenge, transform every challenge into opportunity, seize every opportunity and ensure growth in every aspect of life by utilizing all the technical skills imbibed.

Dr Rajiv Singal
MD, MS (Orthopaedics)
Vice Chairman
RP Educational Trust,
Karnal (Haryana)

Dr Nidhi Singal
MD, MS
(Gynaecologist)

Contributors

Gajendra Singh M Pharm PhD
Dean, Faculty of Pharmaceutical Sciences
Pt. BD Sharma University of Health Sciences, Rohtak

Ravindra Tiwari M Pharm (PhD)
Senior Reserach Scientist
Ranbaxy Research Laboratories, Gurgaon

Subrato Kundu M Pharm
Senior Reserach Scientist
Vergo, Goa

Ish Grover M Pharm
Assistant Professor in Pharmaceutics
Faculty of Pharmacy
RPIIT Technical Campus, Karnal

Bharat Khurana M Pharm
Assistant Professor in Pharmaceutics
DIPM, Karnal

Daisy Arora M Pharm
Assistant Professor in Pharmaceutics
DIPM, Karnal

Pallavi Sharma (M Pharm)
DIPSAR, Delhi University
Delhi

Shubhangi Bhilla (M Pharm)
Faculty of Pharmacy
RPIIT Technical Campus, Karnal

Anshuman Agarwal (B Pharm)
Faculty of Pharmacy
RPIIT Technical Campus, Karnal

Preface

"Pharmaceutical Technology I" is designed and written intentionally for newcomers to the design of dosage form. The subject matter of the book remains the same in essence but the details have been changed significantly because pharmaceutics has changed. It contains a comprehensive description, an overview of existing knowledge of Pharmaceutics and making it appropriate for introductory and institutional purposes.

Being an interdisciplinary subject, it is today covering a wide range of interest both among the students and teaching communities. Taking this increasing interest into account, this book gives a comprehensive introduction to the subject. The book is primarily intended as a text for students of Pharmacy for degree and diploma courses. The structure and the content of the book have changed to reflect modern thinking and current university curricula throughout the world. The involvement of wide range of authors in this edition, all are accepted experts in the field on which they have written and, just as importantly, all have experience and ability in conveying that information to undergraduate pharmacy and pharmaceutical sciences students.

The book contains numerous specimens, vivid illustrations, tables, diagrams and flow diagrams to present the ideas. The distinguishing feature is practical experiment related to subject at the end of the book. In spite of great care there might be some mistakes and deficiencies. We will be grateful for getting suggestions to improve upon the text material. So go through the content and do mail to us at *gbitsian@rediffmail.com*.

Gaurav Agarwal
Atul Kaushik

Acknowledgments

It is a moment of great pleasure and immense satisfaction for me to express deep gratitude and gratefulness to **Prof. (Dr) Gajendra Singh, Dean**, Faculty of Pharmaceutical Sciences, Pt B.D. Sharma University of Health Sciences, Rohtak for inspiring me to bring out this book.

I am specially thankful to **Shri RP Singal, Chairman, RP Educational Trust**, for his all-time support and encouragement.

My special thanks to Er Bharat Singal, Secretary, RP Educational Trust for inspiring us to bring out this book.

I am indebted to Dr Saurabh Gupta, Director RPIIT Technical Campus. Dr GS Sharma, Executive Director, RPIIT Technical Campus, Dr PK Karar, Principal, Faculty of Pharmacy, RPIIT Technical Campus, for their motivation.

Special thanks to my peers Ish, Nitika, Nidhi, Anju, Renu, Nitesh, Jasvinder, Ravinder, Sandeep for their moral support.

I express my gratefulness to Shri YN Arjuna, Senior Director—Publishing, Editorial and Publicity, CBS Publishers and Distributors and special thanks to Shri Satish K Jain, Proprietor, CBS Publishers and Distributors for their sincere efforts.

Last but not least, I express my love to my wife Shilpi and regards to my parents for their all time inspiration and dedication. They are the major driving force in bring out this achievement!

To my numerous students, whom I cannot possibly name individually, I say thanks for their class interactions which have been the guiding spirit in selection of the subject matter and its logical arrangement.

Gaurav Agarwal

I would like to acknowledge the large heartedness of my family and colleagues. My family was supportive from the beginning and encouraged me to write this book. I would like to appreciate the critical eyes and viewpoints of my friends Dhawal, Haripriya, Puthoori and Munish, who read the drafts and kept me on the correct path. I thank Dr Ravindra Tiwari and Mr Subrato Kundu who spent a good deal of time in writing the text for the chapters. I would also like to thank Mr Praveen Raheja, Mr Kamal Mehta and Mr. Rakesh Kumar Bhasin who have always been inspirational to me.

This book is dedicated to all the students to whom I have taught in IFTM, Moradabad and ITS, Ghaziabad. I hope students of pharmaceutics will appreciate this book.

At last I would like to thank the almighty.

Atul Kaushik

Contents

Preformulation Studies

DEFINITION

Preformulation (pre+formulation, i.e. prior to formulation) as the name depicts before initiating formulation development, preformulation is the step to understand physicochemical (physical and chemical) properties of drug substance. Preformulation studies help the formulation scientist to develop in-depth understanding about physicochemical parameters of drug substance, which leads to design optimum drug delivery system without significant barriers during development. In other words, preformulation studies describe as the process of optimizing the delivery of drug through determination of physicochemical properties of the new compound that could effect drug performance and development of an efficacious, stable and safe dosage form.

Before beginning the formal preformulation programs, the preformulation scientist must consider the following factors:

- The amount of drug available.
- The physicochemical properties of the drug already known.
- Therapeutic category and anticipated dose of compound.

Objectives of Preformulation Studies

The primary objectives of preformulation studies are as follows:

1. Establish the identity and physicochemical parameters of a new drug substance.
2. Establish chemical stability profile of drug substance.

3. Bulk characterization.
4. Establish drug substance compatibility with common excipients.
5. Establish relation between physicochemical properties of drug substance and formulation stability. Preformulation studies give preliminary idea about selection of excipients, which makes the formulation stable.
6. Establish relation between physicochemical properties of drug substance and bioavailability. Preformulation studies give preliminary idea about selection of excipients, selection of particle size and morph of drug substance, which can affect bioavailability of drug.
7. Preformulation studies give preliminary idea about selection of manufacturing process. For example, if drug substance has fine particle size, then it is advisable to use granulation process instead of direct compression because there is possibility of blend non-uniformity, if direct compression method is used.

Studies Involved in Preformulation

Following studies are conducted as basic preformulation studies; special studies are conducted depending on the type of dosage form and the type of drug molecule:

1. Organoleptic properties
2. Purity
3. Bulk characterization
   - Particle size distribution
   - Surface area
   - Density
   - Wettability
   - Hygroscopicity
   - Compression property
   - Crystallinity and polymorphism
   - Powder flow property
     a. Bulk density
     b. Angle of repose
4. Physicochemical properties
   - Solubility analysis

- Intrinsic solubility
- pH solubility profile
  - Common ion effect (ksp)
  - Solubilization
  - pKa determination
  - Solvent
  - Partition coefficient
  - Dissolution
  - Effect of temperature
5. Assay developments
6. Stability analysis
   - Solution stability
   - Solid state stability
     - Hydrolysis
     - Oxidation
     - Pyrolysis/elevated temperature studies
     - Photolysis
   - Stability under high humidity condition
7. Active drug compatibility with excipients or excipient compatibility.

Organoleptic Properties

Organoleptic properties provide useful information mainly color, odor and taste of the drug substance. A few examples of these three organoleptic properties are tabulated in Table 1.1.

Table 1.1: Organoleptic properties of drug substance

Color	Odor	Taste
White	Pungent	Acidic
Off white	Sulfurous	Bitter
Cream yellow	Fruity	Intense
Tan	Aromatic	Sweet
Shiny	Odorless	Bland (smooth)

Organoleptic properties help in identification of the drug substance as well as they help to identify any degradation. For example, when oxidation reaction produces a colored degraded product, it will often be detected by human eye. Smell can be an effective method by which chemical and microbiological instabilities can be detected.

Purity

The preformulation scientists must have knowledge of the purity of a drug substance. Thin layer chromatography (TLC) and high pressure liquid chromatography (HPLC) are of very wide ranging applicability and are excellent tools for characterizing the chemical homogeneity of many types of materials. Paper chromatography and gas chromatography can also be used in the determination of chemical homogeneity. All of these techniques can be designed to give a quantitative estimate of purity.

Bulk Characterization

Particle Size Distribution

Bulk flow, formulation homogeneity, and surface area controlled processes such as dissolution and chemical reactivity are directly affected by size, shape and surface morphology of the drug particles. In general, each new drug candidate should be tested during preformulation with the smallest particle size as is practical to facilitate preparation of homogeneous samples and maximize the drug's surface area for interactions.

Various chemical and physical properties of drug substances are affected by their particle size distribution and shapes. The effect is not only on the physical properties of solid drugs but also, in some instances, on their biopharmaceutical behavior. It is generally recognized that poorly soluble drugs showing a dissolution-rate limiting step in the absorption process will be more readily bioavailable when administered in a finely subdivided state rather than as a coarse material. Gibbs-Kelvin has explained the relationship between particle size and solubility.

Gibbs-Kelvin relation: It is a relationship between particle size and apparent solubility of a drug.

$$\log\left(\frac{S_r}{S_\alpha}\right) = \frac{2\gamma_{SL}M}{2.303\ RT\ \rho r}$$

where, S_r = apparent solubility of a drug

S_α = true equilibrium solubility

γ_{SL} = interfacial energy that exists between solid and liquid

r = radius of particle

M = molecular weight

R = gas constant

T = absolute temperature

ρ = density of the solid

In case of tablets, size influences the flow and the mixing efficiency of powders and granules. Size can also be a factor in stability; fine materials are relatively more open to attack from atmospheric oxygen, the humidity, and interacting excipients than coarse materials.

Particle Size Determination (Table 1.2)

1. Simple method—microscopy with help of light microscope and sieving (but sieving is a less useful technique at preformulation stage due to lack of bulk material)
2. Instrument based on light scattering—ROYCO
3. Instrument based on light blockage—HIAC
4. Instrument based on blockage of electrical conductivity path—Coulter counter
5. Based on rate difference of sedimentation of different particle—Anderson pipette method

Table 1.2: Common techniques for measurement

Technique	Particle size (μm)
Microscopic	1–100
Sieve	>50
Sedimentation	>1
Permeability	>1
Centrifugal	<50
Light scattering	0.5–50

Surface Area

Reason for controlling the particle size is that changes will alter the available surface area and consequently affect dissolution and potentially bioavailability.

Methods of determination

BET nitrogen absorption: A precise measurement of surface area is based on Brunaver, Emette, Teller (BET) theory of adsorption. Most substances adsorb a monomolecular layer of gas under certain conditions of partial pressure of gas and temperature. Here nitrogen absorption in which a layer of nitrogen molecule is absorbed to the sample surface at $-196°C$. Once surface absorption reached equilibrium, the sample is heated to room temperature, the nitrogen gas is desorbed and its volume is measured and converted to the number of absorbed molecule via the ideal gas low.

SEM (scanning electron microscope): Surface morphology can be observed by an SEM which serves to confirm qualitatively a physical observation related to surface area.

Density

Bulk density of a compound varies substantially with the method of crystallization, milling or formulation. It is of great importance when one considers the size of high capsule product or the homogeneity of a low dose formulation in which there are larger difference in drug and excipient densities.

Bulk density = mass of powder/bulk volume

Wettability

Wetting is an adsorption process in which an intimate contact of the solid phase is achieved. The process is important in the following ways:

1. Intimate contact of solids with liquid or liquids with liquid is an initial step towards the preparation of suspension and emulsion.

2. In granulation prior to tabletting, the powders are mixed with a liquid binding agent. The success of this process in part depends on the wetting and spreading of the liquid over the solid.

3. Film coating requires the wetting and spreading of liquids (containing coating material) over the tablet surface.

4. Dissolution of a tablet or a capsule requires the penetration of liquid into pores of the dosage form.

Surfactants are used to aid wetting of powders, because of their following properties:

a. Lowering the interfacial tension
b. Lowering of contact angle between the solids and liquids
c. Displacing air and permit the intimate contact

Contact angle (Fig. 1.1) is used as an indicator to evaluate the efficiency of a wetting agent. Contact angle can be defined as angle between the liquid droplets and surface over which they spread.

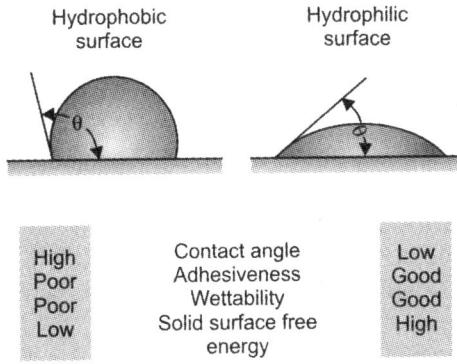

Hydrophobic surface   Hydrophilic surface

High	Contact angle	Low
Poor	Adhesiveness	Good
Poor	Wettability	Good
Low	Solid surface free energy	High

Fig. 1.1: Contact angle, an indicator of adhesiveness, wettability and surface free energy

At equilibrium, Young's equation (Fig. 1.2) defines relationship between contact angle, solid/liquid interfacial free energy, solid free energy and liquid free energy. According to Young's equation

$$\gamma^{sv} = \gamma^{sl} + \gamma^{lv} \cos\theta$$

θ is the contact angle
γ^{sl} is the solid/liquid interfacial free energy
γ^{sv} is the solid surface free energy
γ^{lv} is the liquid surface free energy

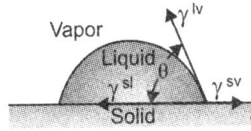

Fig. 1.2: Young's equation and relationship

Examples, with contact angle values;

$\theta = 0°$ a drop of water on a glass surface

$\theta > 90°$ a drop of fatty acid on a clean glass surface or a drop of water on a paraffin coated surface

$\theta = 109°$ a drop of water on Teflon

Hygroscopicity

Many drug substances, particularly water-soluble salt form, have tendency to adsorb atmospheric moisture. Adsorption and equilibrium moisture can depend upon the atmospheric humidity, temperature, surface area, exposure and mechanism for moisture uptake.

Deliquescent material adsorbs sufficient water to dissolve completely, e.g. sodium chloride on a humid day. Other hygroscopic substances adsorb water because of hydrate formation or specific site adsorption.

With most hygroscopic materials, changes in moisture level can greatly influence many important parameters, such as chemical stability, flowability and compatibility.

Analytical methods for monitoring the moisture level are:

a. Gravimetry

b. TGA (thermogravimetric analysis)

c. Karl-Fischer titration

d. Gas chromatography

Compression Characteristics

Benefit to be derived from compression testing is an indication of whether the drug is elastic, plastic or brittle. In order to make a good tablet, there is a need for brittle fracture and plastic flow, elasticity is also often present, but it is not a desirable property. For example, if the drug is plastic material, the diluent should compact by brittle fracture (e.g. lactose). If the drug is brittle material, it is best to mix it with a plastic excipient such as microcrystalline cellulose.

There are three processes by which we can formulate the drug substance into tablets:

1. Direct compression

2. Wet granulation

3. Slugging/dry granulation

Method (A): Shows tablet formed by direct compression,

Method (B): Shows tablet formed by wet granulation and

Method (C): Shows tablet formed by dry granulation respectively.

Method of compression testing

Based on evaluation, process will be selected.

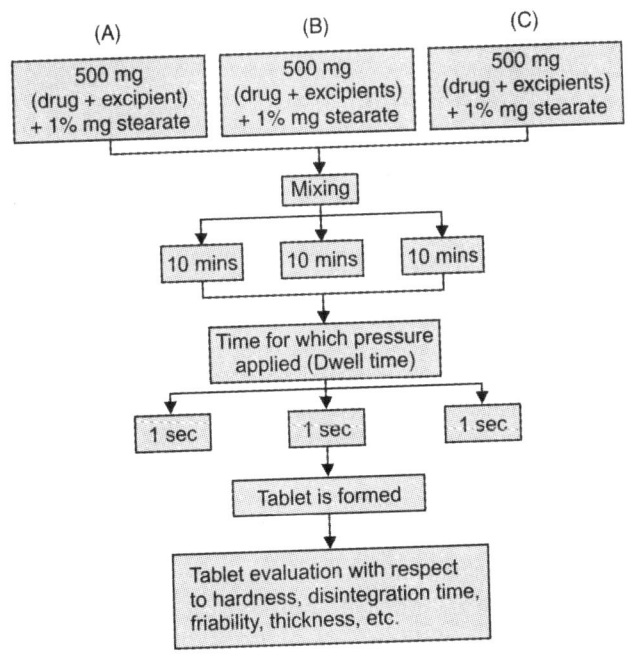

Crystallinity and Polymorphism

Crystal habit and internal structure of a drug can affect bulk and physicochemical properties which ranged from flowability to chemical stability.

Habit is described as the outer appearance of a crystal's internal structure in molecular arrangement within the solid.

Changes with internal structure usually alter the crystal habit. Chemical changes as conversion of a sodium salt to its free acid form produce both a change in internal structure and crystal habit.

Characterization of a solid volume

1. Verifying that the solid is the expected chemical compound.
2. Characterizing the internal structure.
3. Describing the habit of the crystal.

The internal structure of a compound can be classified as given in Table 1.3.

Table 1.3: Various crystal systems (Fig. 1.3)

Sr. no.	Crystal system	Angle of axis	Length of axis	Example
1	Cubic (regular system)	$\alpha = \beta = \gamma = 90°$	$a = b = c$	NaCl
2	Tetragonal	$\alpha = \beta = \gamma = 90°$	$a = b \neq c$	Nickel sulfide
3	Orthorhombic	$\alpha = \beta = \gamma = 90°$	$a \neq b \neq c$	$KMnO_4$
4	Monoclinic	$\alpha = \gamma = 90°$ and $\beta \neq 90°$	$a \neq b \neq c$	Sucrose
5	Triclinic (asymmetric)	$\alpha \neq \beta \neq \gamma \neq 90°$	$a \neq b \neq c$	$CuSO_4$
6	Trigonal (rhombohedral)	$\alpha = \beta = \gamma \neq 90°$	$a = b = c$	Sodium nitrate
7	Hexagonal	$\alpha = \beta = 90°$ and $\gamma = 120°$	$a = b \neq c$	$AgNO_3$

Polymorphism

When a substance exists in more than one crystalline form, the different forms are designated as polymorphs and the phenomenon as polymorphism. Polymorphism also influences biopharmaceutical behavior of drug. A pure more soluble B form of chloramphenicol palmitate was more available after oral administration as compared to less soluble pure A form and their mixture.

Amorphous forms are typically prepared by rapid precipitation, lyophilization or rapid cooling of liquid melts. Since amorphous forms are usually of higher thermodynamic energy than corresponding crystalline forms, solubility as well as dissolution rates are generally greater.

Polymorphisms are of two types:

1. *Enantiotropic:* It is the one which can be reversibly change into another form by altering the temperature or pressure, e.g. sulfur.

2. *Monotropic:* It is the one in which transition from one polymorph to another will be irreversible.

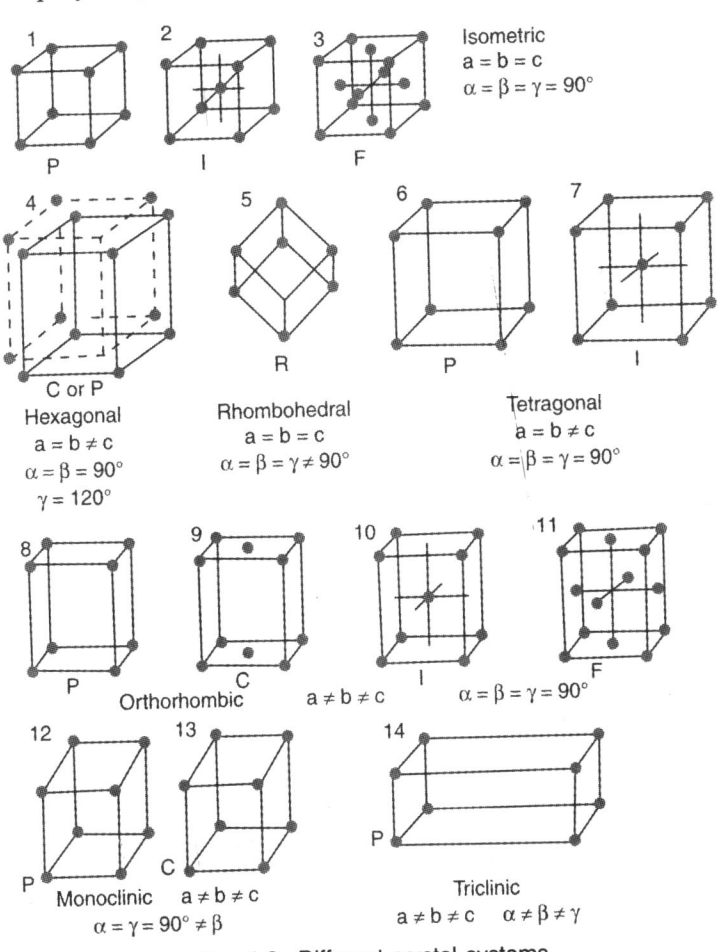

Fig. 1.3: Different crystal systems

Depending upon their relative stability, one of the several polymorphic forms will be physically more stable than others. Stable polymorph represents lowest energy state, has highest melting point and least aqueous solubility. The remaining polymorphs are called metastable forms which represent the higher energy state, have low melting point and high aqueous solubility. Because of their higher energy state, the metastable forms have a thermodynamic tendency to convert to the stable form.

Order of dissolution

Amorphous > Metastable > Stable

Detection: Morph compound can be detected by following techniques:

- Optical crystallography
- X-ray diffractions
- Differential scanning calorimetry

Pseudopolymorphism

A crystalline compound may contain either a stoichiometric or non-stoichiometric amount of crystallization solvent.

Non-stoichiometer adducts such as inclusion or clathrates, involve entrapped solvent molecules within the crystal lattice. Usually, this adduct is undesirable, owing to its lack of reproducibility and should be avoided for development.

Stoichiometric adduct, commonly referred to as solvate is a molecular complex that has incorporated the crystallizing solvent molecules into specific sites within the crystal lattice. The solvate can exist in different crystalline forms called pseudopolymorph and phenomenon called pseudopolymorphism.

When the incorporated solvent is water, the complex is called a hydrate and the terms hemihydrate, monohydrate and dihydrate describe various hydrate forms. A compound not containing any water is called anhydrous compound. Generally, the anhydrous form of a drug has a greater aqueous solubility than the hydrates. This is because the hydrates are already in interaction with water and, therefore, has less energy for crystal break-up in comparison to anhydrates (thermodynamically higher energy state) for further interaction of water, e.g. ampicillin and theophylline anhydrous forms have more aqueous solubility. Pseudopolymorphs should be identified since most polymorphs can be obtained by changing the recrystallizing solvent. Solvent including polymorphic changes are: water, methanol, ethanol, acetone, chloroform, n-propanolol, isopropyl alcohol, n-butanol, n-pentanol, benzene and toluene.

The presence of traces of solvent (either water or organic) is usual in early batches of new drug candidates, as residue from the precipitation process in the final crystalli-zation. These can become molecular addition to the crystal and change in its habit.

These hydrates and solvates (e.g. methanolate, ethanolate) have been confused with the true polymorphism. The distinction between these false forms and true polymorphs can be obtained by observing the melting behavior of the compound dispersed in silicon oil using hot stage microscopy. Pseudopolymorphs will evolve a gas (steam or solvent vapor) causing bubbling of the oil. True polymorphs merely melt, forming a second globular phase. The temperature at which the solvent volatilizes will be close to the boiling point of the solvent and can be used for identification.

Powder Flow Properties

Assessment of flow properties of a drug powder is important to the formulator. When limited amounts of drug are available, then it can be evaluated simply by measurement of: (a) bulk density; and (b) angle of repose.

a. *Bulk density:* Bulk density of the drug substance is very useful in having some idea as to the size of final dosage form. Carr's compressibility index and Hausner index can be used to predict the flow property based on density measurement (Tables 1.4 and 1.5).

Car index (%) or consolidation index

$$= \frac{\text{Tapped density} - \text{Poured density}}{\text{Tapped density}} \times 100$$

$$\text{Hausner index} = \frac{\text{Tapped density}}{\text{Poured density}}$$

Fluff (poured) density is the ratio of mass of powder to the fluff volume. Fluff volume is the volume occupied by a certain mass, when gently poured into a measuring cylinder. Tapped density is the ratio of mass of powder to the tapped volume. Tapped volume is the volume occupied by the same mass of powder after a standard tapping.

Table 1.4: Grading of the powder for their flow properties, according to Carr index

Consolidation index (Carr index, %)	Flow
5–15	Excellent
12–16	Good
18–21*	Fair to passable
23–35*	Poor
33–38	Very poor
>40	Very very poor

*Adding the glidant, e.g. 0.2% aerosil should improve the flow

Table 1.5: Compressibility and flowability of pharmaceutical excipients

Material	% compressibility	Flow
Celutab	11	Excellent
Emcompress	15	Excellent
Star X-1500	19	Fair passable
Lactose monohydrate	19	Fair passable
Maize starch	26–27	Poor
Dicalcium phosphate dihydrate (coarse)	27	Poor
Magnesium stearate	31	Poor
Titanium dioxide	34	Very poor
Dicalcium phosphate dihydrate (fine)	41	Very poor

b. *Angle of repose:* Angle of repose is defined as the maximum angle possible between the surface of pile of the powder and the horizontal plane (Fig. 1.4 and Tables 1.6 and 1.7).

$$\tan\theta = \frac{h}{r}$$

$$\theta = \tan^{-1}\frac{h}{r}$$

Where, θ = angle of repose, h = height of pile, and r = radius of the base of pile.

The lower the angle of repose, the better the flow property. Certain observations are made:

• Decrease in particle size leads to a higher angle of repose.

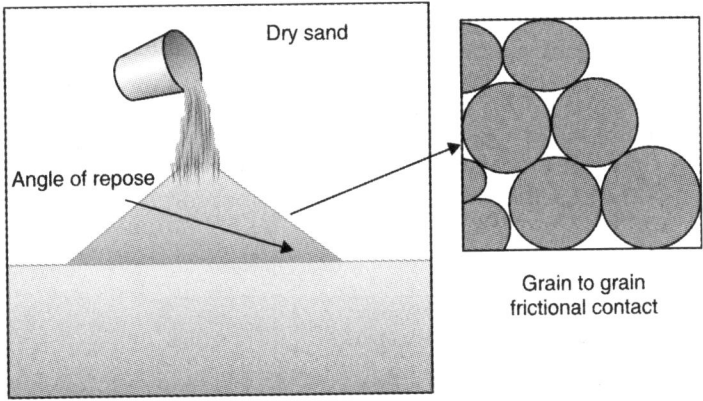

Fig. 1.4: Showing angle of repose of dry sand. Spherical the particle lesser the angle of repose and better will be the flow.

Table 1.6: Relationship between angle of repose (θ) and powder flow

Angle of repose (θ) (degrees)	Flow
<25	Excellent
25–30	Good
30–40*	Passable
>40	Very poor

*Adding glidant, e.g. 0.2% aerosil, may improve flow.

Table 1.7: Angle of repose of some pharmaceutical excipients

Substance	Angle of repose (θ)
Calcium state N.F.	10
Dextrose	25
Lactose USP	15
Lactose (spray dried) USP	20
Magnesium oxide	20
Microcrystalline cellulose USP	15
Starch NF	15
Stearic acid NF	15
Talc USP	15
Sodium bicarbonate USP	20

- Lubricant at low concentration decreases the angle of repose. At high concentration, this enhances the angle of repose.
- Fines (passed through 100 mesh) increase the angle of repose.

Physicochemical Parameters

Solubility

Solid drugs administered orally for systemic activity must dissolve in the gastrointestinal fluids prior to their absorption. Thus the solubility and rate of dissolution of drugs in GIT fluids could influence the rate and extent of their absorptions (Fig. 1.5).

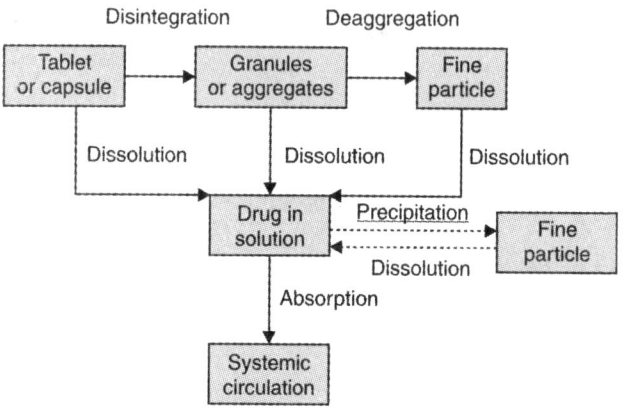

Fig. 1.5: Solubility or dissolution as critical step during absorption

Kaplan (1972) suggested that unless a compound has an aqueous solubility in excess of 1% (10 mg/ml) over the pH range 1–7 at 37°C, then potential bioabsorption problem may occur.

Analytical methods that are particularly useful for solubility measurements include HPLC, UV spectroscopy, fluorescence spectroscopy and gas chromatography. For most drugs, reverse phase HPLC offers an efficient and accurate means of collecting solubility data. Its major advantages are direct analysis of aqueous samples, high sensitivity and specific determination of drug concentration due to chromatographic separation of drug from impurities or degradation products.

Intrinsic Solubility (C₀)

An increase in solubility of a new drug in an acidic solution compared with its aqueous solubility suggested a weak base and an increase in alkali, a weak acid. In both cases, a dissociation constant (pKa) will be measurable and salt should form. An increase in both acidic and alkaline solubility suggests either amphoteric or zwitter ion behavior; in this case there will be two pKa, one acidic and one basic. No change in solubility suggests a non-ionizable neutral molecule with no measurable pKa. Here solubility manipulations will require either solvents or complexation.

Intrinsic solubility (true solubility) C_0 is the solubility due to unionized form of drug. When the purity of drug sample can be assured, then the solubility value obtained in acid for a weak acid or alkali for a weak base can be assumed intrinsic solubility.

The solubility should ideally be measured by two temperatures:

a. 4 or 5°C to ensure good physical stability and to extend short-term storage and chemical stability until more definitive data is available.

b. 37°C to support biopharmaceutical evaluation.

pH Solubility Profile

The degree of ionization and, therefore, the solubility of acidic and basic compounds depend upon the pH of the media. The saturation solubility for such compounds at a particular pH is sum total of solubility of ionized and unionized forms.

$$S_t = [BH^+] + [B]$$

BH^+ is protonated species, B is free base, S_t = total molar solubility.

The pH at which both base and salt species are simultaneously saturated is defined as the pH_{max} or

$$S_t, pH = pH_{max} = [BH^+]_s + [B]_s$$

Where the subscript (s) denotes saturation. For weak bases in the pH region where the solubility of protonated form is limiting, the molar solubility is

$$S_t, pH < pH_{max} = [BH^+]_s + [B]$$

$$= [BH^+]_s \left(1 + \frac{Ka}{H^+}\right)$$

Similarly, the solubility in pH region where free base is limiting is expressed as:

$$S_t, \text{pH} > \text{pH}_{max} = [BH^+] + [B]_s$$

$$= [B]_s \left(1 + \frac{H^+}{Ka}\right)$$

Corresponding equation for acidic compounds

$$S_t \text{ pH} < \text{pH}_{max} = [AH]_s \left(1 + \frac{Ka}{[H^+]}\right)$$

$$S_t \text{ pH} > \text{pH}_{max} = [A^-]_s \left(1 + \frac{H^+}{Ka}\right)$$

Since ionizable compounds may be available in free or salt form, one could use either in solubility experiments, e.g. phenazopyridine, free base, having pKa of 5.2, exhibits maximum solubility at pH 3.45 (pH$_{max}$) over pH range of total solubilities at pH$_{max}$ region.

Solubility product/common ion effect

In a saturated solution of a salt with some undissolved solid, there exists an equilibrium between the excess solid and the ions resulting from the dissociation of the salt in solution. For a hydrochloride salt represented as BH^+Cl^-, the equilibrium is

$$BH^+Cl^- (s) \rightleftharpoons BH^+ + Cl^-$$

Where, B is the base compound, BH^+ and Cl^- represent hydrated ions in solution. The corresponding equilibrium constant K is given by

$$K = \frac{[BH^+][Cl^-]}{[BH^+Cl^-]_{solid}} \qquad \ldots (1)$$

As a solid, the activity of $[BH^+Cl^-]_{solid}$ is constant, then equation becomes

$$K_{sp} = [BH^+] [Cl^-] \qquad \ldots (2)$$

For an ionizable drug as mentioned earlier, total solubility S_T is sum total of $[BH^+]_s$ and $[B]$ since $[BH^+]_s \gg [B]$, equation (2) becomes,

$$K_{sp} = S_T [Cl]^- \qquad \ldots (3)$$

Equation (3) indicates that total solubility of a hydrochloride salt would decrease with an increase in the chloride ion concentration. This phenomenon is known as common ion effect.

Since the gastric contents are high in Cl⁻ ion concentration, the common ion effect phenomenon suggests that one should use salts other than the hydrochloride to benefit fully from the enhanced solubility due to a salt form. Despite this, many drugs are used as hydrochloride salts. This is because solubility of most hydrochloride salts is so high that the suppression of solubility due to common ion effect under *in vivo* conditions is not of sufficient magnitude to affect dissolution or bioavailablity of these compounds.

Solubilization

When the drug substance under consideration is not an acidic or basic compound, or when the acidic or basic character of the compound is not amenable to the formation of a stable salt, other means of enhancing the solubility may be explored like use of co-solvent. A general means of increasing solubility is the addition of a co-solvent to the aqueous system. The solubility of poorly soluble non-electrolytes can often be improved by orders of magnitude with suitable co-solvent such as ethanol, propylene glycol and glycerin. These co-solvents solubilize drug molecule by disrupting the hydrophobic interactions of water at the non-polar solute/water interface. The extent of solubilization due to the addition of co-solvent depends on the chemical structure of the drug, i.e. the more non-polar the solute, the greater is the solubilization achieved by co-solvent addition. Take example of hydrocortisone and hydrocortisone-21-heptonate. The liphophilic ester (i.e. hydrocortisone-21-heptonate) is solubilized to more extent by addition of propylene glycol than by the more polar parent compound (hydrocortisone).

pKa determination/dissociation constant

The amount of drug that exists in unionized form is a function of dissociation constant (pKa) of drug and pH of the fluid at the absorption site.

It is customary to express the dissociation constants of both acidic and basic drugs by pKa values. The lower the pKa of an acidic drug, stronger the acid, i.e. greater the proportion of ionized form at a particular pH. The higher the pKa of basic drug the stronger the base. Thus, from the knowledge of pKa of the drug and pH at the absorption site (or biological fluid), the relative amount of ionized and unionized drugs in solution at a particular pH and the percent of drug ionized at this pH can be determined by Henderson and Hasselbalch equation.

For weak acid:

$$pH = pKa + \log \frac{\text{Ionized drug concentration}}{\text{Unionized drug concentration}}$$

$$\% \text{ drug ionized} = \frac{10^{pH-pKa}}{1+10^{pH-pKa}} \times 100$$

For weak base:

$$pH = pKa + \log \frac{\text{Unionized drug concentration}}{\text{Ionized drug concentration}}$$

$$\% \text{ drug ionized} = \frac{10^{pKa-pH}}{1+10^{pKa-pH}} \times 100$$

The above equations used:

- To determine the pKa by finding/drug ionized at particular pH.
- To allow the prediction of solubility at any pH provided that the intrinsic solubility (C_0) and pKa are known.
- To facilitate the selection of suitable salt forming compounds and predicts the solubility and pH properties of the salts.

A pKa value can be determined by a variety of analytic methods:

- Buffer, temperature, ionic strength and co-solvent affect the pKa value and should be controlled for these determinations.
- The preferred method is the detection of spectral shifts by UV or visible spectroscopy, since dilute solution can be analyzed directly.

- A second method, potentiometric titration, offers maximum sensitivity for compounds with pKa values in the range of 3 to 10 but is often hindered by precipitation of the unionized form during the titration since a high drug concentration is usually required to obtain a significant titration curve.
- To prevent precipitation, a cosolvent such as methanol or dimethyl sulphoxide can be incorporated.

General information: 75% of the all drugs are weak bases (20% are weak acid and the remaining 5% are non-ionic, amphoteric or alcohols).

Salt formation

Most drugs are either weak acids or weak bases. One of the easiest approach to enhance the solubility and dissolution rate of such drugs is to convert them into their salt forms. Generally, with weakly acid drugs, a strong base salt is prepared as the sodium or potassium salts of barbiturates and sulfonamide. In case of weakly basic drug, a strong acid salt is prepared like the HCl or sulfate salts of several alkaloidal drugs, e.g. consequences of changing chlordiazopoxide to various salts form (Table 1.8).

The dissolution rate of a particular salt is usually much greater than the parent drug. Sodium and potassium salts of weak acids dissolve much rapidly than the parent acid. Some comparative data are shown in Table 1.9.

Table 1.8: Solubility of chlordiazopoxide and its various salts			
Salts	*pKa*	*Salt pH*	*Solubility*
Chlordiazopoxide base	4.80	8.30	2.0
Hydrochloride	–6.10	2.53	2165 (1)
Sulfate	–3.00	2.53	Freely soluble
Besylate	0.70	2.53	Freely soluble
Malate	1.92	3.36	57.1
Tartrate	3.00	3.90	17.9
Benzoate	4.20	4.50	6.0
Acetate (2)	4.76	4.78	4.1

(1) Maximum solubility of chlordiazopoxide hydrochloride achieve at pH 2.89 is governed by crystal lattice energy, a common ion.

(2) Chlorodiazopoxide acetate may not form. pKa too high and close to drug.

Table 1.9: Solubility of sodium salts of weak acid

Drug	pKa	pH at (C_s)	Dissolution rate (mg cm^{-2}/min)×10^2 dissolution media	
			0.1 M HCl (pH 1.5)	Phosphate buffer (pH 6.8)
Salicylic acid	3.0	2.40	1.7	27
Sodium salicylate		8.78	1870	2500
Benzoic acid	4.2	2.88	2.1	14
Sodium benzoate		9.35	980	1770
Sulfathiazole	7.3	4.97	<0.1	0.5
Sodium sulfathiazole		10.75	550	810

Solvents

The first choice for a solvent is obviously water. However, although the drug may be freely soluble, some are unstable in aqueous solution. Accordingly water miscible solvents can be used:

- As cosolvents in formulation to improve solubility or stability.
- In analysis to facilitate extraction and separation (chromatography).

Oils are used in emulsions, topicals (creams and ointments), intramuscular injection and liquid-fill oral preparation (soft and hard gelatin capsules) when aqueous pH and cosolvent solubility and stability are unpalatable.

Aqueous methanol is widely used in HPLC and is the standard solvent in samples extraction during analysis and stability testing (Table 1.10).

Partition coefficient

Partition coefficient (oil/water) is a measure of a drug's lipophilicity and an indication of its ability to cross cell membranes. It is defined as the ratio of drug distributed between the organic and aqueous phases at equilibrium.

$$P_{o/w} = (C_{oil}/C_{water})_{equilibrium}$$

For series of compounds, the partition coefficient can provide an empiric handle in screening for some biologic properties.

Table 1.10: Recommended solvents for preformulation screening

Solvent	Dielectric constant	Solubility parameters (δ)	Applications
Water	80	24.4	Formulation
Methanol	32	14.7	Extraction and separation
0.1 M HCl (pH 1.07)	–	–	Dissolution (gastric), basic extraction
0.1 M NaOH (pH 13.1)	–	–	Acidic extraction
Buffer pH (7)	–	–	Dissolution (intestinal)
Ethanol	24	12.7	Formulation, extraction
Propylene glycol	32	12.6	Formulation
Glycol	43	16.5	Formulation
PEG 300 or 400	35	–	Formulation

For drug delivery, the lipophilic/hydrophilic balance has been shown to be a contributing factor for the rate and extent of drug absorption. Although partition coefficient data alone does not provide understanding of *in vivo* absorption, it does provide a means of characterizing the lipophilic/hydrophilic nature of the drug.

Since biological membranes are lipoidal in nature, the rate of drug transfer for passively absorbed drugs is directly related to the lipophilicity of the molecule. The partition coefficient is commonly determined using an oil phase of octanol or chloroform and water.

Drugs having values of partition coefficients much greater than 1 are classified as lipophilic, whereas those with partition coefficients much less than 1 are indicative of a hydrophilic drug.

Although it appears that the partition coefficient may be the best predictor of absorption rate, the effect of dissolution rate, pKa, and solubility on absorption must not be neglected.

Applications of partition coefficient: Partition coefficient (solvent water quotient of drug distribution) has a number of applications which are relevant to preformulation.

- Solubility both in aqueous and in mixed solvents.

- Drug absorption *in vivo.* Applied to a homologous drug series for structure activity relationship.

- Partition chromatography: Choice of column (HPLC) or TLC and choice of miscible phase (eluent).

- Extraction of crude drugs.

- Recovery of antibiotics from fermentation broth.

Dissolution

The dissolution rate of the drug is only important where it is rate limiting step in the absorption process. It has been suggested that the solubility of drug exceeded 10 mg/ml at pH 7 then no bioavailability problem were to be expected.

An equation which describes the process of dissolution is the Noyes Whitney equation.

$$\frac{dC}{dt} = KS(C_s - C_t)$$

where $\frac{dC}{dt}$ = rate of dissolution, K = dissolution rate constant, S = surface area of the dissolved solid, C_t = concentration at time 't', and C_s = saturation solubility.

The constant 'K' has been shown to be equal to D/h where D is the diffusion coefficient of the dissolving solid and 'h' is the thickness of the diffusion layer. The diffusion layer is a thin stationary film of solution adjacent to the surface of the solid. The layer is saturated with drug. Thus the drug concentration in the layer is equal to C_s. The term C_s-C_t represents the concentration gradient between the diffusion layer and the bulk solution. In dissolution rate limited absorption, C_t is negligible, then equation becomes:

$$\frac{dC}{dt} = \frac{DSC_s}{h}$$

Intrinsic dissolution: When dissolution is solely controlled by the diffusion, the rate of dissolution is directly proportional to the dissolution rate of a solid in its own solution is adequately described by Noyes-Nerest equation.

$$\frac{dC}{dt} = \frac{SD(C_s - C)}{hV}$$

where dC/dt= dissolution rate, S = surface area of dissolved solid, D = diffusion coefficient, C = solvent concentration in the bulk medium, h = diffusion layer thickness, V = volume of dissolved medium, C_s = solute concentration in the diffusion layer.

During early phase of dissolution, $C_s \gg C$ and is essentially equal to satura :on solubility C_s, surface area A and volume V can be held constant under this condition and at a constant temperature and agitation above equation becomes

$$\frac{dC}{dt} = KC_s \text{, where, } K = SD/hV = \text{constant}$$

Intrinsic dissolution rate is generally expressed as mg dissolved $\times$ $(min^{-1}cm^{-2})$

This constant rate differs from the dissolution from conventional dosage form which is known as total dissolution (mg/min) where the exposed surface area (S) is uncontrolled as disintegration, deaggregation and dissolution process. According to the intrinsic dissolution rate, it is independent of formulation effects and measures the intrinsic properties of the drug and salt as a function of dissolution media effects, e.g. pH, ionic strength and counter ions.

Influence of some parameters on dissolution rate of drug:

- Diffusion coefficient of drug.
- Surface area of solid drug.
- Water/oil partition coefficient of drug.
- Concentration gradient.
- Thickness of stagnant layer.

Effect of temperature

The heat of solution, ΔH_s, represents the heat released or absorbed when a mole of solute is dissolved in a large quantity of solvent. Most commonly, the solution process is endothermic, or ΔH_s is positive, and thus increasing the solution temperature increases the drug solubility. For such solutes as lithium chloride and other hydrochloride salts that are ionized when dissolved, the process is exothermic (negative ΔH_s) such that higher temperature suppresses the solubility.

Heat of the solution is determined from solubility values for saturated solutions equilibrated at controlled temperatures over the range of interest. Typically, the temperature range should include 5°C, 25°C, 37°C and 50°C. The working equation for determining ΔH_s is

$$\ln S = \frac{-\Delta H_s}{R}\left(\frac{1}{T}\right) + C$$

S = molar solubility, R = Carr's constant, T = temperature (°K)

Over elevated temperature ranges, a semi-logarithmic plot of solubility against reciprocal temperature is linear and ΔH_s is obtained from the slope.

Assay Development

The majority of preformulation method development is chromatographic with differing detection mechanisms.

- HPLC (high performance liquid chromatography): It is of two types: (i) normal phase HPLC: Chromatographic method that uses polar stationary phase and (ii) reversed phase HPLC: Chromatographic method that uses non-polar stationary phase
- GC (gas chromatography)
- TLC (thin layer chromatography)

Specialized method development can also be performed using capillary electrophoresis and supercritical fluid chromatography.

The analyted program consists of:

- Method development
- Forced degradation studies
- Validation

Stability Studies

The stability studies are done to determine shelf-life, and co-related specifications, and it must be taken into account of the chemistry of the active ingredient and its likely vulnerability to degrade by oxidation, hydrolysis, isomerization, polymerization, decarboxylation, moisture, heat and light. Properly conducted stability study must also include an examination of specific decomposition products by appropriate techniques to establish identity and relative toxicity of the decomposition products and the concentrations in which they are formed. Stability studies should not only take the account of the physical state in which the compound is likely to be used, but also the immediate biological environment likely to be met on administration. The substance for tablet, encapsulation and preparation of suspension, should be examined primarily in solid state. Substances for injection, which must be subjected to some form of sterilization procedure, must be examined particularly for stability at elevated temperature for possible hydrolysis or rearrangement in aqueous media and effects of exposure to CO_2 and light. Similarly all substances intended for oral administration must be chemically stable to the pH and enzymatic conditions likely to be met in the gastro-intestinal tract.

Hence, stability studies must be conducted on the drug substance in the solid state over a range of temperature, at varying degrees of humidity, and in both light and dark. Also, if a product is to be used in multiple dose form in the tropics with fluctuation in temperature, which should be stored ideally in cool or refrigerated conditions, then the stability tests should include a study of the effects of fluctuating temperature. Stability studies are an integral part of the drug development program and are of the most important area in the registration of pharma products. Stability assessment started with studies on the substance to determine degradation products and degradation pathway. Stability studies can influence the specification, limits and control method for drug.

The physicochemical parameters, such as the presence of additives as well as the storage conditions, which may affect the stability of drugs, have received considerable attention in the field of pharmaceutics. The formulation of a stable dosage form is essential for the patient's safety and drug efficacy.

In the ICH harmonized tripartite guidelines on stability testing of new drug substances and products, fundamental recommendations are summarized. According to the ICH guideline, long-term (12 months) and accelerated stability studies (least 6 months) have to be carried out (Table 1.11).

Table 1.11: Long-term, accelerated and where appropriate, intermediate storage conditions for the drug substances

Study	Storage conditions	Time period
Long-term*	25°C ± 2°C/60% RH ±5% RH	
	or 30°C ± 2°C/65% RH ± 5% RH	12 months
Intermediate**	30°C ± 2°C/65% RH ± 5% RH	6 months
Accelerated	40°C ± 2°C/75% RH ± 5% RH	6 months

* Long-term stability studies are performed at 25°C ± 2°C/60% RH ± 5% RH or 30°C ± 2°C/65% RH ±5% RH

** If 30°C ±2°C/65% RH ± 5% RH is the long-term condition, there is no intermediate condition

Preformulation stability studies are usually the first quantitative assessment of chemical stability of a new drug. These studies include both solution and solid state experiments under conditions typical for the handling, formulation, storage and administration of a drug candidate.

Stability analysis can be done by:
- UV spectroscopy
- Thin layer chromatography (TLC)
- High performance liquid chromatography (HPLC)
- Differential scanning calorimetry (DSC)

Chemical stability analysis includes:
1. Solution stability
2. Solid state stability
   - Hydrolysis
   - Oxidation
   - Pyrolysis/elevated temperature studies
   - Photolysis
3. Stability under high humidity condition

Solution Stability

The primary objective of this phase of preformulation research is identification of conditions necessary to form a stable solution. These studies should include the effect of pH, ionic strength, cosolvent, light, temperature and oxygen.

Solution stability investigations usually commence with probing experiments to confirm decay at the extreme pH and temperature (e.g. 0.1 N HCl, water and 0.1 N NaOH all at 90°C). These intentionally degraded samples may be used to confirm assay specificity as well as to provide estimate for maximum rates of degradation.

Since most solution in pharmaceutics are intended for parenteral root of administration, this initial pH-rate study should be conducted at a constant ionic strength that is compatible with physiological media.

Ionic strength can be calculated as:

$$\mu = \frac{1}{2} \sum m_i Z_i^2$$

Where, m_i is the molar concentration of the ion, Z_i is the valency.

All ionic species (even the drug molecule) in the buffer solution must be considered in computing ionic strength. The apparent pH of a buffer solution also varies, when there is co-solvent is present.

Solid State Stability

The primary objectives of this investigation are identification of stable storage conditions for drug in the solid state and identification of compatible excipient for a formulation.

Chemical unstability normally results form either of the following reactions:

- Hydrolysis
- Oxidation
- Pyrolysis
- Photolysis

Hydrolysis: The most likely cause of drug instability is hydrolysis, partially in solid dosage form. Hydrolysis may be defined as the reaction of a compound with water. It is of two types, i.e. **ionic** and **molecular forms** of hydrolysis.

Ionic hydrolysis: It occurs with salt of weak acids, e.g. potassium acetate and bases of codeine phosphate interact with water to give alkaline and acidic solutions, respectively.

Molecular hydrolysis: Slower irreversible process involving cleavage of the drug molecule. This form of hydrolysis is mainly responsible for the decomposition of pharmaceutical products ester, e.g. the local anesthetics—amethocaine and benzocaine and amines.

A number of conditions catalyzes the breakdown:

- Presence of OH⁻ ion
- Presence of H_3O^+ ion
- Presence of divalent metal ion is quicker than molecular ion
- Ionic hydrolysis (protolysis)
- Heat
- Light
- Solution polarity and ionic strength
- High drug concentration

Oxidation: Oxidation is a loss of electrons and an oxidizing agent must be able to take electrons. In organic chemistry, oxidation is synonymous with dehydrogenation (the loss of hydrogen). There are two types of oxidation:

- Oxidation processes that produced slowly under the influence of atmospheric oxygen.
- Oxidation processes that involve the reversible loss of electron without the addition of oxygen, e.g. oxidation of morphine, adrenaline, fixed oils, fats, volatile oils and phenol compounds.

Oxidation can be avoided by the use of antioxidant, e.g. hydroquinone, butylated hydroxy anisole, butylated hydroxy to have vitamin E, citric acid, etc. Most antioxidant function by providing electrons or labile H⁺, which will be accepted by any free radical to terminate the chain reaction.

Pyrolysis/elevated temperature studies: The elevated temperatures most commonly used are 40°, 50° and 60° C in conjunction with ambient humidity. Occasionally, higher temperatures are used. The samples stored at the highest temperature should be examined for physical and chemical changes at weekly intervals, and any change, when compared to an appropriate control (usually a sample stored at 5°C), should be noted. If a substantial change is seen, samples stored at lower temperatures are examined. If no change is seen after 30 days at 60°C, the stability prognosis is excellent. Corroborative evidence must be obtained by monitoring the samples stored at lower temperatures for longer durations. Samples stored at room temperature and at 5°C may be followed for as long as 6 months. The data obtained at elevated temperatures may be extrapolated using the Arrhenius treatment to determine the degradation rate at a lower temperature.

Not all solid-state reactions are amenable to Arrhenius treatment. Their heterogeneous nature makes elucidation of the kinetic order and prediction difficult. Long-term lower temperature studies are, therefore, an essential part of a good stability program.

Arrhenius equation

$$K = A\, e^{-E_a / RT}$$

E_a: activation energy; R: Gas constant

$$log K = log A - (E_a / 2.303 RT)$$

Plotting the rate of reaction (K) against $1/T$ allows the calculation of rate at any temperature and, therefore, a prediction of shelf-life (t_{90}, time to 90% potency). This forms the basis of many accelerated stability tests.

Photolysis: Photolysis catalyzes oxidation and to some extent hydrolysis. This energy associated with the radiation increases as its wavelength decreases, so that the energy of UV > Visible > IR and is independent of temperature (Table 1.12).

Table 1.12: Energy associated with different radiations

Types of radiation	Wavelength	Energy (Kcal mol^{-1})
UV	50–400	287–72
Visible	400–750	72–36
IR	750–10,000	36–1

When molecules are exposed to electromagnetic radiations they absorb light (photons) at characteristic wavelengths which causes an increase in the energy state of the compound. This energy can:

- Cause decomposition
- Be retained or transferred

- Converted to heat
- Result in emission of light at a new wavelength (fluorescence, phosphorescence)

Natural sunlight lies in the wavelength range 290–780 nm of which only the higher energy (UV) (290–320 nm) cause

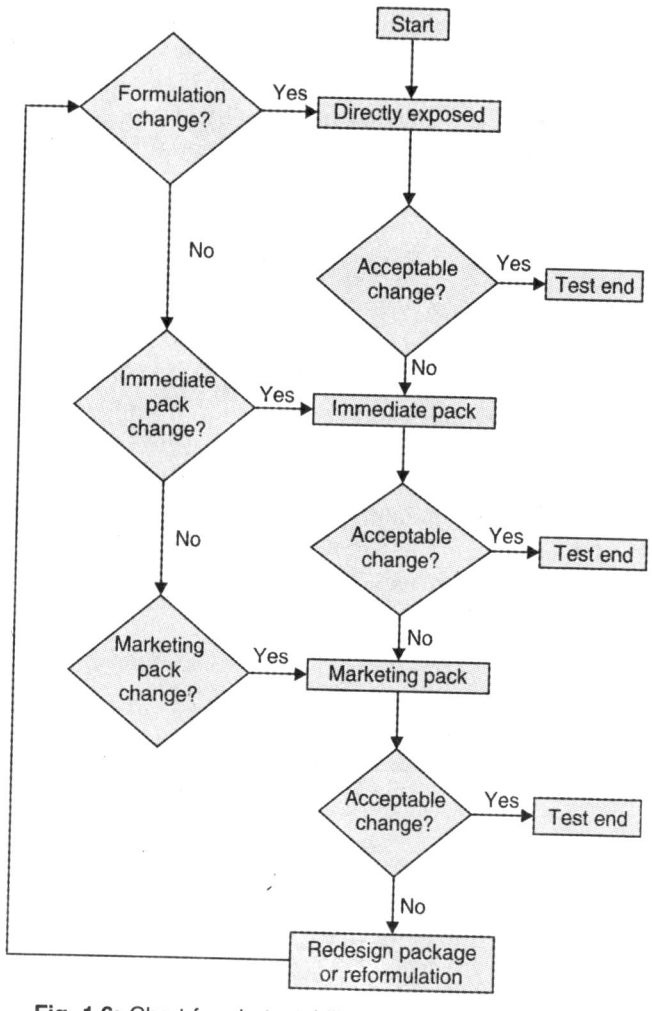

Fig. 1.6: Chart for photostability testing of drug products

photodegradation of drugs. These photolysis can be prevented by:

- Suitable packing: Using amber-colored glass bottles, card board outers and aluminum foil overwraps and blisters.
- Clean flint glass absorbs around 80% in the 290–320 nm range, whereas amber glass absorbs more than 95% in the range of 290–320 nm.

Photostability testing (Fig. 1.6): Exposure of the drug substance to 400 and 900 footcandles of illumination for 4- and 2-week periods, respectively, is adequate to provide some idea of photo-sensitivity. Over these periods, the samples should be examined frequently for change in appearance and for chemical loss, and they should be compared against samples stored under the same conditions but protected from light.

Stability Under High Humidity Conditions

In the presence of moisture, many drug substances hydrolyze, react with other excipients, or oxidize. These reactions can be accelerated by exposing the solid drug to different relative humidity conditions. Controlled humidity environments can be readily obtained using laboratory desiccators containing saturated solution of various salts. The closed desiccators in turn are placed in an oven to provide a constant temperature, e.g. decarboxylation of *p*-aminosalicylic acid shows a dependence on the ambient moisture. So preformulation data of this nature are useful in determining, if the material should be protected and stored in controlled low-humidity environment or if the use of an aqueous-based granulation system should be avoided. They may also caution against the use of excipient that adsorb moisture.

Percentage relative humidity using different saturated salt is tabulated in Tables 1.13 and 1.14.

Drug Excipient Compatibility Studies

The successful formulation of a stable and effective solid dosage forms depends on the careful selection of the excipients which are added to facilitate administration, promote the consistent release and bioavailability of drug and protect it from degradation.

Table 1.13: Saturated salt with % RH below 40%

Temperature °C	Relative humidity (% RH)		
	Lithium chloride	Potassium acetate	Magnesium chloride
0	11.23 ± 0.54		33.66 ± 0.33
5	11.26 ± 0.47		33.60 ± 0.28
10	11.29 ± 0.41	23.28 ± 0.53	33.47 ± 0.24
15	11.30 ± 0.35	23.40 ± 0.32	33.30 ± 0.21
20	11.31 ± 0.31	23.11 ± 0.25	33.07 ± 0.18
25	11.30 ± 0.27	22.51 ± 0.32	32.78 ± 0.16
30	11.28 ± 0.24	21.61 ± 0.53	32.44 ± 0.14
35	11.25 ± 0.22		32.05 ± 0.13
40	11.21 ± 0.21		31.60 ± 0.13
45	11.16 ± 0.21		31.10 ± 0.13
50	11.10 ± 0.22		30.54 ± 0.13
55	11.03 ± 0.23		29.93 ± 0.16
60	10.95 ± 0.26		29.26 ± 0.18
65	10.86 ±0.29		28.54 ± 0.21
70	10.75 ± 0.33		27.77 ± 0.25
75	10.64 ± 0.38		26.94 ± 0.29
80	10.51 ± 0.44		26.05 ± 0.34
85	10.38 ± 0.51		25.11 ±0.39
90	10.23 ± 0.59		24.12 ± 0.46
95	10.07 ± 0.67		23.07 ± 0.52
100	9.90 ± 0.77		21.97 ± 0.60

Incompatibility between excipient and drug substance can be detected by:

1. Differential scanning chromatography.
2. By evaluating organoleptic characteristics like change in color.
3. By checking purity of drug substance using HPLC method.

1. Differential scanning chromatography. Differential scanning chromatography can be used to investigate and predict any physicochemical interaction between components in a formulation and, therefore, can be applied to the selection of suitable chemically compatible excipients. For example, in one of the studies, compatibility of oxcarbazepine (OXC) with excipients was done using DSC analysis. DSC compatibility

Table 1.14: Saturated salt with % RH above 40%

Relative humidity (% RH)

Temperature °C	Potassium carbonate	Magnesium nitrate	Sodium chloride	Potassium chloride	Potassium nitrate	Potassium sulfate
0	43.13 ± 0.66	60.35 ± 0.55	75.51 ± 0.34	88.61 ± 0.53	96.33 ± 2.9	98.77 ± 1.1
5	43.13 ± 0.50	58.86 ± 0.43	75.65 ± 0.27	87.67 ± 0.45	96.27 ± 2.1	98.48 ± 0.91
10	43.14 ± 0.39	57.36 ± 0.33	75.67 ± 0.22	86.77 ± 0.39	95.96 ± 1.4	98.18 ± 0.76
15	43.15 ± 0.33	55.87 ± 0.27	75.61 ± 0.18	85.92 ± 0.33	95.41 ± 0.96	97.89 ± 0.63
20	43.16 ± 0.33	54.38 ± 0.23	75.47 ± 0.14	85.11 ± 0.29	94.62 ± 0.66	97.59 ± 0.53
25	43.16 ± 0.39	52.89 ± 0.22	75.29 ± 0.12	84.34 ± 0.26	93.58 ± 0.55	97.30 ± 0.45
30	43.17 ± 0.50	51.40 ± 0.24	75.09 ± 0.11	83.62 ± 0.25	92.31 ± 0.60	97.00 ± 0.40
35		49.91 ± 0.29	74.87 ± 0.12	82.95 ± 0.25	90.79 ± 0.83	96.71 ± 0.38
40		48.42 ± 0.37	74.68 ± 0.13	82.32 ± 0.25	89.03 ± 1.2	96.41 ± 0.38
45		46.93 ± 0.47	74.52 ± 0.16	81.74 ± 0.28	87.03 ± 1.8	96.12 ± 0.40
50		45.44 ± 0.60	74.43 ± 0.19	81.20 ± 0.31	84.78 ± 2.5	95.82 ± 0.45
55			74.41 ± 0.24	80.70 ± 0.35		
60			74.50 ± 0.30	80.25 ± 0.41		
65			74.71 ± 0.37	79.85 ± 0.48		
70			75.06 ± 0.45	79.49 ± 0.57		
75			75.58 ± 0.55	79.17 ± 0.66		
80			76.29 ± 0.65	78.90 ± 0.77		
85				78.68 ± 0.89		
90				78.50 ± 1.0		
95						
100						

studies were carried out by comparing the thermal curve of pure OXC with the curves obtained from pure OXC at 1:1 w/w individual mixtures with each excipient under consideration.

The DSC curve of OXC was typical of a pure crystalline substance, showing a sharp endothermic peak at its melting point, with an onset temperature of 221.13°C. No significant degradation was seen to occur before 240°C.

Table 1.15: DSC data on drug and excipients

Sample	Melting endotherm on set (°C)
OXC	221.13
OXC/microcrystalline cellulose	223.66
OXC/starch	218.81
OXC/talc	224.50
OXC/sodium lauryl sulfate	–
OXC/mannitol	208.63
OXC/colloidal silica	206.11
OXC/lactose	199.40
OXC/magnesium stearate	206.64

Inference: OXC was found to be compatible with microcrystalline cellulose, starch and talc. Interaction between OXC and mannitol, monohydrate lactose, colloidal silica, magnesium stearate and sodium lauryl sulfate (SLS) was observed and the extent of interaction varied from only a shift in the OXC melting endotherm to total abolition of the peak (refer to Table 1.15). The absence of the melting endotherm of OXC from the mixture with SLS may be due to the dissolution of the drug in the melting of the SLS.

2. By evaluating physical characteristics like change in color: This is the simplest method, where mixtures of drug substance and excipients are charged for 2 and 4 weeks at accelerated condition (40°C/75% RH) under fixed ratios and change in color is evaluated. For example, in one of the studies, physical compatibility study was done with cephalaexin, observation tabulated in Table 1.16.

3. By checking purity of drug substance using HPLC method: Formulation scientist can use HPLC method to detect impurities generated because of incompatibility between

Table 1.16: Physical compatibility studies

Composition	Description		
	Initial	*2 weeks*	*4 weeks*
Cephalexin	White to off white powder	No color change	No color change
Cephalexin + microcrystalline cellulose	White to off white powder	No color change	No color change
Cephalexin + lactose	White to off white powder	No color change	No color change
Cephalexin + HPMC15cps	White to off white powder	No color change	No color change
Cephalexin + HPMC K4M	White to off white powder	No color change	No color change
Cephalexin + HPMC KIOOM	White to off white powder	No color change	No color change
Cephalexin + HPMC K15M	White to off white powder	No color change	No color change
Cephalexin + colloidal silicon dioxide	White to off white powder	No color change	No color change
Cephalexin + magnesium stearate	White to off white powder	No color change	No color change

excipients and drug substance. This is the most effective method for evaluating incompatibility. Similar to physical compatibility studies, mixtures of drug substances and excipients are charged for 2 and 4 weeks at accelerated condition (40°C/75% RH) under fixed ratios. After two and four weeks, mixtures are evaluated with respect to impurities generated because of interaction between excipients and drug substances.

Conclusion

Preformulation studies, properly carried out, have a significant part to play in anticipating formulation problem and identifying logical paths in both liquid and solid dosage form technology. The need for adequate drug solubility cannot be overemphasized. The availability of sufficient solubility data should allow the selection of the most appropriate salt for development.

Stabilities studies in solution will indicate the feasibility of parenteral or other liquid dosage forms and can identify methods of stabilization. In parallel, solid state stability by DSC, TLC and HPLC and in the presence of tablet and capsule excipient will indicate the most acceptable vehicles for solid dosage formulations.

Finally, by physicochemical property of drug, the scientist can assist the synthetic chemist to identify the optimum molecule, provides the biologists with suitable vehicle to elicit pharmacological response and advise the bulk chemist about the selection and production of the best salt with appropriate particle size and morphology for subsequent processing.

ISOLATED KEY POINTS

- *Introduction:* Preformulation studies begin when a new chemical entity shows sufficient pharmacological promise and it may be a viable candidate for studies in man. Preformulation studies primarily include the study of the relevant physicochemical parameters for that dosage form and extensive stability studies so that the appropriate dosage form can be designed.

- *Aim:* To establish the physicochemical properties of a new drug (API); to establish the data on drug–excipient compatibility; to establish its (API) kinetic rate profile.

- *Stability studies:* Some commonly evaluated parameters: Organoleptic properties; purity; particle size, shape and surface area; solubility; dissolution; partition coefficient, ionization constant and Kp; crystal properties and polymorphism; density, hygroscopicity, flowability, wettability, etc.

- *Organoleptic properties:* Color–stability problems, improve appearance by including dye in body or coating. Taste–palatability problems, flavors and excipients may be added. Odor–degradation products, e.g. aspirin, stable form of drug to be used, flavors and excipients may be used.

- *Purity studies are essential for further studies to be carried out safely:* Impurities may make a compound toxic or render it unstable. TLC, HPLC, GC and paper chromatography used. HPLC–impurity index (II) and homogeneity index (HI), DTA, gravimetric analysis and melting point by hot stage microscopy are other techniques.

- *Techniques used for characterizing purity*: Thin layer chromatography (TLC), high pressure liquid chromatography, gas chromatography (GC). Impurity index (II) defined as the ratio of all responses (peak areas) due to components other than the main one to the total area response. Homogeneity index (HI) defined as the ratio of the response (peak area) due to the main component to the total response.

- *Particle size, shape and surface area:* Various chemical and physical properties of drug substances are affected by their particle size distribution and shapes. Size and shape also influence the dissolution of poorly soluble drugs which in turn influence bioavailability.

- Particle size determination microscopy is the simplest technique of estimating size ranges and shapes, e.g. light microscope, electron microscope. Andreason pipette is based on the rate difference of sedimentation of different particles, but techniques like this are seldom used due to their tedious nature. Seiving methods are also used to measure particle size. Instruments based on light scattering, (Royco), light blockage (HIAC) and blockage of electrical conductivity path (coulter counter) are available.

- *Common techniques for measuring fine particles of various sizes:* Technique particle size (mm) microscopic 1–100, sieve > 50, sedimentation > 1, elutriation 1–50, centrifugal < 50, permeability > 1, light scattering 0.5–50.

- *Solubility determinations:* The solubility of drug is an important physicochemical property because it effects the rate of drug release into dissolution medium and consequently, the bioavailabilty of the drug, and therapeutic efficiency of the pharmaceutical product.

- *Common solvents used for solubility determination:* Benzyl alcohol, isopropyl alcohol, tweens, polysorbates, castor oil, peanut oil, sesame oil, buffer at various pHs, water, polyethylene glycols, propylene glycol, glycerin, sorbitol, ethyl alcohol, methanol.

- *Intrinsic solubility:* The solubility should ideally be measured at two temperatures. The minimum density of water occurs at 4°C. This leads to a minimum aqueous solubility. 37°C to support biopharmaceutical evaluation.

- *pKa determination:* It is the negative logarithm of dissociation constant. It describes about the chemical nature of API/NCE. It is mainly determined by using the Henderson-Hasselbalch equation. For acidic compounds, pH = pKa + log (unionized drug)/(ionized drug). For basic compounds, pH = pKb + log (ionized drug)/(unionized drug).

- *Partition coefficient:* It is defined as the ratio of unionized drug distributed between the organic and aqueous phases at equilibrium. $P_{o/w} = (C_{oil}/C_{water})_{equilibrium}$. Partition coefficient (oil/water) is a measure of a drug's lipophilicity and an indication of its ability to cross cell membranes. The partition coefficient is commonly determined using an oil phase of octanol or chloroform and water. If P much greater than 1 are classified as lipophilic, whereas those with partition coefficient much less than 1 are indicative of a hydrophilic drug.

- Many drug substances can exist in more than one crystalline from with different space lattice arrangements. This property is known as polymorphism. Polymorphs generally have different melting points, X-ray diffraction patterns and solubility even though they are chemically identical. Different polymorphs also lead to different morphology, tensile strength and density of power bed which all contribute to compression characteristics of materials.

- *Powder flow properties:* When limited amounts of drugs are available, powder flow properties can be evaluated by measurements of bulk density and angle of repose. Changes in particles size, and shape are generally very important. An increase in crystal size or a more uniform shape will lead to a small angle of repose and a smaller Carr's index.

- *Bulk density:* Knowledge of absolute and bulk density of the drug substance is very useful in having some idea on the size of final dosage form, the density of solids also affects their flow properties. Carr's compressibility index can be used to predict the flow properties based on density measurement. Carr's index (%) = (Tapped density–Poured density) *100/Tapped density.

- *Angle of repose:* "The maximum angle which is formed between the surface of a pile of powder and horizontal surface is called the angle of repose".

- *Elevated temperature studies:* The elevated temperatures commonly used are 40°C, 50°C, and 60°C with ambient humidity. The samples are stored at highest temperature are observed weekly for physical and chemical changes and compared to an appropriate control. If a substantial change is seen, samples stored at lower temperature are examined. If no changes are seen after 30 days at 60°C, the stability prospect is excellent.

- *Stability under high humidity conditions:* The preformulation data of this nature are useful in determining, if the material should be protected and stored in controlled low humidity environment or if non-aqueous solvent be used during formulation.

- *Photolytic stability:* Many drugs fade on exposure light. Though the extent of degradations small and limited to the exposed surface area, it presents an aesthetic problem. Exposure of drug 400 and 900 foot-candles of illumination for 4 and 2 week periods respectively is adequate to provide some idea of photosensitivity. Resulting data may be useful in determining, if an amber-colored container is required or if color masking dye should be used in the formulation.

- *Stability to oxidation:* Drug's sensitivity to oxidation can be examined by exposing it to atmosphere of high oxygen tension. Usually, a 40% oxygen atmosphere allows for rapid evaluation. A shallow layer of drug exposed to a sufficient headspace volume ensures that the system is not oxygen limited. Samples are kept in desiccators equipped with three-way stop cocks, which are alternatively evacuated and flooded with desired atmosphere. The process is repeated 3 or 4 times to ensure 100% desired atmosphere. Results may be useful in predicting, if an antioxidant is required in the formulation or if the final product should be packaged under inert atmospheric conditions.

- *Compatibility studies:* The knowledge of drug excipients interaction is useful for the formulation to select appropriate excipients. Mixtures should be examined under nitrogen to estimate oxidation and paralytic effect at a standard heating rate on DSC, over a temperature range, which will encompass any thermal changes due to both the drug and appearance or disappearance one or more peaks in thermograms of drug excipient mixtures are considered of indication of interaction.

LONG ANSWER TYPE QUESTIONS

Q 1. What do you understand by the term preformulation? Discuss in brief about the objectives of preformulation studies.

Q 2. Enumerate the various factors involved in preformulation studies. Discuss in detail about organoleptic properties.

Q 3. Write short notes on following in context to preformulation studies.
   a. Bulk characterization
   b. Gibbs-Kelvin relation
   c. Crystallinity and polymorphism

Q 4. Discuss in detail about physicochemical parameters related to preformulation.

Q 5. How solubility and common ion effect play role in preformulation studies?

Q 6. Discuss in brief the significance of pKa determination and dissociation constant in preformulation studies.

Q 7. Make a chart for drug X, which is to be formulated in the form of tablet and carry out its preformulation studies at ambient condition for two months.

Q 8. What are various methods of drug excipient compatibility studies? How these incompatibility between excipient and drug can be detected?

Q 9. Write in brief about assay development and stability analysis used for preformulation studies.

Q 10. Write short notes on:
   a. Contact angle
   b. Surface area
   c. Young's equation
   d. Method of compression testing.

OBJECTIVE TYPE QUESTIONS

1. Gibbs-Kelvin is relationship between .... and apparent solubility of a drug.

2. When a substance exists in more than one crystalline form, then the phenomenon is called ....

3. Preformulation studies include all the studies except the following factors.
   a. The amount of drug available.
   b. The physicochemical properties of the drug already known.
   c. Therapeutic category and anticipated dose of compound.
   d. Route of drug administration
   e. None of the above

4. The primary objectives of preformulation studies are as follows:
   a. Establish the identity and physicochemical parameters of a new drug substance.
   b. Establish chemical stability profile of drug substance.
   c. Establish drug substance compatibility with common excipients.
   d. Preformulation studies give preliminary idea about selection of excipients, which make the formulation stable.
   e. All of the above

5. Compatibility stability analysis can be done by:
   a. DSC
   b. By evaluating organoleptic characteristics
   c. High performance liquid chromatography (HPLC)
   d. All of the above

6. Match the following based on particle size determination:

S. No	Method		Instrument
1	Simple visual method	A	Based on rate difference of sedimentation of different particle
2	Anderson pipette	B	Microscopy
3	ROYCO	C	Based on light scattering
4	HIAC	D	Based on light blockage

7. Match the following based on grading of the powder for their flow properties and Carr index

S. No	Carr index		Flow
1	5–15	A	Poor
2	18–21	B	Very poor
3	23–35	C	Excellent
4	33–38	D	Good

8. Match the following between angle of repose (θ) and powder flow

S.No	Angle of repose (θ) (degrees)		Flow
1	<25	A	Very poor
2	25–30	B	Excellent
3	30–40*	C	Good
4	>40	D	Poor

ANSWERS

1. Particle size
2. Polymorphism
3. e
4. e
5. d
6. 1-A, 2-A, 3-C, 4-D,
7. 1-C, 2-D, 3-A, 4-B
8. 1-B, 2-C, 3-D, 4-A

Liquid Dosage Form

INTRODUCTION

These are the pharmaceutical dosage forms that are designed to provide maximum therapeutic response in population with difficulty of swallowing of tablets or capsules or to produce rapid therapeutic response. Water is the major ingredient used in these dosage forms. Maintenance of both physical and chemical stability of formulation is the main challenge in designing a liquid dosage form. In this the physical form of the dosage form is pourable in nature and conforms to the shape of the container at room temperature. Based on the physical characteristics, the liquid dosage form is divided into two types: Solutions and dispersed systems (suspensions and emulsions). Solutions are the liquid dosage forms in which the one or two active ingredients are dissolved in a solvent. In case of dispersed systems, one phase of the system is distributed in other phase. If a solid phase is suspended in a liquid phase, it is termed a 'suspension', whereas if one liquid phase is dispersed in other liquid phase, it is termed an 'emulsion'.

Advantages and Disadvantages of Liquid Dosage Forms

Advantages

1. They are more effective than solid dosage forms as they eliminate the dissolving step of solid drug in the GIT.
2. They are easier to swallow than solid dosage forms especially in case of geriatric and pediatric populations.
3. Certain drugs have to be administered in liquid form only. It may be due to the large dose of the drug that is difficult to administer in solid dosage form.

4. Some drugs cause gastric irritation when administered in solid dosage form, e.g. potassium iodide and bromide. Hence they are to be administered in liquid dosage form.

Disadvantages

1. They undergo deterioration and loss of potency more frequently than solid dosage forms.
2. They show many flavoring and sweetening problems. It is difficult to mask the bitter taste and unpleasant odor of some drugs.
3. Many incompatibility problems occur between the dissolved ingredients of the dosage form.
4. More chances for microbial contamination of the product as water provide a major means for mold and bacterial growth. Hence preservatives are added. But the liquid dosage forms with preservatives are not intended for neonates as the antimicrobial preservatives cause serious acute and long-term adverse effects.
5. Inaccuracy of measuring dose may occur. It needs a accurate measuring device for administration.
6. These are bulkier to carry than solid dosage forms. There are chances for breakage of the container.

SOLUTIONS

Solutions are the homogenous mixtures in which one or more active ingredients are dissolved in one or mixture of solvents which may be aqueous or non-aqueous in nature. These are the oldest dosage forms used in the treatment of patients, which afford rapid and high absorption of soluble active ingredients.

Advantages and Disadvantages of Solutions

Advantages

- Easier to swallow: Especially for pediatrics, geriatrics and unconscious people.
- Quick onset of action: As it eliminates the step of disintegration and dissolution.
- Flexible dosing
- No need to shake the container
- Can be designed for different routes of administration.

Disadvantages

- Difficult to mask the unpleasant taste and odor of active ingredient.
- Need a measuring device (like graduated bottle caps, or a spoon) to measure accurate dose on administration.
- Less stable than solid dosage forms.
- Bulky, difficult to transport and they may prone to breakages.

Classification of Solutions According to Route of Administration

- Oral dosage forms: Syrups, elixirs, drops, mixtures, linctuses, draughts, spirits, pediatric drops.
- In mouth and throat: Mouth washes, gargles, throat sprays.
- In body cavities: Douches, enemas, otic solutions, ophthalmic solutions and nasal solutions.
- External solutions: Collodions, lotions and liniments.

Important aspects of solution preparation: Although different solutions are prepared with different methods, different additives, different drugs, two main aspects are considered majorly while preparing the solution. They are solubility and stability of the active ingredient in the solution.

Solubility: The solubility of the active ingredient in the formulation is a major aspect and the following points are to be checked before preparing a solution.

- The solubility of the drug in the solvent system
- Quantity of the drug to be dissolved
- Dissolution time of the drug in that solvent
- Whether the drug remains in solution and how long it remains as such?
- pH of the solvent required for dissolution

Stability

- The physical stability of the solution towards temperature fluctuations and photosensitivity should be considered
- The chemical stability with respect to the additives and shelf-life should be considered.
- The microbiological stability of the solutions is considered and there is need for addition of preservative.

Major signs of instability

- Color change
- Precipitation or crystal growth appearance
- Microbial growth
- Chemical gas formation

Additives Used in the Preparation of Solutions

Vehicle: It is the medium in which the active ingredient dissolves, which is generally described as solvent in case of solutions. Choice of the vehicle depends on the nature and physicochemical properties of the active ingredient and its usage.

Types of vehicles

Aqueous vehicle: Water is the most widely used vehicle in the preparation of pharmaceutical solutions. It acts as a universal solvent in solubilizing many active ingredients.

Advantages

- Widely available, inexpensive
- Palatable
- Non-toxic and non-irritable both for oral use and external use.
- Acts as a solvent for many drugs

Different Types of Water

Potable Water

It is the normal drinking water that is palatable and safe for drinking. But this water is not used in the preparation of pharmaceutical dosage forms as they may contain micro-organisms and the presence of dissolved mineral salts may contaminate the product.

Purified Water

- It is the water prepared from the potable water by distillation, by the use of ion exchange resin method, or by reverse osmosis.
- Hard waters are those that contain the Ca^{++} and Mg^{++} cations and alkaline waters are those that contain bicarbonates as the major impurity. These can be purified by using the above methods.

- To purify the water form microorganisms, ultraviolet energy, heat or filtration (millipore filtration) methods can be used.
- Distilled water is the purified water prepared by distillation process.

Freshly Boiled and Cooled Water

This water is used for preparations intended for oral and external solutions. In this the boiling removes the dissolved gases like oxygen and CO_2 from the water. Stored water of this type is not used as it may act as source for contamination with microorganisms.

Aromatic Water

- These are the clear saturated solutions of volatile oils, or other aromatic or volatile substances. These are mainly used as vehicles in oral solutions as they are flavored or perfumed vehicles.
- These are generally prepared from concentrated ethanolic solution, in dilution with 1 part of concentrated water with 39 parts of water.
- Chloroform water is a type of aromatic waters which adds sweetness to the preparation and also acts as a preservative.
- Some aromatic waters show mild carminative action, e.g. aromatic waters of Dill.
- Aromatic waters of volatile oils show salting out effect when a very soluble salt is added to the solution.

Storage conditions

- They should be protected from intensive light and heat and so they should be stored in light-resistance air-tight containers.
- They will deteriorate with time, so they should be made in small quantities. Deterioration may be due to volatilization, microbial contamination or decomposition. Cloudy appearance of the solution is considered as deterioration and it should be discarded.

Preparation of aromatic waters: There are two official methods for preparation of aromatic waters.

Distillation Process (Stronger Rose Water NF)

- In this, the drug is coarsely grounded and mixed with sufficient quantity of purified water in the distillation unit.
- After distillation, any excess oil in the distillate is removed by filtration.
- During distillation, drug should not be exposed to the action of direct heat, as the odor of the carbonized substance will be noticeable in the distilled aromatic water.
- If the volatile principle is present in small quantities in the water, the distillate is returned several times with fresh portions of the drug.

Solution Process (Peppermint Water)

- In this the volatile substance is shaked vigorously with purified water. Then the mixture is kept aside for 12 hours and then filtered.
- Talc may be added to increase the surface of the volatile substance, and it ensures more rapid saturation of the water and acts as a filter aid.

Water for Injection

It is pyrogen free distilled water which is then sterilized and used in the preparation of parenteral solutions.

Other Vehicles Used in Pharmaceutical Solutions

- *Syrup BP:* It is a solution of 66.7% w/v of sucrose in water. Syrup BP may be replaced by mannitol, xylitol, sorbitol, hydrogenated glucose syrups, as syrup BP causes dental decay and also not suitable for diabetic patients.
- *Ethanol:* It is mainly used in the preparation of external solutions and rarely in case of internal solutions.
- *Glycerin (glycerol):* It is viscous and miscible both with water and ethanol. It is used as a vehicle for external solutions. It can also be added as a stabilizer and sweetener in internal solutions.
- *Propylene glycol:* It is less viscous and more preferred to glycerin.
- *Oils:* Fractionated coconut oils and groundnut oils are used as a vehicle for fat-soluble compounds, e.g. calciferol oral solution BP.

- *Acetone:* It is used as a co-solvent in case of external solutions.

- *Ether:* It is also used as a co-solvent in case of external solutions for preparing skin preparations. But its usage is limited as it shows risk of fire and explosion and it also shows extreme volatility.

Buffering Agents

These are the agents which are added to maintain different ranges of pH of the solution. They resist the change in pH of the solution, e.g. Sorenson's modified phosphate buffer, sodium acetate buffer.

Isotonicity Modifiers

These are the agents added to maintain the isotonicity of the solutions similar to that of various body cavities. These are mainly added for ophthalmic solutions, injectable solutions and solutions applied for mucous membrane, e.g. Dextrose and 0.9% NaCl solution.

Viscosity Modifiers

In order to increase the residence time of the aqueous based solutions that are intended for skin, eye, and ears, some jelling agents, in low concentrations are added to increase the viscosity of the product. Syrups may also be added to increase the viscosity of the product. They also improve palatability and ease pourability of the product, e.g. hydroxypropylmethylcellulose, hydroxyethylcellulose, methylcellulose, polyvinyl alcohol, and polyvinyl pyrrolidine.

Solubilizing Agents

These are the agents which enhances the solubility of the active ingredient in the solvent, e.g. glycerin, sorbitol, polyethylene glycol, and polysorbate. For external solutions, soaps are used for phenolic disinfectants.

Preservatives

These are the agents added to prevent the contamination of the solution either due to the growth of microorganisms or due to oxidation of the active ingredient. Preservatives may be used alone or in combination.

Causes of Contamination

- The additives like jelling agents, sweetening agents, and flavors are causes for microbial growth.
- In case of multiple dose containers due to opening and closing of the container results in contamination due to exposure of the product for many times.
- Raw materials, equipment, environment and personnel may contribute for the product contamination.
- Extemporaneous dispensing

Ideal Characteristics of a Preservative

- Effective against broad spectrum of microorganisms
- Stable for its shelf-life
- Non-toxic and non-irritable
- Should not affect the stability of the active ingredient
- Free of taste and odor

Classification of Preservatives

- Ethanol (>10% v/v)
- Propylene glycol (15–30% v/v)
- Glycerin (>20% v/v)
- Benzoic acid and sorbic acid (0.1–0.5% w/v)
- Chloroform water BP (0.25% v/v)
- Methyl, ethyl, propyl and butyl parabens (up to 0.2%). These are stable over a pH range of 4 to 8. Generally combination of parabens is used in the formulations in order to achieve a higher total concentration and to be active against a wider range of microorganisms.
- Quarternary ammonium compounds: Benzalkonium chloride (0.002 – 0.02%). It shows optimal activity over the pH range of 4 to 10. This shows incompatibility with most of anionic compounds due to its cationic nature.

Preservatives used in external solutions:

- Chlorocresol (0.1% w/v) is used for external solutions.
- Chlorbutanol (0.5%)

- Parahydroxybenzoate (up to 0.2%)
- Phenylmercuric nitrate.

Antioxidants

- These are agents used to prevent the products like vitamins, essential oils and fats from oxidation. The oxidation reaction may be due to heat, light and heavy metals.
- To prevent from heat and light, they should be stored at cool temperature and in light-resistance container, respectively.
- EDTA or citric acid is mostly used to prevent oxidation by heavy metals like Fe, Cu.
- Other antioxidants: Ascorbic acid, citric acid, propyl and octyl esters of gallic acid, tocopherols, sodium metabisulfite, and sodium sulfite.

Sweetening Agents

These are the agents added to mask the bitter taste of the active ingredient.

- Sucrose is widely used sweetening agent.

  Advantages: Colorless, highly water soluble, stable over a wide pH range (4–8), increase the viscosity, masks both salty and bitter taste, has soothing effect on throat.

  Disadvantages: Prolonged usage of the product with sucrose cause dental caries and it is also not suitable for diabetic patients.

- Polyhydric alcohols such as sorbitol, mannitol and glycerol also act as sweeteners and can be used for diabetic preparations.

Flavors and Perfumes

- These are the agents added to mask the unpleasant taste or odor and make the preparation more acceptable to take.
- Enable the easy identification of the product.
- Natural products: Fruit juices (raspberry), extracts (liquorice), spirits (orange and lemon), syrups (black current), tinctures (ginger), and aromatic water (anise and cinnamon).

- Some flavors are associated with special preparations, e.g. peppermint is associated with antacid preparations.
- Artificial perfumes are cheaper, more readily available and more stable than natural products.

Coloring Agents

These are the agents added to enhance the appearance of the preparation. They should be non-toxic, non-irritant and should not show any therapeutic activity. Both natural and artificial coloring agents are available.

Natural coloring agents: These include materials extracted from plants and animals. Due to their low solubility mineral, pigments like iron oxide are not added to the preparation, e.g. carotenoids, chlorophylls, saffron, red beet root extract, caramel, and cochineal.

Synthetic colors: Azo compounds. These are widely used as they give wide range of bright and stable colors.

Methods of Preparation of Solutions

Solutions are prepared by the following methods.
- a. Simple solution
- b. Solution by chemical reaction
- c. Solution by extraction

a. Simple Solution

- In this, the solute is dissolved in a suitable solvent either by stirring or heating.
- Other additives may be added along with the solvent in order to enhance the stability and solubility of the active ingredient, e.g. in the preparation of strong iodine solution USP (Lugol's solution), KI is added to the mixture of iodine and water, as it forms more soluble polyiodies ($KI.I_2$ $KI.2I_2$ $KI_3.I_3$ $KI.4I_4$).

b. Solution by Chemical Reaction

In this, two or more solutes with each other in a suitable solvent, e.g. calcium carbonate and lactic acid used in the preparation of calcium lactate mixture.

c. Solution by Extraction

Plant or animal products are prepared by suitable extraction process. Preparations of this type may be classified as solutions but more often, are classified as extractives. Extractives will be discussed separately.

Pharmaceutical Solutions

Aqueous Solutions

- Douches
- Enemas
- Gargles
- Mouthwashes
- Otic solutions
- Nasal solutions

Sweet and/or Viscid Solutions

- Syrups
- Honeys
- Mucilages
- Jellies
- Linctuses

Non-aqueous Pharmaceutical Solutions

- Elixirs
- Spirits
- Collodions
- Glycerins
- Liniments
- Lotions
- Oleo vitamin

Aqueous Pharmaceutical Solutions

Douches

- These are the aqueous solutions which are administered into the body cavity or a part of body (like vagina or nasal cavity).
- It acts as a cleansing or antiseptic agent.

- These are frequently dispensed in the form of a powder with directions for dissolving in a specified quantity of water.
- The volumes of these preparations may vary from 5 ml to much larger volumes. It is necessary to warm the solutions to body temperature, if they are used in larger volumes.
- Eye douches are used to remove foreign particles and discharges from the eyes. It is administered gently at an oblique angle and is allowed to run from the **inner cornea** to the **outer** corner of the eye.
- Pharyngeal douches are used to cleanse the interior of the throat for an operation and to cleanse it in supportive conditions.
- Similarly, nasal and vaginal douches are also available.

Enemas

These are the liquid preparations that are intended to administer into the rectum.

Types and their Uses

- Evacuation enemas: They are used to evacuate the bowel.
- Retention enemas: They influence the absorption power of GIT, e.g. nutritive, sedative or stimulating properties. These are used in small quantities of about 30 ml and so they are called retention microenemas.
- Some enemas are prepared for anti-helminthic property which shows their effect locally at the site of disease.
- Some enemas contain radiopaque substances which are used for roentgenographic examination of the lower bowel.

Draughts

This is the older term used to describe the pharmaceutical solution which is dispensed in volumes of about 50 ml in a unit dose container.

Pediatric Drops

These are the oral pharmaceutical solutions that contain potent drugs that are intended for administration to pediatric patients. These are also used for patients suffering with difficulty of swallowing. This is usually dispensed in low dose volumes which are to be administered by using a dropper.

Gargles

- These are the concentrated aqueous solutions that contain antiseptics, antibiotics and/or anesthetics that are used in the treatment of pharynx and nasopharynx disorders, by forcing air from the lungs through the gargle, which is held in the throat and subsequently, the gargle is expelled out.
- These are generally diluted before use.
- The product should be labeled properly such that the container should be easily distinguishable from those preparations intended for swallowing.
- For example, phenol Gargle BPC.

Mouthwashes

These are the aqueous solutions intended for the treatment of mouth disorders. They can be used for both therapeutic and cosmetic purposes, e.g. sodium chloride mouthwash BP, chlorhexidine mouthwash, povidone-iodine mouthwash (betadine).

Therapeutic mouthwashes: These are formulated to reduce plaque, gingivitis, dental caries and stomatitis.

Examples of drugs formulated as mouthwashes:
- Combination of antihistamines, hydrocortisone, nystatin and tetracycline is used for the treatment of stomatitis, a painful side effect of cancer therapy.
- Allopurinol is used in the treatment of stomatitis
- Pilocarpine for xerostoma (dry mouth)
- Tranexamic acid for the prevention of bleeding after oral surgery.
- Carbenoxolone for the treatment of orofacial herpes simplex infections.

Cosmetic mouthwashes: These are formulated to reduce bad breath through the use of antimicrobial and/or flavoring agents.

Additives used in mouthwashes are described below.

Alcohols

- Used in the concentrations of 10–20% in the preparation of mouthwashes.
- They may function as a preservative.
- They also aid in masking the unpleasant taste of active ingredients.
- Also act as a solubilizing agent for some flavoring agents.

Humectants

- Used in the concentrations of 5–20%.
- They increase the viscosity of the preparation.
- Enhance the sweetness of the product.
- They improve the preservative qualities of the product, e.g. glycerin and sorbitol.

Surfactants

- These are used in the solubilization of flavors and they also remove the debris by providing foaming action.
- Generally, non-ionic and anionic surfactants are preferred.
- Cationic surfactants like cetylpyridinium chloride are used for their antimicrobial properties, but these tend to impart a bitter taste, hence their usage is limited.

Flavors: These are used along with alcohol and humectants to overcome disagreeable tastes. The principal flavoring agents are peppermint, cinnamon, menthol or methyl salicylate.

Coloring agents: These are also used in mouthwashes for good pleasant appearance of the product.

Nasal Solutions

Nasal solutions are the aqueous solutions intended to administer into the nasal passages in the form of drops or spray.

- Nasal decongestant solutions are employed in the treatment of common cold and for allergic rhinitis (hay fever) and for **sinusitis**. Their frequent use may lead to chronic edema of the nasal mucosa, i.e. rhinitis medicainentosa. Thus, they are best used for short periods of time (not longer than 3 to 5 days).

- Nasal solutions are prepared so that they are similar in many respects to nasal secretions and normal ciliary action is maintained. Thus aqueous nasal solutions are isotonic in nature and slightly buffered to maintain a pH of 5.5 to 6.5.
- The current route of administration of peptides and proteins is limited to parenteral injection because of inactivation within the GIT. As a result, there is considerable research on intranasal delivery of these drugs such as insulin.
- Drops spread more extensively than the spray and three drops cover most of the walls of the nasal cavity, with the patient in a supine position and head tilted back and turned left and right.

Examples

- Ephedrine sulfate or naphaxoline hydrochloride nasal solution USP shows local effect is used to reduce nasal congestion.
- Lypressin nasal solution USP shows systemic effect is used for the treatment of diabetes insipidus.
- Normal saline drops and ephedrine nasal drops are used generally for treatment of allergic rhinitis.
- Commercial nasal preparations include antibiotics, antihistamines and drugs for asthma prophylaxis.

Sprays

Sprays are solutions of drugs in aqueous vehicles along with a propellant. These are applied to the mucous membrane of the nose and throat by means of a specially designed devices like metered dose inhaler or nebulizer. If the action of the drug is intended at upper respiratory tract, then coarse droplets are to be produced. Fine droplets tend to move to lower respiratory tract, e.g. desmopressin (desmospray), used in the treatment of pituitary diabetes insipidus.

Otic Solutions

These are the aqueous solutions of drugs that are intended to treat disorders of ear.

Drugs intended for administration to the ear include:

- Local anesthetics, e.g. benzocaine;
- Antibiotics, e.g. neomycin; and
- Anti-inflammatory agents, e.g. cortisone.

In this, water or glycerin is used commonly as solvents. Addition of glycerin increases the residence time of the solution at the place of administration. Glycerin also reduces the swelling of the tissue by removing the excess moisture from the surrounding tissue. It also helps in the removal of cerumen (ear wax).

In order to provide sufficient time for aqueous preparations to act, it is necessary for the patient to remain on his side for a few minutes so the drops do not run out of the ear.

Ophthalmic Solutions

These are the aqueous solutions that are instilled into the eye. These are sterile in nature. The pH of these solutions may range from 4.5 to 11.5. pH range of 6.5 to 8.5 is more preferred which prevents the corneal damage. Other additives like buffers, isotonic agents, and viscosity modifiers are added.

Sweet and/or Viscid Pharmaceutical Solutions

These include syrups, honeys, mucilages, and jellies. All of these preparations are viscous liquids or semisolids. The sweetness and viscid appearance are given by sugars, polyols, or polysaccharides (gums).

Syrups

These are concentrated, viscous solutions of single or combination of sugars in water or with other aqueous liquid. These mask the bitter and saline taste of many drugs, e.g. epilim syrup containing sodium valproate.

Classification of Syrups

- Simple syrup: In this, only water is used for making syrup.
- Medicated syrup: In this, medicinal substance is added to the syrup.

- Flavored syrup: In this, aromatic or pleasantly flavored substance is added to the syrup that is used as a vehicle or flavor for other liquid preparations.

- Polyols (e.g. glycerin or sorbitol): These are added to the syrup to prevent crystallization of sucrose and also to increase the solubility of other ingredients.

- Alcohol: It is used as a solvent for volatile oils and it also acts as a preservative.

Invert syrup: It is prepared by hydrolyzing sucrose with hydrochloric acid and neutralizing the solution with $CaCO_3$ or Na_2CO_3. The sucrose in the 66.7% w/v solution must be at least 95% inverted. The invert syrup, when mixed in suitable proportions with syrup, prevents the deposition of crystals of sucrose under storage conditions.

Preparation of Simple Syrups

a. *Solution with heat:* This is the usual method of making syrups, when there are no volatile agents and when the syrup is to be prepared rapidly. The sucrose is added to the purified water or aqueous solution and heated until it dissolves. Then strained and sufficient purified water is added to make the desired weight or volume. Excess heating is avoided while preparing syrups to prevent inversion of sucrose that leads to increased tendency of fermentation. Syrups cannot be sterilized by autoclaving without caramelization (yellow color). Specific gravity is an important property to identify concentration of the syrup. Syrup has a specific gravity of about 1.313 that means each 100 ml of syrup weighs 131.3 g.

b. *Agitation without heat:* This method is used when there is presence of volatile constituents in the syrup. In this, the syrup is prepared by adding sucrose to the aqueous solution in a bottle of about twice the size required for the syrup. This permits active agitation and rapid solution. No heat is applied in this method as it leads to volatilization of the volatile constituents of the syrup. To prevent the product from contamination and from loss, the bottle is to be stoppered.

c. *Addition of a medicating liquid to syrup:* This method is used to those syrups in which fluid extracts, tinctures, or other liquids are added to medicate the syrup. In this, the medicated substance is added to the syrup. This generally develops precipitate as the extracts (dissolved in alcohol), when added to the syrup cause precipitation of the medicated substance. A modification of this process consists of mixing the fluid extract or tincture with the water, allowing the mixture to stand in order to permit the separation of insoluble constituents, if any and then the mixture is filtered and then the sucrose is dissolved in the filtrate. This method is not preferred when the precipitated ingredients are the valuable medicinal agents.

d. *Percolation:* In this procedure, purified water or an aqueous solution is permitted to pass slowly through a bed of crystalline sucrose, thus dissolving it and forming syrup with a pledge of cotton placed in the neck of the percolator. If necessary, a portion of the liquid is repassed through the percolator to dissolve the remaining sucrose, if any. This method is used for the preparation of syrup USP.

Preservation of Syrups

- The USP suggests that syrups should be kept at a temperature not above 25°C.

- Preservatives such as glycerin, methyl paraben, benzoic acid and sodium benzoate may be added to prevent bacterial and mold growth, especially when the concentration of sucrose in the syrup is low.

- The concentration of preservative is proportional to the free water.

- The official syrups should be preserved in well dried bottles and stored in a cool dark place.

Dextrose-based syrups: Dextrose may be used as a substitute for sucrose in syrups containing strong acids in order to eliminate the discoloration associated with inversion. Dextrose forms a saturated solution in water at 70% w/v that is less viscous than simple syrup. It dissolves more slowly than sucrose and is less sweet. Preservatives are required to improve the quality of such syrups. Glycerin is added in concentration of 30 to 45% v/v as preservative.

Artificial syrups (non-nutritive syrups): These act as substitutes for syrups and are to be administered to persons suffering from diabetes mellitus, e.g. "Diabetic Simple Syrup" that contains compound sodium cyclamate (6% cyclamate sodium and 0.6% saccharin sodium).

However, some studies showed that the cyclamate could produce cancer in animals and, as a result, its usage is stopped. Similar studies have been carried out on saccharin. Much research has been done to find a safe synthetic substitute for sucrose. Nowadays, aspartame which is about 200 times sweeter than sucrose is being used in many commercial preparations as the sweetening agent.

Sorbitol-based syrups: Sorbitol which is hexahydric alcohol made by hydrogenation of glucose is used in the preparation of syrups. It is used mostly in the form of a 70% w/w aqueous solution. Sorbitol solution is not irritating to the membrane of the mouth and throat and does not contribute to the formation of dental carries. Sorbitol is metabolized and converted to glucose; however, it is not rapidly absorbed from the GIT as sugars. No significant hyperglycemia has been found and it may also be used as component of non-nutritive vehicles. Sorbitol solution does not support mold growth. Preservative should be used in solution containing less than 60% w/w sorbitol.

Linctuses

These are the liquid oral preparations used for demulcent, sedative or expectorant action. These are formulated as viscous solutions containing high concentrations of sucrose or polyhydric alcohol or alcohols. These are intended to be sipped slowly and are allowed to trickle down through the throat in an undiluted form, e.g. Simple Linctus BP, Diamorphine Linctus.

Honeys

These are thick liquid preparations in which honey is used as a base, instead of syrup. Only few official preparations are available containing honey, e.g. oxymel, or acid honey which is a mixture of acetic acid, water and honey

Mucilages

These are thick, viscid, adhesive liquids, produced by dispersing gum in water. Mucilages are used as suspending agents for insoluble substances in liquids. Their colloidal character and viscosity prevent immediate sedimentation of the insoluble ingredients, e.g. gum acacia, gum tragacanth. Synthetic agents like carboxymethylcellulose (CMC) or polyvinyl alcohol are nonglycogenetic in nature and are be used for diabetic patients.

Jellys

These are preparations having jelly-like consistency. They are also prepared from gums. These are also used as lubricants for surgical gloves and catheters, e.g. lidocaine HCl Jelly USP is used as a topical anesthetic.

Non-aqueous Pharmaceutical Solutions

These are the pharma-ceutical solutions in which non-aqueous solvents are used either alone or in combination with water depending on the type of preparation and its usage. These solvents are used for drugs that are insoluble or incompletely soluble in water. Oily solutions of drugs are often used for depot therapy.

Important aspects to be considered for selection of non-aqueous solvent: The toxicity, irritancy, flammability, stability, compatibility and cost of the solvents used in the preparation of non-aqueous solutions are to be checked before its use.

- Solvents such as acetone, benzene and petroleum ether are not used for internal products.
- Internal products may contain ethanol, glycerol, propylene glycol, certain oils.
- For parenteral products, the choice is very limited.

Non-aqueous Solutions Include

- Alcoholic or hydroalcoholic solutions—the elixirs and spirits
- Ethereal solutions—the collodions

- Glycerin solutions—the glycerites
- Oleaginous solutions—the liniments, medicated oils, oleo-vitamins, sprays, and toothache drops.

Elixirs

These are clear, pleasantly flavored, sweetened hydro alcoholic liquids that have potent or unpleasant tasting drugs, intended for oral use. They are used as flavors and vehicles. The main ingredients in elixirs are ethanol and water but glycerin, sorbitol, propylene glycol, flavoring agents, preservatives, and syrups are often used in the preparation of the final product. Pediatric elixirs generally contain fruit syrup that acts as a flavoring agent, e.g. dexamethasone elixir USP and phenobarbital elixir USP, terpin hydrate elixir USP and chlorol elixir.

Incompatibility of Elixir

- Alcohol precipitates water-soluble substances like tragacanth, acacia, agar and many inorganic salts from aqueous solutions.
- If an aqueous solution is added to an elixir, a partial precipitation of ingredients may occur. This is due to the reduced alcoholic content of the final preparation.

Preparation of elixirs: Simple solution is the general process employed in the preparation of elixirs. In this, the medicinal substances are added directly to aromatic elixir that acts as elixir base. They are simple to mix but difficult to filtrate. Hence suction filtration is recommended.

Spirits: These are alcoholic or hydroalcoholic solutions of volatile substances. The active ingredient may be gas, liquid or solid dissolved in absolute or diluted ethanol. They may be used internally for their medicinal value, by inhalation. Mostly used as flavoring agents. These are stored in air-tight, light-resistant containers and in a cool place.

Collodions: These are mainly solutions with pyroxylin (a nitrocellulose) in a vehicle of ethyl ether and ethanol. They are applied to the skin by means of a soft brush or other suitable applicator. When it becomes dry, the collodion leaves a thin flexible film of cellulose on the surface of the skin. This is used to cover the minor injuries on the skin which retains the dissolved drug in contact with the skin for extended period. Addition of castor oil and camphor enhances the flexibility of the collodion, e.g. salicylic acid collodion USP, contains 10% w/v of salicylic acid is used as a keratolytic agent in the treatment of corns and warts.

Glycerins: These are solutions or mixtures of medicinal substances which contain not less than 50% by weight of glycerin. These are extremely viscous. Glycerin is a valuable pharmaceutical solvent which can form permanent and concentrated solutions. These are hygroscopic in nature and are to be stored in tightly closed containers, e.g. glycerin is used as the sole solvent for the preparation of antipyrine and benzocaine otic solution USP. Glycerin alone is used as an aid in the removal of cerumen.

Liniments: These are solutions or mixtures of various substances in oil, alcoholic solutions of soaps, or emulsions. They are intended for external application and should be so labeled properly. They are applied with rubbing to the affected area, the oil or soap base provides ease of application and massage. Alcoholic liniments are used generally for their rubefacient and counter irritant effects. Such liniments penetrate the skin more readily than those with an oil base. The oily liniments are milder in their action and may function solely as protective coatings. These are not applied to skin that are bruised or broken.

Lotions: These are the solutions which may also be suspensions or emulsions, which are intended to be applied on to the skin smoothly without any friction. Some lotions, in which the vehicle for the medicament is alcohol based, are applied on to the scalp which allows for rapid drying of the hair. This makes the product more acceptable by the patient. In these cases, proper labeling is done to avoid problems of flammability, e.g. salicylic acid lotion 2% BPC.

Oleo Vitamins

These are fish liver oils diluted with edible vegetable oil or solutions of the indicated vitamins (usually vitamins A and D). The indicated vitamins are unstable in the presence of rancid oils and, therefore, those preparations are to be stored in small, light resistance, air-tight containers, preferably under vacuum or under an atmosphere of an inert gas and should be protected from light, e.g. Abidec vitamin drops.

Mixtures

Mixtures are the pharmaceutical oral solutions, e.g. chloralhydrate mixture, ammonia and ipecacuanha mixture BP.

Packaging of Pharmaceutical Solutions

The route of adminis-tration is the major criteria while selecting the type of packaging of the pharmaceutical solutions. The bottles used for packaging are available in different sizes and it is important to choose a suitable container to match the volume of the product to be dispensed.

Containers Used for Dispensing Oral Solutions

- Amber-colored bottles are used with a child-resistance closure.
- A measuring device like spoon or an oral syringe of 5 ml capacity should also be provided.

Containers for Mouthwashes and Gargles

- These are generally packed in fluted amber bottles which have vertical ridges or grooves.
- By this it can be easily identified by both touch and sight that these preparations are not intended for oral administration.

Table 2.1 represents the packaging of pharmaceutical solutions.

SUSPENSIONS

Suspensions are class of liquid dosage forms in which the finely divided solid particles (internal phase) are dispersed uniformly in a liquid dispersion medium (external phase). These forms one of the major classes of liquid dosage forms. A pharmaceutical suspension is a suspension in which the dispersed particles show therapeutic activity. The formulation, manufacturing, stability and packaging are the important aspects to be considered in the designing of pharmaceutical suspensions.

Table 2.1: Packaging of pharmaceutical solutions

Type of preparation	Bottle type	Typical sizes	Examples of pharmaceutical products
Oral solutions	Amber, flat medical bottle	50 ml, 100 ml, 200 ml, 300 ml, 400 ml, 500 ml	Elixirs Linctuses Draughts Mixtures Spirits Syrups
	Amber round medical bottle with dropper	10 ml	Pediatric drops
External solutions	Amber fluted medical bottle	50 ml, 100 ml, 200 ml	Collodions Enemas Douches Mouthwashes Gargles Liniments Lotions
	Amber fluted medical bottle with dropper	10 ml	Ear drops and Nose drops

Phases of a Suspension

Two phases form a suspension: Internal phase and external phase.

- The internal phase consists of finely divided insoluble solid particles which have a specific range of size that are maintained uniformly throughout the dispersion medium with aid of single or combination of suspending agent.
- The external phase is the dispersion medium in which the finely divided solid particles are suspended. It is generally aqueous in nature. Organic or oily liquids are also used for preparation of external suspensions.

Advantages and Disadvantages of pharmaceutical Suspensions

Although suspensions have many advantages, they suffer with certain disadvantages.

Advantages

- Insoluble derivatives of certain drugs are more palatable than soluble forms and these derivatives are formulated in the form of suspensions.
- Some insoluble derivatives of drugs are more stable in aqueous solvents than in the soluble salts.
- Suspension can improve chemical stability of certain drug, e.g. procaine penicillin G.
- Suspended insoluble powders are easy to swallow. Bulky powders such as kaolin BP and chalk BP can be administered in suspension form which acts as adsorbents of toxic substances in the gastrointestinal tract.
- Drug in suspension exhibits higher rate of bioavailability than other solid dosage forms. The decreasing order of bioavailability of drug in the dosage form is as follows:
  Solution > Suspension > Capsule > Compressed tablet > Coated tablet
- Duration and onset of action can be controlled, e.g. protamine zinc-insulin suspension.
- Suspension can mask the unpleasant/bitter taste of drug, e.g. chloramphenicol palmitate.

Disadvantages

- They should be shaked well prior to administration.
- Physical stability, sedimentation and compaction can causes problems.
- Care should be taken while handling and transport due to its bulky nature.
- Formulation of an ideal suspension is difficult.
- Uniform and accurate dose cannot be achieved unless suspension is packed in single dosage form.

Types of pharmaceutical suspensions: The common pharmaceutical products that are administered in the form of surfactants include ear drops, enemas, inhalations, lotions and mixtures for oral use.

Desired Features of an Ideal Pharmaceutical Suspension

- The sediment formed should be easily re-suspended by the use of moderate shaking.

- It should be easy to pour.
- It should have pleasant odor, color and palatability.
- It should have good syringeability.
- It should be physically, chemically and microbiologically stable.
- Parenteral/ophthalmic suspension should be sterile.

CLASSIFICATION OF SUSPENSIONS

- *Based on route of administration:*
  - Oral suspensions
  - Parenteral suspensions
  - Topical suspensions

- *Based on proportion of solid particles:*
  - Dilute suspension (2 to 10% w/v solid)
  - Concentrated suspension (50% w/v solid)

- *Based on electrokinetic nature of solid particles:*
  - Flocculated suspension
  - Deflocculated suspension

- *Based on size of solid particles*
  - Colloidal suspension (< 1 micron)
  - Coarse suspension (>1 micron)

Reasons for the Formulation of a Pharmaceutical Suspension

- The drug is insoluble in the vehicle.
- To mask the bitter taste of the drug
- To increase the stability of the drug
- To make the drug sustained or controlled release

Important Considerations in Formulation of a Suspension

During the formulation of a suspension, the properties both the dispersed phase and dispersion medium should be known well in order to obtain a good suspension. The route of administration, intended application and possible adverse effects of the material should be well studied, and then it is selected for formulating into a suspension. The following are the most important factors that are to be considered during formulation a pharmaceutical suspension.

Nature of the Suspended Material

The suspended particles should possess low interfacial tension so that they are easily wetted by water and hence can be suspended easily. Particles with high interfacial tension are not wetted easily. In this case, surfactants are used which reduces the interfacial tension of the particles and increases their wettability.

Size of the suspended particles: As per the Stoke's law, the sedimentation rate decreases when the particle size is reduced. It is given by the equation

$$\text{Rate of sedimentation, } V = \frac{d^2(\rho_1 - \rho_2)g}{18\eta_o}$$

where,

V	=	terminal velocity of sedimentation (cm/s)
d	=	diameter of the particle (cm)
η_o	=	viscosity of the suspending medium
g	=	acceleration due to gravity
ρ_1 and ρ_2	=	densities of the suspending particles and the medium, respectively.

The particle size reduction can be achieved by milling, grinding, and sieving. The particle size of the suspension affects the drug dissolution, rate and extent of absorption and biodistribution of the drug. The particle size should be maintained as such it should not form a hard cake on sedimentation.

Viscosity of the dispersion medium: Greater viscosity of the medium provides good suspension as it slows the rate of sedimentation of suspending particles. The viscosity of the suspension should be maintained as such it shows good syringeability (parenteral suspensions) and spreadability (topical suspensions). The property of shear thinning is desirable as such high viscosity during storage (low shear) decreases the rate of sedimentation and achieving of low viscosity after agitation (high shear) facilitates the ease of pourability of suspension from the bottle.

Applications of Pharmaceutical Suspensions

1. Suspension is usually applicable for drug which is insoluble or poorly soluble, e.g. prednisolone.

2. To enhance the stability of drug, e.g. oxytetracycline suspension.

3. To mask bitter or unpleasant taste of the drug, e.g. chloramphenicol palmitate suspension.

4. Suspension of drug can be formulated for topical application, e.g. calamine lotion.

5. Suspension can be formulated for parenteral application in order to control rate of drug absorption, e.g. procaine penicillin.

6. Vaccines are often formulated as suspension, e.g. cholera vaccine.

7. X-ray contrast agents can also be formulated as suspension, e.g. barium sulfate for examination of alimentary tract.

Theory of Suspensions

Sedimentation Behavior

Sedimentation means settling of particles or floccules under gravitational force in liquid dosage form. The rate of sedimentation is given by Stokes's law

$$\text{Rate of sedimentation, } V = \frac{d^2(\rho_1 - \rho_2)g}{18\eta_o}$$

where,

V	=	terminal velocity of sedimentation (cm/s)
d	=	diameter of the particle (cm)
η_o	=	viscosity of the suspending medium
g	=	acceleration due to gravity
ρ_1 and ρ_2	=	densities of the suspending particles and the medium, respectively.

Factors Affecting Sedimentation

Particle size diameter (d): Sedimentation velocity (V) is directly proportional to the square of diameter of particle (d).

$$V \propto d^2$$

Density difference between dispersed phase and dispersion media $(\rho_1 - \rho_2)$*:* The velocity of sedimentation is directly proportional to the difference between the dispersed phase and dispersion medium.

$$V \alpha (\rho_1 - \rho_2)$$

Generally, the density of the suspended particles is greater than dispersion medium. But in certain cases particle density is less than dispersion medium, so suspended particle floats and hence uniform dispersion of the particles is difficult. If density of the dispersed phase and dispersion medium are equal, the rate of settling becomes zero.

Viscosity of dispersion medium (η_o): Sedimentation velocity is inversely proportional to viscosity of dispersion medium.

$$V \alpha 1/\eta_o$$

Increase in viscosity of medium decreases settling, so that the particles achieve good dispersion system. But increase in viscosity should not be such that it gives rise to problems like pouring, syringeability and redispersibility of suspension.

Advantages of the Viscosity of Medium

- High viscosity inhibits the crystal growth.
- High viscosity prevents the transformation of metastable crystal to stable crystal.
- High viscosity enhances the physical stability.

Disadvantages of the Viscosity Medium

- High viscosity hinders the redispersibility of the sediment.
- High viscosity retards the absorption of the drug.
- High viscosity creates problems in handling of the material during manufacturing.

Sedimentation parameters: There are two important parameters that are to be considered in the formulation of suspensions.
1. Sedimentation volume (F)
2. Degree of flocculation (B)
3. Sedimentation velocity (V_s)

Sedimentation volume (F): It is the ratio of final or ultimate volume (V_u) of the sediment to original volume of the suspension (V_o). The sedimentation volume gives only a qualitative account of suspension. It is given by the equation;

$$F = V_u/V_o$$

Sometimes sedimentation volume is represented as height of suspension (H) when measuring cylinder is used to measure the volume of sediment. It is given by the equation;

$$F = H_u/H_o$$

where,

H_u = Final or ultimate height of the sediment;

H_o = Initial or original height of the sediment;

The following diagrammatic representation (Fig. 2.1) shows the sedimentation volumes of flocculated and deflocculated suspensions.

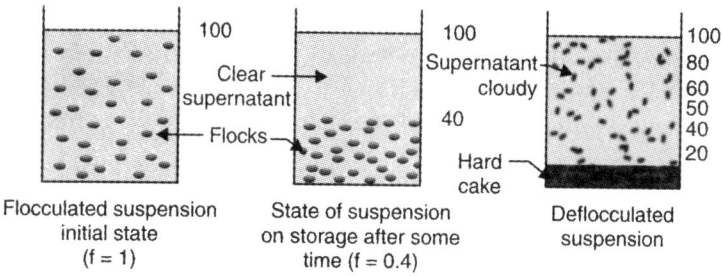

Flocculated suspension
initial state
(f = 1)

State of suspension
on storage after some
time (f = 0.4)

Deflocculated
suspension

Fig. 2.1: Sedimentation volume of flocculated and deflocculated suspensions

Ranges of Sedimentation Volume

- Sedimentation volume can have values ranging from < 1 to >1
- F is normally less than 1.
- When F = 1, the suspension is said to be in flocculation equilibrium and it shows no clear supernatant on standing. It is said as an ideal suspension.

Degree of flocculation (B): It is the ratio of ultimate volume of sedimentation (F) of the flocculated suspension to the ultimate volume of sedimentation (F_∞) of the deflocculated suspension.

Degree of flocculation, $B = F/F_\infty$

Sedimentation velocity (V_s)

Sedimentation behavior of flocculated and deflocculated suspensions

Flocculated suspensions: In the flocculated suspension, the flocks or loose aggregates formed increase the rate of sedimentation of particles. Hence the sediment will form at a faster rate. In this the sedimentation depends not only on the size of the flocks but also on the porosity of flocks. In this the loose structure of the rapidly sedimenting flocks tends to preserve in the sediment, which contains an appreciable amount of entrapped liquid (Fig. 2.2). In this case, the volume of the final sediment is relatively large. This type of suspensions is easily redispersed upon little agitation.

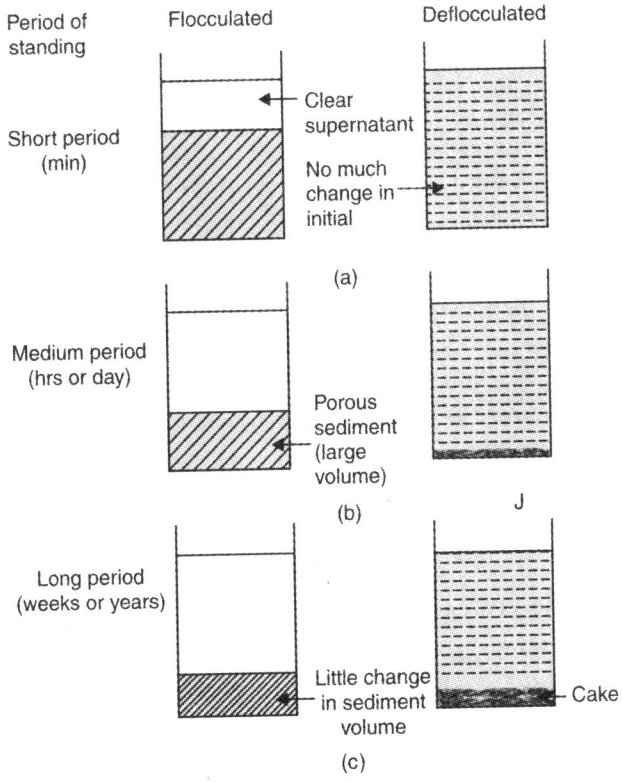

Fig. 2.2: Rate of sedimentation of flocculated and deflocculated suspensions

Deflocculated suspensions: In deflocculated suspension, the particles of the suspension settle separately without formation of any flocks or aggregates. If the rate of sedimentation is slow that prevents entrapping of liquid medium in between the particles and hence it forms a hard cake upon standing for longer period. The sediment cannot be redispersed by little agitation. This phenomenon is also called 'cracking' or 'claying'. In deflocculated suspension, larger particles settle faster and the smaller particles remain in supernatant liquid. Hence supernatant appears cloudy. Whereas in flocculated suspension as the smaller particles are also involved in formation of flocks or aggregates, the supernatant does not appear cloudy.

Brownian movement: Brownian movement of the particle prevents the sedimentation of the particles by keeping them in random motion. This depends on the density of the dispersed particles and density and viscosity of the suspending medium. The molecules of the suspending medium help in kinetic bombardment of the particles, which makes them suspended in the medium. This phenomenon is carried out only when the particle size of the dispersed phase is below the critical radius (r).

When the density and viscosity of the suspending medium are favorable and when the particle size of the dispersed phase is in the range of 2–5 mm, Brownian motion can be observed. This phenomenon can be observed under a microscope or the light scattering of the bombarded particles can be observed under an ultra-microscope, when the particle is about 2 μ in diameter.

The distance (Di) moved by the particles due to Brownian motion is given by,

$$Di^2 = \frac{RTt}{N_3 \pi \eta r}$$

where,

R = Molar gas constant
T = Temperature in Kelvin
N = Avogadro's number
η = Viscosity of the suspending medium
r = Radius of the suspended particle
t = Time

As the radius of the particles increases, the Brownian motion becomes less and this leads to sedimentation of the particles. No sedimentation diameter (NSD) refers to the diameter of the particles in which there will be no sedimentation of the particles. This also depends on the density and viscosity of that particular system.

Zeta Potential

It is the difference in the potential between the surface of the tightly bound layer (shear plane) and electro-neutral region of the suspension. Figure 2.3 shows a rapid potential drop at first, followed by gradual decrease, as the distance from the surface increases. This is because the counterions that are close to the surface act as a screen that reduces the electrostatic attraction between the charged surface and those counter-ions that are away from the surface.

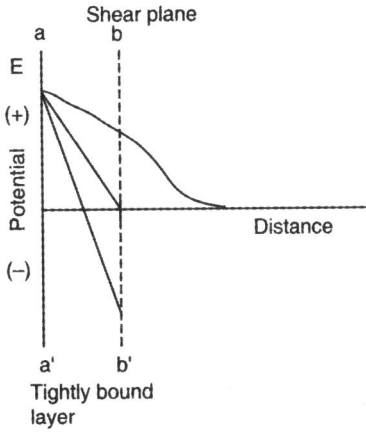

Fig. 2.3: Zeta potential behavior of a suspension

Zeta potential governs the degree of repulsion between the similarly charged, adjacent dispersed particles and it maintains the stability of the dispersed systems. If the zeta potential is reduced below a certain value, attractive forces exceed the repulsive forces and the particles come closer. This phenomenon is called flocculation. When the zeta potential is between +20 to –20 mv, the system forms a flocculated suspension. Thus zeta potential determines the flocculation or deflocculation behavior of the suspension. The zeta potential is measured by using zeta meter.

The charge carried by the particles can be obtained from the adjuvants used as well as during processes like crystallization, grinding processing, and adsorption of ions from solution having ionic surfactants.

Flocculating agents: Flocculating agents are the substances that decrease zeta potential of the suspended particle and thus cause aggregation (flock formation) of the particles. For example:

- Neutral electrolytes such as KCl and NaCl.
- Calcium salts, sulfates, citrates and phosphate salts, and alum.

Applications

- Neutral electrolytes like NaCl and KCl also reduce the interfacial tension of the surfactant solution besides acting as a flocculating agent.
- For particles having less surface charge, e.g. monovalent ions are sufficient to cause flocculation, e.g. for steroidal drugs.
- For particles having high surface charge divalent or trivalent ions are used as flocculating agents, e.g. for insoluble polymers and polyelectrolyte species.

Approaches of floccule formation: The different substances employed in the floccules formation are as follows:

1. *Electrolytes:* Electrolytes decrease electrical barrier between the particles and bring them together to form floccules. They reduce zeta potential near to zero value that results in formation of bridge between adjacent particles so that they arrange together as loose structures, e.g. addition of monobasic potassium phosphate to the bismuth subnitrate suspension results in the formation of a flocculated suspension due to the decrease in the zeta potential of the suspended particles.

2. *Surfactants:* Both ionic and non-ionic surfactants in optimum concentrations can be used to bring about flocculation of suspended particles. The addition of surfactants reduces the surface free energy by reducing the surface tension. This causes the particles to attract each other by van der Waals forces and hence forms loose agglomerates, e.g. polysorbate 80, etc.

Disadvantages of surfactants:

- They have foaming tendencies.
- They are bitter in taste (except poloxamers).

- Some surfactants interact with preservatives such as methyl parabens, e.g. polysorbate 80.

3. *Polymers:* Polymers possess long chain in their structures. The part of the long chain is adsorbed on to the surface of the particles and remaining part projects out into the dispersed medium. Bridging between these later portions, also leads to the formation of flocs, e.g. starch, alginates, cellulose derivatives, carbomers, tragacanth.

4. *Viscosity of suspensions:* Viscosity of suspensions is of great importance for stability and pourability of suspensions. As the viscosity of the dispersion medium increases, the dispersed phase settles at a slower rate and it remains dispersed for longer time and hence increases the stability of the suspension. The viscosity of suspension should be maintained within optimum range to yield stability and pourability.

Different Approaches to Increase the Viscosity of Suspensions

Various approaches have been suggested to enhance the viscosity of suspensions.

1. *Viscosity enhancers:* These are the agents that increase the viscosity of the suspension, e.g. some natural gums (acacia, tragacanth), cellulose derivatives (sodium CMC, methylcellulose), clays (bentonite, veegum), carbomers, colloidal silicon dioxide (aerosil), and sugars (glucose, fructose) are used to enhance the viscosity of the dispersion medium. They are known as suspending agents.

2. *Cosolvents:* Some solvents which themselves have high viscosity are used as cosolvents to enhance the viscosity of dispersion medium, e.g. glycerol, propylene glycol, sorbitol.

Thixotropy: It is the phenomenon of conversion of gel to sol. Thixotropic substances on applying shear stress convert to sol (fluid) and on standing they slowly turn to gel (semisolid).

Other components of a suspension

1. *Wetting agents:* Hydrophilic materials are easily wetted by water than hydrophobic materials. However, hydrophobic

materials are easily wetted by non-polar liquids. The extent of wetting by water is dependent on the hydrophilicity of the materials. Inability of wetting reflects the higher interfacial tension between material and liquid. The interfacial tension must be reduced so that air is displaced from the solid surface by liquid. For example:

- *Non-ionic surfactants:* The surfactants having HLB value between 7–10 are best as wetting agents with concentration of less than 0.5.

- *Hydrophilic colloids:* Hydrophilic colloids coat hydrophobic drug particles in one or more than one layer. This enhances the hydrophilicity of the drug particles and hence facilitates wetting, e.g. acacia, tragacanth, alginates, guar gum, pectin, gelatin, wool fat, egg yolk, bentonite, veegum, methylcellulose, etc.

- *Solvents:* The most commonly used solvents are alcohol, glycerin, polyethylene glycol and polypropylene glycol. They reduce liquid air interfacial tension and hence improve the wettability of the suspended particles.

Quality control of suspensions: The following tests are carried out in the final quality control of suspension:

- Color, odor and taste
- Physical characteristics such as particle size determination and microscopic photography for crystal growth
- Sedimentation volume
- Sedimentation rate
- Zeta potential measurement
- Redispersibility and centrifugation tests
- Rheological measurement
- Stress test
- Freeze-thaw temperature cycling
- Compatibility with container and cap liner

Packaging of Suspensions

Pharmaceutical suspensions are generally packaged in wide mouth container that has adequate space above the liquid to ensure proper mixing. Generally, glass and plastic materials are used as packaging material. The guidelines for packaging of suspensions are summarized in Table 2.2.

Table 2.2: Packaging of pharmaceutical suspensions

Suspension type	Bottle type	Typical size	Examples
Oral suspensions	Amber flat medical bottle	50 ml, 100 ml, 150 ml, 200 ml, 300 ml and 500 ml	Mixtures for oral (suspension) use
External suspensions	Amber fluted medical bottle	50 ml, 100 ml and 200 ml	Inhalations, applications, lotions
	Amber fluted medical bottle with dropper top	10 ml and 20 ml	Ear drops and nasal drops

The ideal requirements of packaging material should comply with the following requirements;

- It should be inert.
- It should effectively preserve the product from light, air, and other contamination throughout the shelf life.
- It should be cheap.
- It should effectively deliver the product without any difficulty.

Labeling requirements: The labeling of pharmaceutical suspensions is important for ease of patient administration.

They are as follows:

- Shake well before use
- Not to taken: In case of inhalation suspensions
- For external use only: In case of external suspensions that are not intended for oral administration.
- Do not freeze
- Protect from direct sunlight.

EMULSIONS

Emulsion is a thermodynamically unstable liquid preparation containing at least two immiscible liquids, in which one liquid phase is dispersed as globules (dispersed or internal phase) in other liquid phase (continuous or external phase) stabilized with the aid of an emulsifying agent (Fig. 2.4). General types of pharmaceutical emulsions include lotions, liniments, ointments, creams, and vitamin drops.

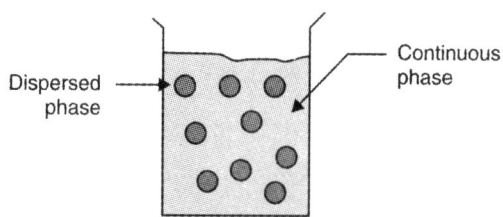

Fig. 2.4: Dispersed phase and continuous phase of an emulsion

Advantages and Disadvantages of Pharmaceutical Emulsions

Advantages

- Unpalatable drugs can be administered in palatable form.
- Oil sensation of oil-soluble drugs can be masked as aqueous phase can easily disperses the flavors in it.
- Improve the rate of absorption of drugs.
- Two incompatible ingredients can be included one in each phase of an emulsion.

Disadvantages

- The emulsion should be shaked every time prior to administration.
- It needs an accurate measuring device for measuring the dose for administration.
- Proper storage conditions are required.
- Bulky and difficult to transport and may prone to breakage.
- Easily contaminated by microorganisms that lead to emulsion instability.

Types of Emulsions

- Macroemulsion or simple emulsion
- Microemulsion
- Multiple emulsion

Macroemulsions (Simple Emulsions)

In this type of emulsion, one phase of emulsion gets dispersed in the other phase generally water in oil (w/o type) or oil in water (o/w type) (Fig. 2.5). The size of the droplets is approximately 5 μm.

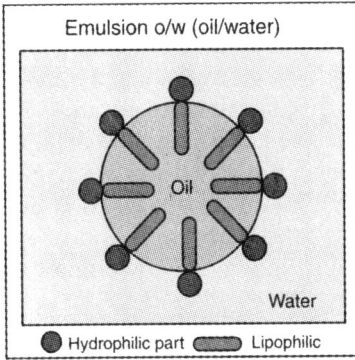 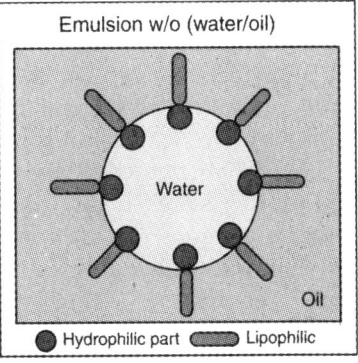

Fig. 2.5: A simple emulsion: o/w type and w/o type

Oil in water (o/w): In this, the oil droplets are dispersed in a continuous aqueous phase. This emulsion is generally formed if the aqueous phase constitutes more than 45% of the total weight. In this, a hydrophilic emulsifier is used. The globule size is 0.25 to 10 microns. These are generally used for oral administration. These are useful as water-washable drug bases.

Water in oil (w/o): In this case, the aqueous phase is dispersed in a continuous oily phase. This emulsion is generally formed, if the oily phase constitutes more than 45% of the total weight and a lipophilic emulsifier is used. These are generally used for cosmetics. These are employed for treatment of dry skin and emollient applications.

Microemulsions

These are the clear, homogenous emulsions in which one insoluble liquid is dispersed in a second liquid. Droplets sizes range from 0.01 to 0.1 µm. These are generally referred to as solubilized systems or transparent emulsions, micellar solutions as they appear as true solutions to the naked eye. Microemulsions are believed o be thermodynamically stable. These are used for drug adn inistration and toiletry products.

Pharmaceutical applications of microemulsions

- Increase the bioavailability of poorly water-soluble drugs.
- Topical drug delivery systems.

Multiple emulsions: These emulsions consist of three phases that are developed with a view to delay the release of an active ingredient. They may be oil-in-water-in-oil (o/w/o) or of water-in-oil-in-water (w/o/w) (Fig. 2.6). Lipophilic (oil-soluble, low HLB) surfactants are used to stabilize w/o emulsions, whereas hydrophilic (water-soluble, high HLB) surfactants are used to stabilize o/w systems. In these types of emulsions, the drug is present in innermost phase so that is has to cross two phase boundaries to reach the external continuous phase. In some cases, inversion of such emulsions take place such that they form simple emulsions by converting from a w/o/w emulsion to o/w emulsion.

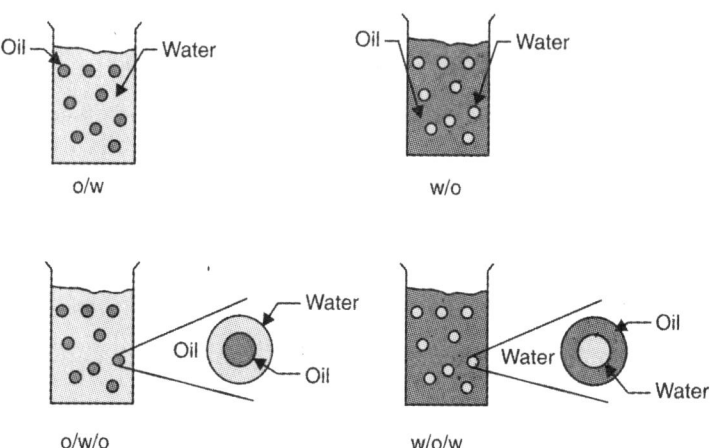

Fig. 2.6: Multiple emulsions

Preparation of Multiple Emulsions

In this, the aqueous phase is added to oily phase, containing a lipophilic surfactant by continuous mixing. This results in the formation of primary w/o emulsion. This w/o emulsion is then poured into a second aqueous solution that has a hydrophilic surfactant by continuous mixing. This results in the formation of a w/o/w multiple emulsion.

Pharmaceutical applications

- Multiple emulsions are widely used in cosmetics, pharmaceuticals and foods.
- They sustained the release of active ingredient as it has to pass from the internal phase (w/o or o/w phase) to the continuous phase (either water or oil). They can also improve dissolutions or solubilization of insoluble materials.
- These types of emulsions are used to protect sensitive and active molecules such as vitamin C and E from undergoing oxidation.

Factors Affecting the Type of Emulsion

The type of emulsion produced (o/w or w/o) depends upon following factors.

Type of Emulsifying Agent

Type of emulsion is a function of relative solubility of emulsifying agent. The phase in which the emulsifying agent gets solubilized becomes the continuous phase.

Phase volume ratio, i.e. the relative amount of oil and water

This determines the relative number of droplets formed and hence the probability of number of collision. As the number of droplets becomes more the chance for collision. Thus the phase present in greater amount becomes the external phase. The polar portions of the emulsifying agents are better barriers to coalescence than hydrocarbon counterparts. So o/w emulsions can be formed with relatively high internal phase volume. In w/o emulsion (in which the barrier is of hydrocarbon nature), if the amount of internal phase is increased more than 40%, it inverts to o/w emulsion because hydrocarbon part of surfactant cannot form a strong barrier.

Viscosity of each phase

An increase in viscosity of a phase helps in making that phase the external phase.

Detection of type of emulsion

In general, the emulsion will be diluted only with its continuous phase. Hence o/w can be diluted with water and w/o can be diluted with oil. So when oil is added to o/w emulsion or when water is added to w/o emulsion, separation of internal and continuous phase occurs. This test is used for liquid emulsions (Fig. 2.7).

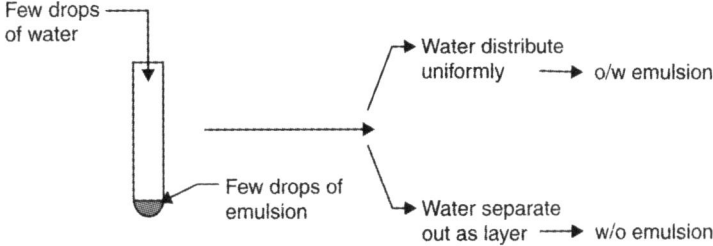

Fig. 2.7: Dilution test for liquid emulsions

Dye Solubility Test

In general, water-soluble dye (e.g. amaranth dye or methylene blue) will be taken up by the aqueous phase where as oil-soluble dye (e.g. scarlet dye) will be taken by oily phase. When it is observed microscopically that water-soluble dye is taken up by the continuous phase, it is o/w emulsion. If the dye is not taken up by the continuous phase, test is repeated with oil-soluble dye. If it is taken up by the continuous phase, it can be confirmed as w/o emulsion. This test can fail, if ionic emulsions are present (Fig. 2.8).

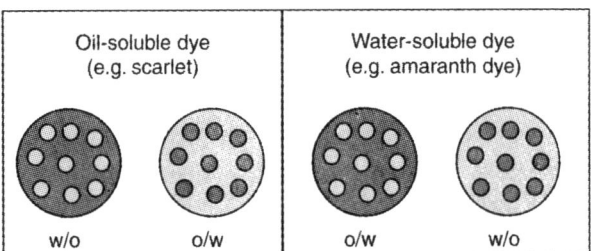

Fig. 2.8: Microscopic examination of type of emulsion by dye solubility test

Conductivity Test

Water is a good conductor of electricity than oil. Hence an emulsion with water as the continuous phase possesses more conductivity than an emulsion with oil as continuous phase. When a pair of electrodes connected to a lamp and an electrical source is dipped into o/w emulsion, the lamp lights because of passage of current between two electrodes. If the lamp does not light, it is assumed to be w/o emulsion (Fig. 2.9).

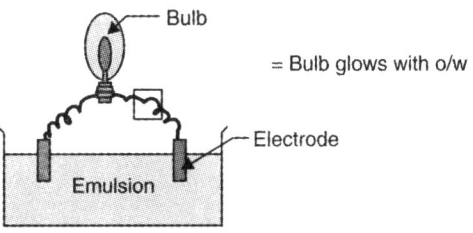

Fig. 2.9: Conductivity test for determination of type of emulsion

CoCl₂ Filter Test

To a filter paper impregnated with $CoCl_2$ and dried (blue), o/w emulsion is added. It changes to pink. It may fail, if emulsion is unstable or breaks in presence of electrolyte.

Fluorescence Test

Since some oils fluoresce under UV light, o/w emulsions exhibit no fluorescence whereas w/o emulsion exhibits fluorescence. But this test is applicable for oils that have fluorescent property.

Pharmaceutical Applications of Emulsions

Emulsions can be used for oral, parenteral or topical pharmaceutical dosage forms.

1. Oral products:
   - It covers the unpleasant taste
   - Increases absorption rate
2. o/w parenteral emulsion:
   - IV lipid nutrients
   - IM depot for water-soluble antigenic material

3. Topical use:
   - Easily washable
   - Acceptable viscosity
   - Less greasy

1. Oral products

Water insoluble drugs are generally administered as o/w emulsions compared to oily solutions, e.g. vitamin capsules.

Advantages of emulsions for oral use

- *More palatability:* Unpleasant taste or texture of medicinal agents gets masked.
- *Better absorption:* Due to small globule size, the medicinal agent gets absorbed faster.

2. Topical Products

Emulsions are widely used for topical application.
- o/w emulsions are more acceptable as they are easily washed by water.
- w/o emulsions are used for the treatment of dry skin.

Advantages of emulsions for topical use

- Patient acceptance due to their elegance
- Washable character
- Acceptable viscosity
- Less greasiness

3. Parenteral Emulsions

- IV route: Lipid nutrients are emulsified and given to patients by IV route. Such emulsions have particle size less than 100 nm, e.g. oil-soluble drugs (like Taxol) can be given parenterally by w/o emulsion.
- Depot injections: w/o emulsions are used to disperse water-soluble antigenic materials in mineral oil for intra-muscular depot injection.

4. Diagnostic Purposes

Radiopaque emulsions are used in X-ray examination.

Theory of emulsification: Stabilization of emulsion is the major step in the preparation of an ideal emulsion that is stable throughout the shelf-life. Droplets can be stabilized by two methods;

1. By reducing interfacial tension
2. By preventing the coalescence of droplets.
   a. By formation of rigid interfacial film
   b. By forming electrical double layer.

By reducing the interfacial tension: The formation of droplets leads to increase in surface free energy, and hence by reducing the surface area of the droplets in emulsion, the interfacial tension can be lowered. Assuming the droplets to be spherical in shape, the energy input is given by;

$$\Delta F = 6 \text{ g V/d}$$

where,

ΔF = energy input required
g = interfacial tension
V = volume of dispersed phase in ml
d = mean diameter of particles

Example: Considered an o/w emulsion which consists of 100 ml of oil, and the mean diameter of the globule is 1 μm (10^{-4} cm) with interfacial tension, g of 50 dynes/cm. The energy input is given by;

$\Delta F = 6 \times 50 \times 100/(1 \times 10^{-4}) = 30 \times 10^7$ ergs = 30 joules or 30/4.184 = 7.2 cal.

In the above example, addition of emulsifier which reduces g from 50 to 5 dynes/cm will reduce the surface free energy from 7.2 to 0.7 cal. This reduction in surface free energy helps in maintaining the surface area generated during the dispersion system thereby increasing the stability of the emulsion.

Preventing the coalescence of droplets: Coalescence of droplets can be prevented by two methods;

• By formation of rigid film around the droplets.
• By formation of electrical double layer.

By formation of rigid interfacial film: Coalescence of droplets can be prevented by formation of films that act as mechanical barrier around each droplet of the dispersed material. This film should possess some degree of surface elasticity, so that it does not breaks when compressed between two droplets. If broken, it should form again rapidly. These films are of three types:

1. *Monomolecular films:* The surface active agents form a monolayer at the oil water interface. This monolayer serves two purposes:
   - Reduces the surface free energy.
   - Forms a barrier between droplets so that they cannot coalesce.

2. *Multimolecular films:* Hydrated lipophilic colloids and finely divided solids form multimolecular films around droplets of dispersed oil. They prevent coalescing by forming a coat around the droplets.

3. *Solid particle films:* Small solid particles which are wetted to some extent by both oily and aqueous phase, can act as emulsifying agent. If the particles are too hydrophilic, they get dispersed in aqueous phase. If they are too hydrophobic, they get dispersed in oily phase. Other requirement is that the particles should be smaller than the droplet size.

By forming electrical double layer: Development of charge on the droplet surface increases stability by causing repulsion between individual droplets. This charge is likely to be greater, if ionized emulsifying agent is employed. In general, intravenous fat emulsions are stabilized with lecithin due to the electrical repulsion.

In an o/w emulsion stabilized by sodium soap, the hydrocarbon tail is dissolved in the oil phase and ionic heads are facing the continuous aqueous phase. As a result, the surface of the droplet is studded with negatively charged carboxylic group. The cations of opposite charge are oriented near the surface, producing a double layer of charge. The potential produced by double layer creates a repulsive effect between the oil droplets and thus prevents coalescence.

Additives Used in the Formulation of Emulsions

1. Emulsifying agents
2. Auxiliary emulsifiers

3. Antimicrobial preservatives
4. Antioxidants

Emulsifying Agents

These are the substances added to an emulsion to prevent the coalescence of the globules of the dispersed phase and hence maintain the stability of emulsion. They are also known as emulgents or emulsifiers. HLB method is indicative of emulsification behavior. An HLB value of 3–6 is used for w/o emulsion and HLB value of 8–18 is used for o/w emulsion. HLB number of a surfactant depends on which phase of the final emulsion it will become. An emulsifying agent mainly acts by the following mechanisms;

- Reduction in interfacial tension: Thermodynamic stabilization
- Formation of a rigid interfacial film: Mechanical barrier to coalescence
- Formation of an electrical double layer: Repulsion of individual droplets.

Ideal requirements of emulsifying agent

- It should be able to reduce the interfacial tension between the two immiscible liquids.
- It should be physically and chemically stable, inert and compatible with the other ingredients of the formulation.
- It should be non-irritant and non-toxic when used in required concentrations.
- It should be organoleptically inert, i.e. should not impart any color, odor or taste to the preparation.
- It should be able to form a coherent film around the globules of the dispersed phase and should prevent the coalescence of the droplets of the dispersed phase.
- It should be able to produce and maintain the required viscosity of the preparation.

Classification of emulsifying agents

a. Synthetic surface active agents (monomolecular films)
b. Semisynthetic polysaccharides
c. Natural hydrophilic colloids (multimolecular films)
d. Finely divided solid particles (particulate film)

Synthetic surface active agents: This group contains surface active agents which act by getting adsorbed at the oil water interface in such a way that the hydrophilic polar groups are oriented towards water and lipophilic non-polar groups are oriented towards oil, thus forming a stable film. This film acts as a mechanical barrier and thus prevents coalescence of the globules of the dispersed phase. The functions of surface active agents to provide stability to dispersed droplets are:

i. Reduction of the interfacial tension

ii. Form coherent monolayer to prevent the coalescence of two droplets when they approach each other (Fig. 2.10)

iii. Provide surface charge which causes repulsion between adjacent particles

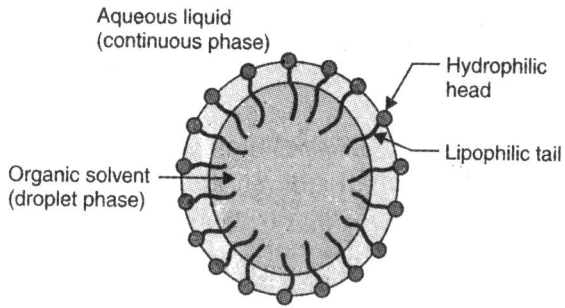

Fig. 2.10: Formation of monomolecular film by surface active agent

Classification of synthetic surface active agents: They are classified according to the ionic charge possessed by the molecules of the surfactant.

• *Anionic surfactants:* These agents are primarily used for external preparations and not for internal use as they have an unpleasant bitter taste and irritant action on the intestinal mucosa, e.g. alkali soaps, polyvalent soaps (metallic soaps), organic soaps, sulfated alcohols and alkyl sulfonates.

• *Cationic surfactants:* They are mainly used in external preparations such as lotions and creams. They have good antibacterial activity and are also used in combination with secondary emulsifying agents to produce o/w emulsions for external application, e.g. quaternary ammonium compounds such as cetrimide, benzalkonium chloride and benzethonium chloride.

- *Non-ionic surfactants:* These are widely used as emulsifying agents to prepare both w/o and o/w emulsions for internal as well as external use, e.g. glyceryl esters, polyoxyethylene glycol esters and ethers, sorbitan fatty acid esters (spans), polyoxyethylene derivatives of sorbitan fatty acid esters (tweens or polysorbates), polyoxyethylene/polyoxypropylene block polymers (poloxamers).

- *Ampholytic surfactants:* These are the substances whose ionic charge depends on the pH of the system. Below a certain pH, these are cationic while above a defined pH, these are anionic. At intermediate pH, these behave as zwitterions, e.g. lecithin.

Semisynthetic polysaccharides: They mainly include cellulose derivatives. They are used for formulating o/w type of emulsions. They primarily act by increasing the viscosity of the system, e.g. methylcellulose, hydroxypropyl cellulose and sodium carboxymethylcellulose.

Natural emulsifying agents: These consist of agents that are derived from either plant or animal source. The emulsifying agents from plant source include mainly of carbohydrates that includes gums and mucilaginous substances. They act as primary emulsifying agents as well as secondary emulsifying agents (emulsion stabilizers). Since carbohydrates act a good medium for the growth of microorganism, the emulsions prepared using these emulsifying agents have to be suitably preserved in order to prevent microbial contamination, e.g. tragacanth, acacia, agar, chondrus (Irish Moss), pectin and starch. The emulsifying agents from animal source include lecithin, cholesterol and wool fat.

Finely dispersed solids: They form particulate films around the dispersed droplets and produce coarse grained emulsions that are stable, e.g. colloidal clays like bentonite, veegum (magnesium aluminum silicate), magnesium trisilicate, metallic hydroxides, magnesium hydroxide and aluminum hydroxide.

Auxiliary (Secondary) Emulsifying Agents

Auxiliary emulsifying agents include those compounds that are normally incapable themselves to form stable emulsion. Their main value lies in their ability to function as thickening agents and thereby helping to stabilize the emulsion. They increase the viscosity of the external phase and restrict the collision of droplets. Some of them prevent coalescence by reducing van der Waals forces between particles or by providing a physical barrier between droplets. Proteins, semisynthetic polysaccharides (methylcellulose, carboxymethylcellulose), clays can be used as auxiliary agents.

Preservatives

These are the agents which are used to prevent the microbial contamination of the emulsion. Once a microbiologically uncontaminated product has been formed, a relatively mild antimicrobial agent is sufficient to protect the product against microbial contamination. The preservative system must be effective against invasion by a variety of pathogenic organisms and protect the product during use by consumer. The microbial contamination may occur due to the following reasons;

- Contamination during development or production of emulsion or during its use
- Usage of impure raw materials
- Poor sanitation conditions
- Invasion by an opportunistic microorganisms
- Contamination by the consumer during use of the product.

Ideal requirements of a preservative

- Less toxic
- Stable to heat and storage
- Chemically compatible
- Reasonable cost
- Acceptable taste, odor and color
- Effective against fungus, yeast, bacteria
- Should be available in oil and aqueous phase at effective level concentration
- Should be in unionized state to penetrate the bacteria
- Should not bind to other components of the emulsion

Types of preservatives

- Chloroform B.P. 50% v/v
- Acids and acid derivatives: Antifungal agent—benzoic acid
- Aldehydes: Broad spectrum—formaldehyde
- Phenols: Broad spectrum—cresol and propyl p-hydroxy benzoate
- Quaternaries: Broad spectrum—chlorhexidine, benzalkonium chloride and cetyl trimethyl ammonium bromide
- Mercurials: Broad spectrum—phenyl mercuric acetate and phenyl mercuric nitrate.

Antoxidants

Many drugs that are incorporated into emulsions are subject to autoxidation resulting in decomposi-tion of the product. Upon autoxidation, unsaturated oils, such as vegetable oils, give rise to rancidity that has unpleasant odor, appearance, and taste. On the other hand, mineral oil and related saturated hydrocarbons rarely undergo oxidative degradation. Since autoxidation is as free radical chain oxidation it can be inhibited by the absence of oxygen, or by a free radical chain breaker, or by addition of an antioxidant or a reducing agent. Antioxidants are generally used at concentration ranging from 0.001 to 0.1%. For example:

- Gallic acid, propyl gallate—pharmaceuticals and cosmetics
- Ascorbic acid—suitable for oral use products
- Sulfites—suitable for oral use products
- L-tocopherol—pharmaceuticals and cosmetics—suitable for oral preparations, e.g. those containing vitamin A.
- Butylated hydroxyl toluene—pharmaceuticals and cosmetics—pronounced odor, to be used at low concentration.
- Butylated hydroxylanisol—pharmaceuticals and cosmetics.

Emulsification Techniques

Two steps of emulsification are to be followed while preparing an emulsion:

1. Breaking of internal phase into droplets by putting energy into the system
2. Stabilization of droplets

Emulsification process can be carried out by four methods:

1. Addition of internal phase to the external phase under high shear or fracture.

2. Phase inversion technique: In this case, inversion of one emulsion to other takes place. For example, if o/w emulsion is to be prepared, first the aqueous phase is added to the oily phase, as a result w/o emulsion is formed. At the inversion point, the addition of more water results in the inversion of the emulsion system and results in an o/w emulsion. This phase inversion technique allows the formation of small droplets with minimal mechanical action and heat.

3. Mixing both phases after warming: This method is used for creams and ointments.

4. Alternate addition of two phases to the emulsifying agent: In this method, the water and oil are added alternatively, in small portions to the emulsifier. This technique is suitable for food emulsions.

Preparation techniques of emulsions

The preparation techniques for emulsion can be divided into laboratory scale production and large-scale production.

Laboratory scale techniques (extemporaneous method of preparation of emulsions): Techniques used on laboratory scale are

- Continental or dry gum method
- Wet gum method
- Bottle or Forbes bottle method
- Auxiliary method
- *In situ* soap method

Continental method or dry gum method: The continental method is used to prepare the initial or primary emulsion from oil, water and an emulsifier (gum usually acacia) in 4:2:1 ratio. The 4 parts of oil and 1 part of gum represent their total amount for the final emulsion.

Method: In this method, 1 part of gum (acacia) is triturated with 4 parts of oil in a mortor, until the powder is thoroughly wetted. Then 2 parts of water is added all at once and the mixture is vigorously and continuously triturated until a creamy white primary emulsion is formed. Additional water may be incorporated after the primary emulsion is formed. Solid substances (like active ingredients, preservatives, colors and flavors) are added as a solution to the primary emulsion, oil- soluble substances in small amounts may be incorporated directly into the primary emulsion. Any substance which might reduce the physical stability of the emulsion, such as alcohol (which may precipitate the gum) is added at the end. When all agents have been incorporated, the emulsion should be transferred to a calibrated vessel, and the final volume is made with water, then homogenized or blended to ensure uniform distribution of ingredients.

Example: Cod liver oil emulsion

Cod liver oil	50 ml
Acacia	12.5 gm
Syrup	10 ml
Flavor oil	0.4 ml
Purified water	up to 100 ml

Method: Weigh accurately all the ingredients. The cod liver oil is placed in dry mortar. Add acacia and mix it quickly. Add 25 ml of water and immediately triturate to form thick white, homogenous primary emulsion. Add flavor and mix. Add syrup and mix. Add sufficient water to make the final volume.

Wet gum method or English method: In this method, the proportion of oil and water and emulsifier (gum) are in the ratio of 4:2:1, but the order and technique of mixing is different from dry gum method. In this 1 part of gum is triturated with 2 parts of water to form mucilage. To this four parts of oil is slowly added in portions, while triturating. After all the oil is added, the mixture is triturated for several minutes to form the primary emulsion. Then other ingredients are added as in continental method. In general, the English method is more difficult to perform successfully, especially with more viscous oils, but it results in a more stable emulsion.

Bottle method: This method is used to prepare emulsions with volatile oils, or oligogenous substances of very low viscosities. This method is a variation of dry gum method. One part of powdered acacia (or other gum) is placed in a dry bottle and

4 parts of oil are added. The bottle is capped and thoroughly shaken. The time of mixing the gum and oil should be less as the gum will tend to imbibe the oil and will become water-proof. To this, required volume of water is added all at once and shaked thoroughly until the primary emulsion is formed.

Auxiliary method: A hand homogenizer is used to improve the emulsion prepared by other methods. In this method, the emulsion is passed through a very small orifice, and hence reduces the dispersed droplet size to about 5 microns or less.

In situ soap method: This contains oils such as olive oil, oleic acid along with lime water (calcium hydroxide solution, USP). These are called calcium soaps. It is prepared by mixing equal volumes of oil and lime water.

Example: Nascent soap which consists of oil phase as olive oil/oleic acid and lime water as aqueous phase. Olive oil can be replaced by other oils but oleic acid must be added. Lime water [$Ca(OH)_2$] should be freshly prepared. The emulsion formed is w/o type emulsion.

Large scale production: Commercially, emulsions are prepared in large volume mixing tanks and refined and stabilized by passage through a colloid mill or homogenizer. The internal phase can be reduced to small droplets by application of energy in the form of heat, agitation, homogenization, milling and ultrasonification.

1. *Heat:* The internal phase can be reduced to small droplets by the application of heat by the following methods:
   - Emulsification by vaporization (condensation method)
   - Emulsification by change in temperature (phase inversion technique)
   - Low energy emulsification

Emulsification by vaporization (condensation method): Vaporization is an effective way of breaking almost all bonds between molecules of a liquid. Emulsions may be prepared by passing vapor of a liquid into an external phase that contains suitable emulsifying agent. This process is called condensation method. But it is a slow and tedious process.

Emulsification by change in temperature (phase inversion technique): Change in temperature can be used as an effective way of making emulsion by phase inversion technique. The temperature at which phase inversion takes place is called phase inversion temperature (PIT). In this method, first the emulsion is prepared at a higher temperature. On cooling, phase inversion takes place and a stable inversion with finely divided internal phase is produced. PIT is generally considered to be the temperature at which the hydrophilic and the lipophilic properties of the emulsifier are in balance and is, therefore, also called the HLB temperature and it depends upon emulsifier concentration.

Low energy emulsification: The emulsification by change in temperature requires considerable expenditure of energy during both heating and cooling cycles. In low energy emulsification, all of the internal phase and only a portion of the external phase are heated. After emulsification of the heated portions, the remainder of the external phase is added to the emulsion concentrate, or the preformed concentrate is blended into the external phase. In those emulsions in which a phase inversion temperature exists, the emulsion concentrate is preferably prepared above PIT which results in emulsion having extremely small droplets size. Good emulsions can be prepared by this method. Variables like emulsification temperature, mixing time, mixing intensity, amount of external phase employed during emulsification and the method of blending are carefully controlled.

2. *Mechanical agitation:* To break up the internal phase into the fine droplets, mechanical agitation is required. In this, the liquid jet at high speed through a small diameter nozzle is introduced into a second liquid or liquid may flow into a second liquid that is agitated vigorously. The degree of shear and turbulence plays an important role in the formation of droplets which further depends on agitation of the dispersion. The degree of agitation depends on total volume of the liquid to be mixed, the viscosity of the system, and the interfacial tension at the oil water interface. Once initial droplets had formed, the droplets are further subjected to additional forces due to turbulence which forms fine droplets. The amount of work depends on the

length of time during which energy is supplied; thus timing becomes another physical parameter.

Timing

- On continuous agitation of the emulsion, it may result in coalescence between the initially formed droplets. Hence excessive period of agitation is avoided during and after the formation of emulsion. The optimum time of agitation has to be determined empirically.

- As it takes some time for the distribution of the emulsifier between the phases, intermittent shaking is the best way in the preparing an emulsion. This film formation on the surface of the droplets may be interrupted by continuous shaking.

- Timing also affects the rate of mixing of two immiscible liquids. The rate at which the oil phase is added to the aqueous phase in o/w emulsion shows effect on the particle size, thereby the stability of emulsion.

- Timing also affects the rate of cooling or heating of the emulsion. The cooling rate of the initial emulsion shows influence on the characteristics of the final emulsion.

Mechanical stirrers: These are generally used for agitation of the liquids. Various impellers are employed for stirring the immiscible liquids that are placed directly into the system that is to be emulsified. Impellers may be of following types.

Propeller type mixers: Simple propeller mixers are generally used for lab scale preparation of emulsion. The degree of agitation is controlled by the speed of propeller. The efficiency of mixing is controlled by the type of impeller, its position in the container, the presence of baffles, and the shape of the container. These stirrers cannot be used when vigorous agitation is needed, and when very fine droplets are needed. These mixers may have paddle blades, counter-rotating blades or planetary blades.

Turbine type mixers: These are employed for vigorous agitation and for liquids that are more viscous.

3. *Homogenization:* In homogenization, the mixture of the two liquids to be emulsified is passed through a small inlet

orifice at big pressure. Homogenizers are used for this purpose.

Homogenizer: This consists of a pump that raises the pressure of the dispersion to a range of 500 to 5000 psi. An orifice through which the fluid impinges is held in place on the valve seat by a strong spring. The spring gets compressed as the pressure increases and hence some of the dispersion escapes between the valve and valve seat. At this point, the energy that has been stored in the liquid as pressure is released instantaneously thereby subjecting the dispersion to intense turbulence and hydraulic shear. These are made with more than one emulsifying stage, and it is possible to recycle the emulsion through the homogenizer more than one time. Cooling of the emulsion is necessary as the temperature raises during homogenization. These are used when monodisperse emulsion of small droplet size of about 1 nm is required.

4. *Milling:* In this type, fine droplets are formed by subjecting the dispersion to high shear. Colloidal mill is generally used for such purpose.

Colloid mill: It operates on principle of high shear that is generated between rotor and stator of the mill. Colloid mill consists of a fixed stator plate with a high-speed rotating rotator plate. The dispersion is pumped through the adjustable gap between the rotor and stator that is homogenized by the physical action and hence fine droplets are formed.

5. *Ultrasonification:* Ultrasonic energy is used to produce pharmaceutical emulsions. In this case, transduced piezoelectric devices are expensive. They are useful for laboratory preparation of emulsions of moderate viscosity and extremely low particle size. Large scale equipment works on principle of Pohlmn liquid whistle. In this case, the dispersion is forced through an orifice at moderate pressure (150–350 psi) and is allowed to impinge on a blade. This pressure causes blade to vibrate rapidly to produce an ultrasonic note. When the system reaches a steady state, a gravitational field is generated at the edge of the blade. This causes the dispersion to form fine droplets of emulsion.

Incorporation of medicinal agents: The active ingredients are generally added in two ways:

- Addition of drug during emulsion formation
- Addition of drugs to a preformed emulsion

Example of manufacturing of oral emulsion using colloidal mill:

Ingredients

A. Cotton seed oil	460 g
Sulfadiazine	200 g
Sorbitan monostearate	84 g
B. Polyoxyethylene(20) and sorbitan monostearate	36 g
Sodium benzoate	2.0 g
Sweetener	q.s
Water	1000 g
C. Flavor oil	q.s.

Method: It involves the following steps:

1. Heat (A) to 50°C and pass through colloidal mill
2. Add (A) to (B) at 65°C and stir while cooling to 45°C
3. Add (C) and continue to stir until room temperature is reached.

Type of emulsion: o/w emulsion is preferred as it has better taste.

Internal phase: Cotton seed oil is used as internal phase to prepare oral o/w emulsion of sulfadiazine. To keep sulfadiazine in suspension, the final product should possess more viscosity. This could be achieved by increasing the internal phase.

Emulsifying agent: HLB value of 10 is needed to prepare o/w cotton seed oil emulsion. A combination of two emulsifying agents [sorbitan monostearate and polyoxythylene (20)] is used to get a net value of HLB 10. This combination gives a better interfacial film around globules.

Procedure: The mixture of oil, drug and emulsifier is warmed and passed through a colloidal mill to reduce the particle size of sulfadiazine. The emulsion is formed by adding the drug suspension to the aqueous phase. In order to avoid settling of sulfadiazine, mixing of two phases is done at low temperature and this low temperature prevents the loss of flavor oil by volatility.

Emulsion Stability (Instability)

The term emulsion stability refers to the ability of an emulsion to resist the changes in the emulsion properties during its shelf-life. The more stable the emulsion, the more slowly its properties change. The instability of the emulsion may be due to either physical instability or chemical instability.

Physical Instability

The physical instability of the emulsion can be assessed by the following phenomena (Fig. 2.11):

1. Aggregation or coalescence
2. Flocculation
3. Creaming or sedimentation
4. Breaking
5. Phase inversion

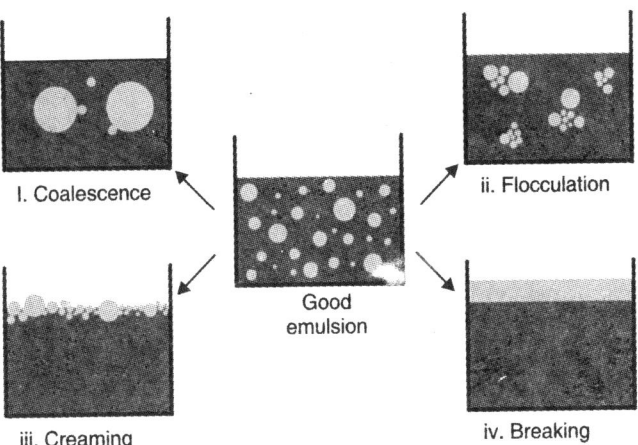

Fig. 2.11: Physical instability of an emulsion

1. Coalescence (Cracking)

In this, the emulsified globules join to form larger particles. The major factor which prevents coalescence is the mechanical strength of electrical barrier. This can be prevented by the addition of natural gums as auxiliary emulsifiers at low concentrations.

Reasons for coalescence (cracking)

Globule size: If globule size is more 1–3 µm, creaming of emulsion takes place followed by cracking. Hence globule size is reduced.

Storage temperature: Extreme of temperature leads to cracking. Freezing of water causes undue pressure on dispersed globules and the emulsifying film that leads to cracking. On the other hand, increase in temperature decreases the viscosity of the continuous phase and disrupts the integrity of interfacial film. An increasing number of collisions between droplets will also occur, leading to increased creaming and cracking.

2. Flocculation

Flocculation is defined as the association of globules within an emulsion to form large aggregates. However, these aggregates can easily be redispersed upon shaking. It is considered as a precursor to the irreversible coalescence. It differs from coalescence mainly in that interfacial film and individual droplets remain intact. Flocculation is influenced by the charges on the surface of the emulsified globules. The reversibility of flocculation depends upon strength of interaction between particles as determined by;
- The chemical nature of emulsifier
- The phase volume ratio
- The concentration of dissolved substances, specially electrolytes and ionic emulsifiers.

3. Creaming and Sedimentation

The upward or downward movement of dispersed droplets is termed creaming and sedimentation, respectively. In any emulsion, creaming or sedimentation takes place depending on the densities of dispersed and continuous phases. Creaming or sedimentation is undesirable as it may lead to coalescence.

Rate of creaming of emulsion: The rate of creaming of an emulsion is governed by Stoke's law. It is given by the following equation

$$Y = 2r^2 (\rho_1 - \rho_2) \, g/9\eta$$

where,

Y = rate of creaming or sedimentation

r = radius of droplets of dispersed phase

ρ_1, ρ_2 = density of dispersed and continuous phase, respectively

g = gravitational rate constant

η = viscosity of continuous phase.

Factors Affecting Rate of Creaming

- *Droplet size:* As per Stoke's law, rate of creaming is directly proportional to the square of radius of the globule or droplet. Smaller is the diameter of the droplet, lesser will be the rate of creaming. Hence reduction in droplet size helps in reducing creaming or sedimentation.
- *Difference in densities of dispersed and continuous phase:* As per Stoke's law creaming is avoided, if densities of the two phases are equal and it can be achieved by adjusting the density of dispersed phase.
- *Viscosity of the continuous phase:* As per Stoke's law, rate of creaming is inversely proportional to viscosity of the continuous phase. Hence increase in viscosity of the continuous phase by viscosity enhancing agents reduces the rate of creaming.

Factors Affecting Viscosity

- *Viscosity of continuous phase:* Clays and gums increase the viscosity of continuous phase. For w/o emulsions, addition of polyvalent metal soaps or high melting waxes and resins in the oil phase can be used to increase the viscosity.
- *Volume of internal phase:* More the volume of internal phase greater is the viscosity.
- *Particle size of dispersed phase:* Smaller the globule size more will be the viscosity and hence enhanced stability of emulsion can be achieved by reduction in globule size.

4. Breaking

It occurs due to coalescence and creaming of an emulsion which results in the complete separation of the oil from the water so that it floats at the top in a single, continuous layer.

5. Phase Inversion

Conversion of one type of emulsion to other type (like w/o type to o/w type and vice versa) is termed phase inversion. The optimum range of concentration of the dispersed phase should be 30–60% of the total volume. If this range exceeds to about 74%, it may result in inversion of the emulsion.

Other factors leading to phase inversion

Temperature of the system: Increased temperature of o/w (with polyoxyethylenated nonionic surfactant) makes the emulsifier more hydrophobic and the emulsion may invert to w/o type.

Addition of strong electrolytes to o/w emulsion (stabilized by ionic surfactants) may invert to w/o emulsion, e.g. addition of polyvalent Ca ions leads to inversion of o/w emulsion (stabilized by sodium cetyl sulfate and cholesterol) to a w/o type emulsion.

Chemical instability: The chemical instability of the emulsion may be due to oxidation, hydrolysis, and microbial growth.

Parameters for assessing the emulsion stability: Both physical and chemical parameters are used to assess emulsion stability.

Physical parameters: The following parameters are commonly measured to assess the effect of stress conditions on emulsions.

1. Phase separation
2. Viscosity
3. Electrophoretic properties
   a. Zeta potential
   b. Electrical conductivity
   c. Dielectric constant
4. Particle size distribution analysis

Phase separation: The rate and extent of phase separation after aging of an emulsion may be observed visually or by measuring the volume of separated phase. The separated phase may be due to coalescence or due to creaming. It is important to differentiate between the coalescence and creaming, since the means of correcting these defects are different. To detect this, small samples of the emulsion are withdrawn from top and the bottom of the preparation after some period of storage and the composition of the two samples are compared by appropriate analysis of water content, oil content or any other suitable constituent.

Viscosity: Changes in viscosity during aging can give an idea about shelf-life of an emulsion. Viscometers of cone and plate type or instruments having co-axial cylinders are used to measure the viscosity. The viscosity changes in first few days are different for w/o and o/w emulsions. The viscosity of w/o emulsion decreases up to certain period (5–15 days) and then remains constant. This is due to the formation of floccules by the oil globules. In case of o/w emulsions, flocculation causes increase in viscosity for some time. After this initial change almost all emulsions show changes in consistency with time, which follow a linear relationship on a log scale. The complete absence of slope (no change in viscosity with age) is ideal. However, slight increase of viscosity between 0.04 and 400 days is acceptable. Other emulsions exhibit much more drastic and sudden nonlinear increases in viscosity after two to three months aging. Such behavior is frequently followed by a drop in viscosity probably associated with phase inversion.

Electrophoretic properties: The following electrophoretic properties are to be determined to evaluate emulsion stability.

a. *Zeta potential:* Stability of emulsions can be evaluated through zeta potential measurement by evaluating the effect of the repulsive forces between globules. It is observed that a minimum zeta potential of ±50 mV is needed to get satisfactory stability of dispersion. Zeta potential of emulsion is useful for assessing flocculation since electrical charges on particles influence the rate of flocculation. Reduction of zeta potential on aging indicates instability of the emulsion. Maximum zeta potential is associated with maximum emulsion stability.

b. *Electrical conductivity:* It is also used to evaluate emulsion stability. The electrical conductivity of o/w or w/o emulsions is determined using platinum electrodes for a short time at room temperature or at 37°C. Conductivity depends on degree of dispersion. o/w emulsions with fine particles exhibit low resistance. If resistance increases, it is a sign of aggregation and instability. A fine emulsion of water in w/o product does not conduct current until droplet coagulation occurs which indicates instability of emulsion.

c. *Dielectric constant:* An inverse relationship existed between log of rate of increase in dielectric constant and the absolute temperature. This can be used as a prediction test.

Particle size distribution analysis: Particle size is inversely proportional to the stability. Changes of the average particle size or size distribution of droplets are important parameters for evaluating emulsion stability. Particle analysis can be carried out by microscopic methods or by electronic counting devices, e.g. Coulter counter method.

Chemical parameters: Emulsifying agents like polyethylene glycols may undergo autoxidation that leads to formation of undesirable odor. Hydrolytic degradation of non-ionic esters may result in changes in dielectric constant of emulsion.

Packaging of emulsions: These are generally packaged in wide mouthed containers made of plastic, glass and metal. Parenteral emulsions are generally stored in glass vials or glass ampoules or glass bottles. Disposable syringes are generally made of plastic material. The stoppers used are made up of elastomeric materials. Metallic containers are used for packaging of topical emulsions. This protects the emulsion from light. Table 2.3 represents the type of packaging of pharmaceutical emulsions.

Table 2.3: Packaging of pharmaceutical emulsions

Emulsion type	Bottle type	Typical size
Oral emulsions	Amber flat medical bottles	50 ml, 100 ml, 150 ml, 200 ml, 300 ml and 500 ml
External emulsions	Amber fluted medical bottles	50 ml, 100 ml and 200 ml

Expiry date of emulsions: The expiry date of oral emulsion is for 4 weeks, if no guidance is available. The preparation should be discarded after the expiry date.

Labeling requirements of emulsions: The labeling of pharmaceutical emulsions is important for ease of patient administration. They are as follows:

- Shake well before use
- For external use only: In case of external emulsions that are not intended for oral use.

- Do not freeze
- Protect from direct sunlight.

EVALUATION TESTS OF LIQUID DOSAGE FORMS

Particle Size Determination of Dispersed Particles in a Suspension

The particle size of the suspension is to be determined as it affects the drug absorption and larger sizes of the particles cause irritation in case of parenteral suspensions. The particle size can be determined by the following methods.

a. *Optical microscopy:* Particle size can be measured microscopically by sizing against a graticule and counting, but for a statistically valid analysis, millions of particles must be measured. This is impossibly arduous when done manually, but nowadays automated analysis of electron micrographs is commercially available. Instruments such as the Retsch camsizer can perform this analysis using standard camera technology.

b. *Coulter counter method (electroresistance counting methods):* In this, the momentary changes in the conductivity of a liquid passing through an orifice is measured when individual non-conducting particles pass through. The particle count is obtained by counting pulses, and the size is dependent on the size of each pulse.

   Technique advantages: Very small sample aliquots can be examined.

   Technique disadvantages: Sample must be dispersed in a liquid medium as some particles may (partially or fully) dissolve in the medium altering the size distribution. The results are only related to the projected cross-sectional area that a particle displaces as it passes through an orifice. This is a physical diameter, not really related to mathematical descriptions of particles.

c. *Acoustic spectroscopy or ultrasound attenuation spectroscopy:* In this method, ultrasound is employed for collecting information on the particles that are dispersed in fluid. Dispersed particles absorb and scatter ultrasound similarly to light. It turns out that instead of measuring *scattered energy versus angle*, as with light, in the case of ultrasound, measuring the *transmitted energy versus frequency* is a better choice. The resulting ultrasound attenuation frequency spectra are the raw data for calculating particle size distribution. It can be measured for any fluid system with no dilution or other sample preparation. Calculation of particle size distribution is based on theoretical models that are well verified for up to 50% by volume of dispersed particles.

d. *Laser diffraction methods:* In this "halo (dark portion)" of diffracted light is produced when a laser beam passes through a dispersion of particles either in air or in a liquid. The angle of diffraction increases as particle size decreases. This method is particularly good for measuring sizes between 0.1 and 3,000 µm. A particular advantage is that the technique can generate a continuous measurement for analyzing process streams.

Tests for Solutions

Clarity of the solution: Retention of clarity of solution is a main concern regarding stability of solution. In this, a microscopic light is projected though a diaphragm into the solution. The solution will remain clear, if there are no undissolved particles. The solution appears hazy due to the scattering of light by undissolved particles. Light scattering instruments are most widely used to test the clarity of the solution.

Test for particulate matter in solutions: Solutions should be essentially free from particulate matter that can be observed on visual inspection. Particulate matter includes mobile, randomly sourced, extraneous substances, other than gas bubbles that cannot quantified by chemical analysis due to less amount and of their heterogeneous compositions. It can be determined by the following two methods:

1. Light obscuration method
2. Microscopic method.

1. Light Obscuration Method

This method applies for solutions, including solutions constituting from sterile solids, for which the test for particulate matter is specified in the individual monograph. The product meets the requirements of the test, if the average numbers of particles present in the units tested does not exceed the appropriate value listed in Table 2.4.

Table 2.4: Light obscuration particle count test		
	Diameter	
	≥ 10 µm	≥ 25 µm
Number of particles	50 per ml	5 per ml

If the average number of particles exceeds this limit, the test article is subjected to microscopic method.

2. Microscopic Method

This method is employed when some particles are not exactly detected by the light obscuration method. This test enumerates the subvisible particles essentially solid particulate matter present in the otic and ophthalmic solutions. The test sample is collected on a microporous membrane filter. The product meets the requirements of the test, if the average number of particles present in the units tested does not exceed the appropriate value listed in Table 2.5.

Table 2.5: Microscopic method particle count test			
	Diameter		
	≥ 10 µm	≥ 25 µm	≥ 50 µm
Number of particles	50 per ml	5 per ml	2 per ml

Test for Sterility

This is used to test the presence of microorganisms in the sterile liquid dosage form intended for parenteral administration. The following tests are performed to determine the sterility of the liquid formulation.

a. Membrane filtration method
b. Direct inoculation (immersion) method

Membrane filtration method: In this method, the test product is first passed through a size exclusion membrane capable of retaining the microorganisms. The concept is that the microorganisms will collect on the surface of a 0.45 micron pore size filter. The filter is rinsed and then the membrane is transferred to appropriate test medium as specified in the monograph.

Direct inoculation (immersion) method: In this method, the test article is directly inoculated into the test medium and then the medium is incubated for the growth of microorganisms, if present.

Test media: The test media generally used include fluid thioglycollate medium (FTM) and soybean casein digest medium (SCDM). FTM is selected based upon its ability to support the growth of anaerobic and aerobic microorganisms. SCDM is selected based upon its ability to support a wide range of aerobic bacteria and fungi (i.e. yeasts and molds).

Incubation time: In both the methods, the test medium after the transferring of the test solution is to be incubated for 3 days in case of bacteria and 5 days in case of fungi and then the growth is compared with that of standard. If no growth is observed, then the sample passes the test and it meets the GMP requirements. Table 2.6 outlines the requirement for sterility testing as per USP.

Table 2.6: Volume of product to be tested

Volume/container	Minimum quantity to test in each media
<1 ml	The entire contents of each container
1–40 ml	Half the contents of each container but not <1 ml
41–100 ml	20 ml
>100 ml	10% of the contents of the container, but not <20 ml

Test for Pyrogens

Pyrogens are the endotoxins produced by microorganisms which are responsible for increase in body temperature. This test is designed to limit to an acceptable level the risks of febrile reaction in the patient to the administration, by injection, of the product concerned. The following tests are performed to check the presence of pyrogens in the liquid dosage forms intended for parenteral administration.

a. Rabbit test and
b. LAL test

Rabbit Test

Unless otherwise specified in the individual monograph, 10 ml of the test solution per kg of body weight has to be injected into an ear vein of each of three rabbits, completing each injection within 10 minutes after start of administration. Assure that the test product is protected from contamination. Perform the injection after warming the test product to a temperature of 37 ± 2°C. Record the temperature at 30-minute intervals between 1 and 3 hours subsequent to the injection.

Test interpretation

Consider any temperature decreases as zero rise. If no rabbit shows an individual rise in temperature of 0.5°C or more above its respective control temperature, the product meets the requirements for the absence of pyrogens. If any rabbit shows an individual temperature rise of 0.5°C or more, continue the test using five other rabbits. If not more than three of the eight rabbits show individual rises in temperature of 0.5°C or more and if the sum of the eight individual maximum temperature rises does not exceed 3.3°C, the material under examination meets the requirements for the absence of pyrogens.

LAL test

Limulus amebocyte lysate (LAL) is an aqueous extract of blood cells (amoebocytes) from the horseshoe crab, *Limulus polyphemus*. LAL reacts with bacterial endotoxin or lipopolysaccharide (LPS), which is a membrane component of gram-negative bacteria. This reaction is the basis of the LAL test.

Method

Blood is removed from the horseshoe crab's pericardium and the blood cells are separated from the serum using centrifugation and are then placed in distilled water, which causes them to swell up and burst ("lyse"). This releases the chemicals from the inside of the cell (the "lysate"), which is then purified and freeze-dried. To test a sample for endotoxins, it is mixed with lysate and water. Coagulation occurs, if endotoxins are present.

Viscosity Measurement

The flow of fluids through the bottle is influenced by viscosity of the product. In order to have a better flow and to maintain residence time in the ear, the viscosity of the formulation should be checked under controlled temperature. In general, viscosity is measured by Brookfield viscometer, and cone and plate viscometer.

Brookfield Viscometer

It measures the shearing stress on a spindle rotating at a definite, constant speed while immersed in the sample (Fig. 2.12). The degree of spindle lag is indicated on a rotating dial. This reading multiplied by a conversion factor based on spindle size and rotational speed, gives a value for viscosity in centipoise.

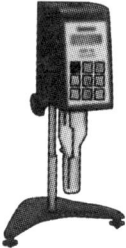

Fig. 2.12: Brookfield viscometer

Cone and Plate Viscometer

It used a cone of very shallow angle in bare contact with a flat plate (Fig. 2.13). With this system, the shear rate beneath the plate is constant to a modest degree of precision and deconvolution of a flow curve. A graph of shear stress (torque) against shear rate (angular velocity) yields the viscosity in a straight forward manner.

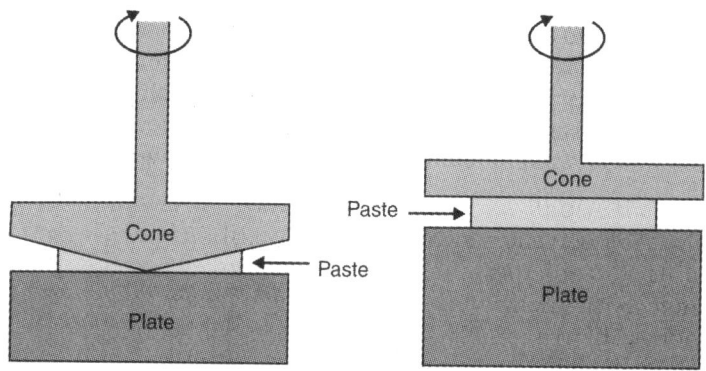

Fig. 2.13: Cone and plate viscometer

Test for Antimicrobial Effectiveness

Generally, an antimicrobial agent is used in multiple dose units of liquid formulations to protect the product from microbial contamination that may occur during the suck back of an unreleased drop, when the pressure is released after withdrawal of the product. So there is need to check the efficacy of the antimicrobial agent against these microorganisms. In this test, cultures of *Candida albicans, Aspergillus niger, Escherichia coli, Pseudomonas aeuroginosa, Staphylococcus aureus* are used. In this, a standardized inoculum of microorganisms is prepared with a count of 10^5–10^6 per ml and added to the test product. They are incubated for 28 days at 20–25°C and observed for the preservative action at 7, 14, 21 and 28 days. The products preservative action is found to be effective, if it satisfies the following:

- There should be reduction of no more than 0.1% of viable bacteria with that of initial concentrations by day 14th.

- There should be decrease in concentration of viable yeasts and molds when compared to initial by day 14th.

- The concentration of remaining viable organisms should be lower as designated at the end of 28th day.

Cidal test

This is another test employed to determine antimicrobial agent efficacy. In this, the formulation is tested against 5–14 species of microorganisms including gram-negative, gram-positive, bacteria, and fungi in previously standardized inoculums. Cidal times (growth of microorganisms) are measured within 24, 48 and 72 hours of contact.

Summary

The liquid dosage forms are one of the major pharmaceutical dosage forms of drug administration. Many drugs are administered through this dosage form especially for geriatric and pediatric patients as it is easy to swallow the liquid than that of solid form. The stability of the liquid dosage form is a main concern in its manufacturing and it is maintained by both physical and chemical parameters. Hence liquid dosage forms offer different routes of drug administration and many products are successfully administered that are intended for both oral and external use.

ISOLATED KEY POINTS

- *Liquid dosage forms solution:* Solutions are clear liquid preparations containing one or more active ingredients dissolved in a suitable vehicle. *Suspension* (solid in liquid dispersion): Liquid preparations containing one or more active ingredients suspended in a suitable vehicle.

- *Emulsion (liquid in liquid dispersion):* Emulsions are two phase system in which one liquid is dispersed throughout another liquid in the form of small particles. *Colloids:* A system in which finely divided particles, which are approximately less than 1 μm in size, are dispersed within a continuous medium in a manner that prevents them from being filtered easily or settled rapidly.

- *Solutions* are liquid preparations that contain one or more chemical substances dissolved in a suitable solvent or mixture of mutually miscible solvents. Dosage forms prepared by dissolving the active ingredient(s) in an aqueous or non-aqueous solvent.

- *Classification of solution:* (i) According to the route of administration: (a) oral solutions—through oral route, (b) otic solutions—instilled in the ears, (c) ophthalmic solution—instilled in the eyes, (d) topical solutions—applied over the skin surface.

- *Solutions* can be formulated for different routes of administration. Orally: Syrups, elixirs, drops. In mouth and throat: Mouth washes, gargles, throat sprays. In body cavities: Douches, enemas, ear drops, nasal sprays. On body surfaces: Lotions.

- *Advantages of solutions:* 1. Easier to swallow, therefore, easier for: children - old age - unconscious people. 2. More quickly effective than tablets and capsules. 3. Homogenous, therefore, give uniform dose than suspension or emulsion which need shaking. 4. Dilute irritant action of some drugs (aspirin, Kl, KBr) minimize adverse effects in the GIT like KCl.

- *Disadvantages of solutions:* 1. Bulky, therefore, difficult to transport and store. 2. Unpleasant taste or odors are difficult to mask. 3. Needs an accurate spoon to measure the dose. 4. Less stable than solid dosage forms. Major signs of instability: Color change, precipitation microbial growth and chemical gas formation.

- *Additives:* 1. Buffers, 2. Isotonicity modifiers, 3. Preservatives, 4. Antioxidants, 5. Sweetening agents, 6. Flavors and perfumes.

- *Buffers:* To resist any change in pH. Isotonicity modifiers *Solutions for injection *Application to mucous membrane *Large-volume solutions for ophthalmic application. Most widely used isotonicity modifiers are: dextrose and NaCl

- *Viscosity enhancement:* It is difficult for aqueous-based topical solutions to remain on the skin or in the eye (why?) therefore, low concentrations of jelling agents are added to increase the viscosity of the product.

- Preservatives solution may become contaminated for a number of reasons: Raw materials used in the manufacture of solutions are excellent growth media for bacterial substances such as gums, dispersing agents, sugars and flavors.

- Preservatives may be used alone or in combination to prevent the growth of microorganisms. Alcohols: Ethanol is useful as a preservative when it is used as a solvent. It needs a relatively high concentration (>10%) to be effective. Propylene glycol also used as a solvent in oral solutions and topical preparations. It can function as a preservative in the range of 15 to 30%. It is not volatile like ethanol.

- *Antioxidants:* Vitamins, essential oils and almost all fats and oils can be oxidized. Oxidation reaction can be initiated by: 1. Heat: Maintain oxidizable drugs in a cool place. 2. Light: Use of light-resistant container. 3. Heavy metals (e.g. Fe, Cu): Effect of trace metals can be minimized by using citric acid or ethylenediamine tetra-acetic acid (EDTA), i.e. sequestering agent. Antioxidants as propyl and octyl esters of gallic acid, tocopherols or vitamin E, sodium sulfite, ascorbic acid (vit. C) can be used.

- *Sweetening agents:* Sucrose is the most widely used sweetening agent. Advantages: Colorless, highly water-soluble, stable over a wide pH range (4–8), increase the viscosity, masks both salty and bitter taste, has soothing effect on throat. Polyhydric alcohols (sorbitol, mannitol and glycerol) possess sweetening power and can be used for diabetic preparations.

- *Flavors and perfumes:* Mask unpleasant taste or odor, enable the easy identification of the product. Natural products: Fruit juices, aromatic oil (peppermint, lemon). Artificial perfumes are cheaper, more readily available and more stable than natural products.

- *Methods of preparation of solutions:* (a) Simple Solution (b) solution by chemical reaction (c) solution by extraction

- *Simple solution:* Solutions of this type are prepared by dissolving the solute in a suitable solvent (by stirring or heating). The solvent may contain other ingredients which stabilize or solubilize the active ingredient, e.g. solubility of Iodine is 1: 2950 in water, however, it dissolves in presence of KI due the formation of more soluble polyiodides (KI.I 2 KI.2I 2 KI3.I 3 KI.4I 4).[Strong Iodine Solution USP (Lugol's solution)].

- *Solution by chemical reaction:* These solutions are prepared by reacting two or more solutes with each other in a suitable solvent, e.g. calcium carbonate and lactic acid used to prepare calcium lactate mixture. calcium lactate used as an antacid and also to treat calcium deficiencies

- *Solution by extraction:* Plant or animal products are prepared by suitable extraction process. Preparations of this type may be classified as solutions but more often, are classified as extractives.

- *Pharmaceutical solutions:* Aqueous 1. Douches, 2. Enemas, 3. Gargles, 4. Mouthwashes, 5. Nasal washes, 6. Juices, 7. Sprays, 8. Otic solutions, 9. Inhalations. Sweet and/or viscid: 1. Syrups, 2. Honeys, 3. Mucilages, 4. Jellies. Non-aqueous: 1. Elixirs, 2. Spirits, 3. Collodions, 4. Glycerins, 5. Liniments, 6. Oleo vitamin.

- *Douches:* Douche is an aqueous solution, which is directed against a part or into a cavity of the body. It functions as a cleansing or antiseptic agent. Eye douches are used to remove foreign particles and discharges from the eyes. It is directed gently at an oblique angle and is allowed to run from the inner to the outer corner of the eye.

- *Enemas:* These preparations are rectal injections employed to: 1. Evacuate the bowel (evacuation enemas), 2. Influence the general system by absorption (retention enemas), e.g. nutritive, sedative, 3. Affect locally the site of disease (e.g. anthelmintic property), 4. They may contain radiopaque substances for roentgenographic examination of the lower bowel.

- *Gargles:* Gargles are aqueous solutions frequently containing antiseptics, antibiotics and/or anesthetics used for treating the pharynx (throat) and nasopharynx by forcing air from the lungs through the gargle, which is held in the throat; subsequently, the gargle is expectorated. Many gargles must be diluted with water prior to use. Although mouthwashes are considered as a separate class of pharmaceuticals, many are used as gargles, either as is, or diluted with water. The product should be labeled so that it cannot be mistaken for preparations intended for internal administration.

- *Mouthwashes* can be used for therapeutic and cosmetic purposes. Therapeutic mouthwashes can be formulated to reduce plaque, gingivitis, dental caries and stomatitis. Cosmetic mouthwashes may be formulated to reduce bad breath through the use of antimicrobial and/or flavoring agents. Mouthwashes are used as a dosage form for a number of specific problems in the oral cavity, e.g. mouthwashes containing: Combination of antihistamines, hydrocortisone, nystatin and tetracycline have been prepared for the treatment of stomatitis, a painful side effect of cancer therapy. Pilocarpine for xerostoma (dry mouth). Tranexamic acid for the prevention of bleeding after oral surgery. Carbenoxolone for the treatment of orofacial herpes simplex infections.

- *Nasal solutions* are usually aqueous solutions designed to be administered to the nasal passages in drops or sprays. Ephedrine sulfate or naphazoline hydrochloride nasal solution USP are administered for their local effect to reduce nasal congestion. Vasopressin (Minirin) nasal solution USP for its systemic effect for the treatment of diabetes insipidus.

- *Sprays:* Sprays are solutions of drugs in aqueous vehicles and are applied to the mucous membrane of the nose and throat by means of an atomizer nebulizer. The spray device should produce relatively coarse droplets, if the action of the drug is to be restricted to the upper respiratory tract. Fine droplets tend to penetrate further into the respiratory tract than is desirable.

- *Otic solutions:* The main classes of drugs used for topical administration to the ear include local anesthetics, e.g. benzocaine; antibiotics, e.g. neomycin; and anti-inflammatory agents, e.g. cortisone. These preparations include the main types of solvents used, namely glycerin or water. The viscous glycerin vehicle permits the drug to remain in the ear for a long time.

- *Preparation of simple syrup:*
  - Solution with heat: This is the usual method of making syrups : in the absence of volatile agents or those injured by heat when it is desirable to make the syrup rapidly. The sucrose is added to the purified water or aqueous solution and heated until dissolved, then strained and sufficient purified water added to make the desired weight or volume.

  - Agitation without heat: This process is used in those cases where heat would cause loss of valuable volatile constituents. The syrup is prepared by adding sucrose to the aqueous solution in a bottle of about twice the size required for the syrup. This permits active agitation and rapid solution. The stoppering of the bottle is important, as it prevents contamination and loss during the process.

  - Percolation: In this procedure, purified water or an aqueous solution is permitted to pass slowly through a bed of crystalline sucrose, thus dissolving it and forming a syrup. A pledget of cotton is placed in the neck of the percolator. If necessary, a portion of the liquid is repassed through the percolator to dissolve all of the sucrose.

- *Honeys:* Are thick liquid preparations. At one time, before sugar was available, honey was used as a base, instead of syrup. There are few official preparations containing honey, e.g. oxymel, or "acid honey" is a mixture of acetic acid, water and honey.

- *Mucilages:* The official mucilages are thick viscid, adhesive liquids, produced by dispersing gum (acacia or tragacanth) in water. Mucilages are used as suspending agents for insoluble substances in liquids; their colloidal character and viscosity prevent immediate sedimentation. Synthetic agents, e.g. carboxymethylcellulose (CMC) or polyvinyl alcohol are nonglycogenetic and may be used for diabetic patients.

- *Non-aqueous pharmaceutical solutions:* Advantages: If the drug is not completely soluble or unstable in aqueous medium, it may be necessary to use an alternative non-aqueous solvent. Oily solutions of drugs are often used for depot therapy, e.g. in muscles. It is essential to test: toxicity–irritancy–flammability–cost–stability and compatibility of solvents to avoid problems. Solvents such as acetone, benzene and petroleum ether are not used for internal products. Internal products may contain ethanol, glycerol, propylene glycol, certain oils. For parenteral products, the choice is very limited.

- *Types of non-aqueous solutions:* 1. Alconolic or hydroalcoholic solutions, e.g. elixirs and spirits, 2. Ethereal solutions, e.g. the collodions 3. Glycerin solutions, e.g. the glycerites, 4. Oleaginous solutions, e.g. the liniments, medicated oils, oleo-vitamins, sprays, and toothache drops.

- *Elixirs:* These are clear, pleasantly flavored, sweetened hydroalcoholic liquids intended for oral use. They are used as flavors and vehicles, e.g. dexamethasone Elixir USP and Phenobarbital Elixir USP. The main ingredients in elixirs are ethanol and water but glycerin, sorbitol, propylene glycol, flavoring agents, preservatives, and syrups are often used in the preparation of the final product. An elixir may contain water and alcohol soluble ingredients.

- *Spirits:* Alcoholic or hydroalcoholic solutions of volatile substances. The active ingredient may be gas, liquid or solid. Generally, the alcoholic concentration of spirits is rather high. Spirits may be used internally for their medicinal value, by inhalation but is mostly used as flavoring agents. Spirits should be stored in air-tight, light-resistant containers and in a cool place. Spirits are preparation of high alcoholic strength and when diluted with aqueous solutions or liquids of low alcoholic content turbidity may occur.

- *Collodions* are liquid preparations containing pyroxylin (a nitrocellulose) in a mixture of ethyl ether and ethanol. They are applied to the skin by means of a soft brush or other suitable applicator and, when the ether and ethanol have evaporated, leave a film of pyroxylin on the surface. The official medicated collodion, salicylic acid collodion USP, contains 10 % w/v of salicylic acid in flexible collodion USP and is used as a keratolytic agent in the treatment of corns and warts. Collodion is made flexible by the addition of castor oil and camphor.

- *Glycerins:* Glycerins or glycerites are solutions or mixtures of medicinal substances in not less than 50% by weight of glycerin. Most of the glycerins are extremely viscous. Glycerin is a valuable pharmaceutical solvent forming permanent and concentrated solutions. It is used as the sole solvent for the preparation of antipyrine and benzocaine otic solution USP. As noted under otic solutions, glycerin alone is used to aid in the removal of cerumen. Glycerins are hygroscopic and should be stored in tightly closed containers.

- *Liniments* are alcoholic or oleaginous solutions or emulsions of various medicinal substances. They are intended for external application and should be so labeled. They are applied with rubbing to the affected area, the oil or soap base providing for ease of application and massage. Alcoholic liniments are used generally for their rubefaciant and counterirritant effects. Such liniments penetrate the skin more readily than do those with an oil base. The oily liniments are milder in their action and may function solely as protective coatings. Liniments should not be applied to skin that are bruised or broken.

- *Rubefacient:* A medicine for external application that produces redness of the skin, e.g. by causing dilation of the capillaries and an increase in blood circulation. Counter-irritant: A medicine applied locally to produce superficial inflammation in order to reduce deeper inflammation.

- *Pharmaceutical suspension:* A pharmaceutical suspension is a coarse dispersion in which internal phase is dispersed uniformly throughout the external phase. The internal phase consisting of insoluble solid particles having a specific range of size which is maintained uniformly throughout the suspending vehicle with aid of single or combination of suspending agent. The external phase (suspending medium) is generally aqueous in some instance, may be an organic or oily liquid for non-oral use.

- *Classification:* 1. Based on general classes: Oral suspension, externally applied suspension parenteral suspension. 2. Based on proportion of solid particles: Dilute suspension (2 to10% w/v solid), concentrated suspension (50% w/v solid). 3. Based on electrokinetic nature of solid particles: Flocculated suspension, deflocculated suspension. 4. Based on size of solid particles: Colloidal suspension (<1 micron), coarse suspension (>1 micron), nano suspension (10 ng).

- *Advantages:* Suspension can improve chemical stability of certain drugs, e.g. procaine penicillin G. Drug in suspension exhibits higher rate of bioavailability than other dosage forms. Bioavailability is in following order, Solution > Suspension > Capsule > Compressed Tablet > Coated tablet. Duration and onset of action can be controlled, e.g. protamine zinc-insulin suspension can mask the unpleasant/bitter taste of drug, e.g. chloramphenicol palmitate.

- *Disadvantages:* Physical stability, sedimentation and compaction can cause problems. It is bulky, sufficient care must be taken during handling and transport. It is difficult to formulate. Uniform and accurate dose cannot be achieved unless suspensions are packed in unit dosage form.

- *Theory of suspensions: Sedimentation behavior:* Sedimentation means settling of particle or floccules occur under gravitational force in liquid dosage form. Theory of sedimentation: Velocity of sedimentation expressed by Stokes equation:

$$V = 2r^2 (\rho_s - \rho_o) g/\eta \text{ or } V = d^2 (\rho_s - \rho_o) g/9\eta$$

where,

V = sedimentation velocity in cm/sec
d = diameter of particle
r = radius of particle
ρ_s = density of disperse phase
ρ_o = density of disperse media
g = acceleration due to gravity
ρ = viscosity of disperse medium in poise.

- *Factors affecting sedimentation:* Particle size diameter (d), $V \propto d^2$. Sedimentation velocity (V) is directly proportional to the square of diameter of particle. Density difference between dispersed phase and dispersion media $(\rho_s - \rho_o)$ $V \propto (\rho_s - \rho_o)$. Generally, particle density is greater than dispersion medium but, in certain cases, particle density is less than dispersed phase, so suspended particle floats and is difficult to distribute uniformly in the vehicle. If densities of the dispersed phase and dispersion medium are equal, the rate of settling becomes zero.

- The sedimentation behavior of flocculated and deflocculated suspensions: Flocculated suspensions: In flocculated suspension, formed flocks (loose aggregates) will cause increase in sedimentation rate due to increase in size of sedimenting particles. Hence, flocculated suspensions sediment more rapidly. Here, the sedimen-tation depends not only on the size of the flocks but also on the porosity of flocks. In flocculated suspension, the loose structure of the rapidly sedimenting flocks tends to preserve in the sediment, which contains an appreciable amount of entrapped liquid. The volume of final sediment is thus relatively large and is easily redispersed by agitation.

- *Deflocculated suspensions:* In deflocculated suspension, individual particles are settling, so rate of sedimentation is slow which prevents entrapping of liquid medium which makes it difficult to redisperse by agitation. This phenomenon also called 'cracking' or 'claying'. In deflocculated suspension, larger particles settle fast and smaller particles remain in supernatant liquid so supernatant appears cloudy whereby in flocculated suspension, even the smallest particles are involved in flocks, so the supernatant does not appear cloudy.

- *Flocculating agents:* Flocculating agents decrease zeta potential of the suspended charged particle and thus cause aggregation (flock formation) of the particles. Examples of flocculating agents are: Neutral electrolytes such as KCl, NaCl, surfactants, polymeric flocculating agents, sulfate, citrates, phosphate salts.

- *Surfactants:* Both ionic and non-ionic surfactants can be used to bring about flocculation of suspended particles. Optimum concentration is necessary because these compounds also act as wetting agents to achieve dispersion. Optimum concentrations of surfactants bring down the surface free energy by reducing the surface tension between liquid medium and solid particles. This tends to form closely packed agglomerates. The particles possessing less surface free energy are attracted towards to each other by van der Waals forces and forms loose agglomerates.

- *Viscosity of suspensions:* Viscosity of suspensions is of great importance for stability and pourability of suspensions. As we know, suspensions have least physical stability amongst all dosage forms due to sedimentation and cake formation. So as the viscosity of the dispersion medium increases, the terminal settling velocity decreases thus the dispersed phase settlit at a slower rate and it remains dispersed for longer time yielding higher stability to the suspension. On the other hand, as the viscosity of the suspension increases, its pourability decreases and inconvenience to the patients for dosing increases. Thus, the viscosity of suspension should be maintained within optimum range to yield stable and easily pourable suspensions.

- *Different approaches to increase the viscosity of suspensions:* Various approaches have been suggested to enhance the viscosity of suspensions. Few of them are as follows:
  1. Viscosity enhancers some natural gums (acacia, tragacanth), cellulose derivatives (sodium CMC, methyl-cellulose), clays (bentonite, veegum), carbomers, colloidal

silicon dioxide (aerosil), and sugars (glucose, fructose) are used to enhance the viscosity of the dispersion medium. They are known as suspending agents.

- *List of suspending agents:* Alginates, methylcellulose, hydroxyethylcellulose, carboxymethylcellulose, sodium carboxymethylcellulose, microcrystalline cellulose, acacia, tragacanth, xanthan gum, bentonite, carbomer, powdered cellulose, gelatin.

- Surfactants decrease the interfacial tension between drug particles and liquid and thus liquid is penetrated in the pores of drug particle displacing air from them and thus ensures wetting. Surfactants in optimum concentration facilitate dispersion of particles. Generally, we use non-ionic surfactants but ionic surfactants can also be used depending upon certain conditions. Disadvantages of surfactants are that they have foaming tendencies. Further they are bitter in taste. Some surfactants such as polysorbate 80 interact with preservatives such as methyl-paraben and reduce antimicrobial activity.

- *Quality control of suspensions:* The following tests are carried out in the final quality control of suspension: Appearance, color, odor and taste, physical characteristics such as particle size determination and microscopic photography for crystal growth, sedimentation rate, and zeta potential measurement, sedimentation volume redispersibility, and centrifugation tests, rheological measurement, stress test, pH, freeze-thaw temperature cycling, compatibility with container and cap liner.

- *Ideal requirements of packaging material:* It should be inert. It should effectively preserve the product from light, air, and other contamination through shelf-life. It should be cheap. It should effectively deliver the product without any difficulty.

- *An emulsion* is mixture of two liquids that would not normally mix. That is to say, a mixture of two immiscible liquids. By definition, an emulsion contains tiny particles of one liquid suspended in another. Chemically, they are colloids where both phases are liquids. They are typically milky in appearance and the suspended material may be colloidal in nature. A classic example of an emulsion is oil and water when mixed slowly under vigorous stirring.

However, when the agitation is stopped, the two liquids separate and the emulsion breaks down. This is an example of an unstable emulsion. Stable emulsions can be formed from two immiscible liquids when an emulsifier is used. Such emulsions do not separate out after a change in conditions like temperature or over time.

- *Emulsion types:* Oil-in-water (o/w), water-in-oil (w/o), oil-in-water-in-oil (o/w/o), water-in-oil-in-water (w/o/w), *determination of o/w or w/o:* Water soluble dye (e.g. methylene blue), dilution of emulsions, conduction of current.

- *Physical stability of emulsion:* Creaming is the upward movement of dispersed droplets of emulsion relative to the continuous phase (due to the density difference between two phases). Stoke's law: $dx/dt = d^2 (S_1 - S_2)g/18\eta_0$, dx/dt = rate of setting; d = diameter of particles; S_1 and S_2 = density of particles and medium; g = gravitational constant; η = viscosity of medium.

- *Physical stability of emulsion:* Breaking, coalescence, aggregation. Breaking is the destroying of the film surrounding the particles. Coalescence is the process by which emulsified particles merge with each other to form large particles. Aggregation: Dispersed particles come together but do not fuse. The major fact preventing coalescence is the mechanical strength of the interfacial film.

- *Physical stability of emulsion: Phase inversion:* An emulsion is said to invert when it changes from an o/w to w/o or vice versa. Addition of electrolyte: Addition of $CaCl_2$ into o/w emulsion formed by sodium stearate can be inverted to w/o. Changing the phase: volume ratio.

- *Preservation of emulsions:* Growth of microorganisms in emulsions. Preservatives should be in aqueous phase. Preservatives should be in unionized state to penetrate the bacteria. Preservatives must not bind to other components of the emulsion.

- *Methods of emulsion preparation: Dry gum method:* The continental method is used to prepare the initial or primary emulsion from oil, water, and a hydrocolloid or "gum" type emulsifier (usually acacia). The primary emulsion, or emulsion nucleus, is formed from 4 parts oil, 2 parts water, and 1 part emulsifier. The 4 parts oil and 1 part emulsifier represent their total amounts for the final emulsion. In a mortar, the 1 part gum (e.g. acacia) is levigated with the 4 parts oil until the powder is thoroughly wetted; then the 2 parts water are added all at once, and the mixture is vigorously and continually triturated until the primary emulsion formed is creamy white. Additional water or aqueous solutions may be incorporated after the primary emulsion is formed. Solid substances (e.g. active ingredients, preservatives, color, flavors) are generally dissolved and added as a solution to the primary emulsion. Oil-soluble substance, in small amounts, may be incorporated directly into the primary emulsion. Any substance which might reduce the physical stability of the emulsion, such as alcohol (which may precipitate the gum) should be added as near to the end of the process as possible to avoid breaking the emulsion. When all agents have been incorporated, the emulsion should be transferred to a calibrated vessel, brought to final volume with water, then homogenized or blended to ensure uniform distribution of ingredients.

- *Wet gum method:* In this method, the proportions of oil, water, and emulsifier are the same (4:2:1), but the order and techniques of mixing are different. The 1 part gum is triturated with 2 parts water to form a mucilage; then the 4 parts oil is added slowly, in portions, while triturating. After all, the oil is added, the mixture is triturated for several minutes to form the primary emulsion. Then other ingredients may be added as in the continental method. Generally speaking, the English method is more difficult to perform successfully, especially with more viscous oils, but may result in a more stable emulsion.

- *Bottle method:* This method may be used to prepare emulsions of volatile oils, or oleaginous substances of very low viscosities. This method is a variation of the dry gum method. One part powdered acacia (or other gum) is placed in a dry bottle and four parts oil are added. The bottle is capped and thoroughly shaken. To this, the required volume of water is added all at once, and the mixture is shaken thoroughly until the primary emulsion forms. It is important to minimize the initial amount of time the gum and oil are mixed. The gum will tend to imbibe the oil, and will become more waterproof.

- *Auxiliary method:* An emulsion prepared by other methods can also usually be improved by passing it through a hand homogenizer, which forces the emulsion through a very small orifice, reducing the dispersed droplet size to about 5 microns or less.

- *Microemulsion:* Microemulsions are thermodynamically stable, optically transparent, isotropic mixtures of a biphasic oil-water system stabilized with surfactants.

LONG ANSWER TYPE QUESTIONS

Q 1. What are the different types of liquid dosage form? Give their advantages and disadvantages.

Q 2. Define the term solutions. Give classification of solution based on the route of the administration.

Q 3. Discuss in detail various additives used in the formulation of solution.

Q 4. Write short notes on following with respect to liquid dosage form:
      A. Viscosity enhancer   B. Preservatives
      C. Antioxidant   D. Flavors and perfumes
      E. Coloring agent

Q 5. What are douches? Give their types and uses.

Q 6. Compare and contrast between gargles and mouthwashes.

Q 7. What are syrups? Discuss in detail about various types of syrup used in liquid dosage form.

Q 8. What are biphasic liquid dosage forms? Compare and contrast between suspension and emulsion.

Q 9. What are different types of phases in suspension? Give advantages and disadvantages of suspension.

Q 10. What are important factors which is to be kept in mind while formulating a suspension? Give pharmaceutical application of suspension.

Q 11. Discuss in brief various theories of suspension. Compare and contrast between flocculated and deflocculated suspension.

Q 12. Write short notes on:
  A. Brownian movement   B. Zeta potential
  C. Flocculating agent

Q 13. Discuss in brief quality control methods, packaging and labeling of suspension.

Q 14. What are emulsion? Give their advantages and disadvantages.

Q 15. Discuss in detail various types of emulsion with suitable examples.

Q 16. How multiple emulsions are prepared give their pharmaceutical application?

Q 17. Write in brief about various test used to differentiate between various types of emulsion.

Q 18. Discuss in detail various theories of emulsification.

Q 19. Write short notes on additives used in formulation of emulsion:
  A. Emulsifying agent   B. Preservatives
  C. Antioxidant   D. Auxiliary emulsifier

Q 20. Give various methods of preparation of emulsion with suitable example.

Q 21. Give various methods of detecting physical instability of emulsion.

Q 22. Discuss in detail various chemical instability occurring in emulsion.

Q 23. Give detailed evaluation test used for liquid dosage form.

OBJECTIVE TYPE QUESTIONS

1. Match the following

S. no	Type of water		Specification
1	Potable water	A	Water prepared by distillation, by ion exchange resin method, or by reverse osmosis.
2	Purified water	B	Safe drinking water
3	Aromatic water	C	Clear saturated solutions of volatile oils, or other aromatic or volatile substances
4	Sterile water	D	Free from microbes

2. Match the following

S. no	Type of agents		Example/Functions
1	Buffering Agents	A	Improve palatability and ease pourability of the product
2	Isotonicity modifiers	B	0.9% NaCl solution
3	Viscosity modifiers	C	Propylparaben
4	Solubilizing agents	D	Resist the change in pH
5	Preservatives	E	Enhances the solubility of the

3. Match the following

S. no	Type of agents		Example
1	Antioxidants	A	Raspberry and ginger
2	Sweetening agents	B	BHA, BHT
3	Flavors	C	Carotenoids, chlorophylls
4	Coloring agents	D	Aspartame

4. Match the following

S. no	Type of preparation		Example/functions
1	Elixirs	A	Alcoholic or oleaginous solutions or emulsions of various medicinal substances.
2	Spirits	B	Alcoholic or hydroalcoholic solutions of volatile substances
3	Collodions	C	Medicinal substances in not less than 50% by weight of glycerin
4	Glycerins	D	Clear, pleasantly flavored, sweetened hydroalcoholic liquids intended for oral use
5	Liniments	E	Liquid preparations containing pyroxylin (a nitrocellulose) in a mixture of ethyl ether and ethanol

5. Which of the following is false regarding preservative
   A. Effective against broad spectrum of microorganisms
   B. Stable for its shelf life
   C. Should be highly toxic.
   D. Should not affect the stability of the active ingredient
   E. Free of taste and odor

6. ....are aqueous solution, which are instilled into a cavity of the body, functions as .... While .... are rectal preparations used to evacuate the bowel.

7. .... are aqueous solutions frequently containing antiseptics, antibiotics and/or anesthetics used for treating the pharynx (throat) and nasopharynx by forcing air from the lungs through the gargle while ....are formulated to reduce plaque, gingivitis, dental.

8. Sprays are solutions of drugs in aqueous vehicles and are applied to the mucous membrane of the nose and throat by means of an ....

9. Medicine for external application that produces redness of the skin are called .... while .... are medicine applied locally to produce superficial inflammation in order to reduce deeper inflammation.

10. When the two phases are immiscible like oil and water they form .... and when two phases are different like one is solid and other is liquid they form ....

11. The particle size of the suspended drug particles in the suspension should be in the range of .... to .... micron.

12. The suspensions which are instilled into the eye should be free from .... particles.

13. The fine particle size of solid in suspension give a .... rate of ....

14. The particles form .... and from a .... like structure in case of flocculated suspension.

15. The flocculating agent reduces the .... and improved the .... of solid particles.

16. In non-flocculated suspension, the particles exist as ....

17. Thickening agents are .... colloids which increase the ....…..... of the continuous phase.

18. In o/w emulsion, ... is in disperse phase, whereas .... is in continuous phase.

19. Emulsifying agents reduce ....between two phases.

20. Emulsions meant for external use should be .... type.

21. Soaps formed from monovalent base produce .... emulsion and soaps from divalent base produce .... emulsion.

22. Bottle method is used for preparation of emulsions of .... and .... oils.

ANSWERS

1. 1-B, 2-A, 3-C, 4-D

2. 1-D, 2-B, 3-A, 4-E, 5-C

3. 1-B, 2-D, 3-A, 4-C

4. 1-D, 2-B, 3-E, 4-C, 5-A

5. C

6. Douche, cleansing or antiseptic agent, enemas

7. Gargles, mouthwashes

8. Atomizer nebulizer

9. Rubefacient, counter-irritant

10. Emulsion, suspension

11. 0.5, 5 micron

12. Gritty

13. Faster, dissolution

14. Loose aggregated, net work

15. Surface tension, dispersion

16. Separate entities

17. Hydrophilic, viscosity

18. Oil, water

19. Interfacial tension

20. o/w type

21. o/w, w/o

22. Volatile, non-viscous

3

Semisolid Dosage Form

DEFINITION

Semisolid dosage forms are dermatological products of semisolid consistency and applied to skin for therapeutic or protective action or cosmetic function. Semisolid formulations which when applied to the skin or accessible mucous membranes tend to alleviate or treat a pathological condition or offer protection against a harmful environment. Because of their peculiar rheological behavior, semisolids can adhere to the application surface for sufficiently long periods before they are washed off. This property helps prolong drug delivery at the application site. A semisolid dosage form is advantageous in terms of its easy application, rapid formulation, and ability to topically deliver a wide variety of drug molecules.

TYPES OF CONVENTIONAL SEMISOLID DOSAGE FORMS AND THEIR PROPERTIES

Conventional semisolid dosage form mainly includes ointments, creams, pastes, gels or jellies, etc. A brief introduction about these is given in Table 3.1.

IDEAL PROPERTIES OF SEMISOLID DOSAGE FORMS

Physical Properties

1. Smooth texture
2. Elegant in appearance
3. Non-dehydrating
4. Non-gritty

Table 3.1: A brief introduction of semisolid dosage forms

Dosage form	Properties
Ointments	• Ointments are soft semisolid preparations meant for external application to the skin or mucous membrane. • They usually contain medicament which is either dissolved or suspended in the base. • They have emollient and protective action.
Creams	• Creams are semisolid emulsions and are generally of softer consistency and lighter than ointments. • They are less greasy and are easy to apply.
Pastes	• Pastes are semisolid preparations for external application that differ from similar products in containing a high proportion of finely powdered medicaments. • They are stiffer and are usually employed for their protective action and for their ability to absorb serous discharges from skin lesions. • Thus when protective, rather than therapeutic action is desired, the formulation pharmacists will favor a paste, but when therapeutic action is required, he will prefer ointments and creams.
Jellies	• Jellies are transparent or translucent, non-greasy, semisolid preparation mainly used externally. • The gelling agent may be gelatin, starch, tragacanth, sodium alginate or cellulose derivative (e.g. carboxy methyl cellulose).

5. Non-greasy and non-staining
6. Non-hygroscopic

Physiological Properties

1. Non-irritating
2. Do not alter membrane/skin functioning
3. Miscible with skin secretion
4. Have low sensitization index

Application Properties

1. Easily applicable with efficient drug release
2. High aqueous washability.

Storage Properties

Ideally, semisolid dosage form should remain stable under various real world storage conditions as per ICH guidelines (Table 3.2). Storage of semisolids should be at temperatures not exceeding 25°C unless otherwise authorized. They should not be allowed to freeze and must be stored in a well-closed container or, if the preparation contains water or other volatile ingredients, store in an air-tight container. The containers are preferably collapsible metal tubes from which the preparation may be readily extruded. If the preparation is sterile, store in a sterile, airtight, tamper-proof container.

Table 3.2: Storage/test conditions for four climatic zones for semisolid dosage form

Climatic zones	Definition	Storage/test conditions	Example
I	Temp. climate	21°C ± 2°C and 45% RH ± 5% RH	Northern Europe, Canada
II	Mediterranean and subtropical climate	25°C ± 2°C and 60% RH ± 5% RH*	Southern Europe, Japan, US
III	Hot dry climate	30°C ± 2°C and 35% RH ± 5% RH*	Egypt, Sudan
IV	Hot, humid	30°C ± 2°C and 75% RH ± 5% RH	Central Africa, South Pacific

*RH = Relative humidity

MECHANISMS OF DRUG PENETRATION AND ROUTE OF ABSORPTION

Skin Anatomy

Semisolid dosage forms are generally used as a topical system for administration of drugs. Thus to understand the mechanism of drug penetration, one should know about the anatomy of skin.

The skin is made up of several layers including stratum corneum, viable epidermis and dermis, and it contains appendages that include sweat glands, sebaceous glands, and hair follicles. The stratum corneum is the outermost desquamating 'horny' layer of skin, comprising about 15–20 rows of flat, partially desiccated, dead, keratinized epidermal cells (Fig. 3.1).

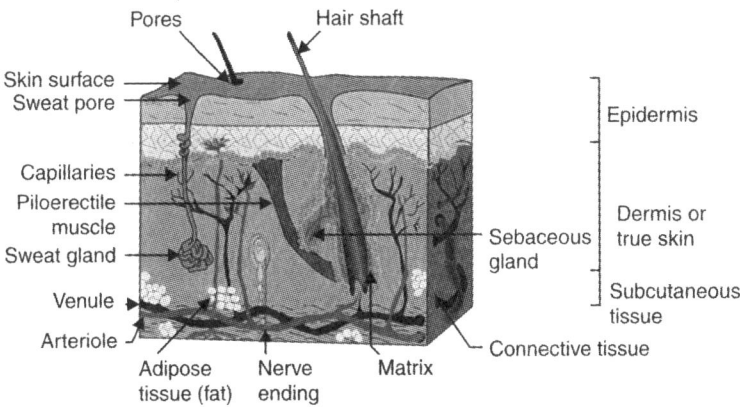

Fig. 3.1: Cross section of skin

Semisolid dosage forms for dermatological drug therapy are intended to produce desired therapeutic action at specific sites in the epidermal tissue. A drug's ability to penetrate the skin's epidermis, dermis, and subcutaneous fat layers depends on the properties of the drug (physicochemical properties), the carrier base and skin condition.

Both topical and transdermal drug products are intended for external use. However, topical dermatologic products are intended for localized action on one or more layers of the skin (e.g. sunscreens, keratolytic agents, local anesthetics, antiseptics and anti-inflammatory agents). Although some medication from these topical products may unintentionally reach systemic circulation, it is usually in subtherapeutic concentrations, and does not produce effects of any major concern except possibly in special situations, such as the pregnant or nursing patient.

When a drug system is applied topically, the drug diffuses out of its vehicle on to the surface tissue of the skin. There are three potential portals of entry:

1. Through the follicular region
2. Through the sweat ducts
3. Through the unbroken stratum corneum between these appendages.

Absorption by the transdermal route, penetration is fairly rapid, although slower than intestinal tract absorption, and is almost always accompanied by some degree of pilosebaceous penetration as well.

Mechanism of Drug Absorption

Generally, drug absorption into the skin occurs by passive diffusion. The rate of drug transport across the stratum corneum follows Fick's law of diffusion,

$$dA/dt = D.C.K/h$$

where,

i. dA/dt is the steady-state flux across stratum corneum,

ii. D is the diffusion coefficient or diffusivity of drug molecules,

iii. C is the drug concentration gradient across the stratum corneum,

iv. K is the partition coefficient of the drug between skin and formulation medium, and

v. h is the thickness of the stratum corneum.

In particular, the transient diffusion that occurs shortly after the application of a substance to the surface of the skin is shown to be potentially far greater through the appendages than through the matrix of stratum corneum. After the steady state has been established, the dominant diffusion mode is probably no longer intra-appendageal, but occurs through the matrix of stratum corneum. The recognition of transient diffusion, occurring primarily via follicles and ducts, and steady state diffusion, occurring primarily through the intact stratum corneum, results in a considerably more self-consistent and orderly treatment of the process of percutaneous absorption.

The concentration gradient ends in the dermal layer at the beginning of the circulation. The systemic circulation acts as a reservoir or "sinks" for the drug. Once in the general circulation, the drug is diluted and distributed rapidly with little systemic build up.

Diffusion through the horny layer is a passive process. The passive process is affected only by the substance being absorbed, by the medium in which the substance is dispersed and by ambient conditions. On the other hand, percutaneous absorption is the more complicated process, of which epidermal diffusion is the first phase and clearance from the dermis the second which depends on effective blood flow, interstitial fluid moment, lymphatic and perhaps other factors that combine with dermal constituents.

Transport of lipophilic drug molecules is facilitated by their dissolution into intercellular lipids around the cells of the stratum corneum. Absorption of hydrophilic molecules into skin can occur through pores or openings of the hair follicles and sebaceous glands, but the relative surface area of these openings is barely 1% of the total skin surface. This small surface area limits the amount of drug absorption.

Factors Affecting Skin Penetration

The factors that influence skin penetration are essentially the same as those for gastrointestinal absorption, with the rate of diffusion depending primarily on the physicochemical property of drug and only secondarily on the vehicle, pH, and concentration.

The principal physicochemical factor in skin penetration is the hydration state of stratum corneum, which affects the rate of passage of all substances that penetrate the skin. The clinical importance of hydration can be found in the use of occlusive plastic film in steroid therapy. Here, the prevention of water loss from the stratum corneum and the subsequent increased water concentration in this skin layer apparently enhances the penetration of the steroid. The temperature of skin and the concentration of the drug play significant roles, but they are secondary to that of hydration.

The solubility of a drug determines the concentration presented to the absorption site, the water or lipid partition coefficient influences the rate of transport. An inverse relationship appears to exist between the absorption rate and the molecular weight. Small molecules penetrate more rapidly than large molecules, but within a narrow range of molecular size, there is little correlation between the size and the penetration rate.

FORMULATION OF SEMISOLID DOSAGE FORMS

Ointments

Ointments are semisolid preparations for external application to skin or mucous membranes. The components of an ointment soften but do not melt upon application to the skin. Ointments are used topically on a variety of body surfaces. These include the skin and the mucous membranes of the eye (an *eye ointment*), vagina, anus, and nose. An ointment may or may not be medicated. Therapeutically, ointments function as skin protective and emollients, but they are used primarily as vehicles for the topical application of drug substances. Since they are greasy nature so they stain cloths. Ointments are usually very moisturizing, and good for dry skin, have low risk of sensitization because of having few ingredients. The vehicle of an ointment is known as the ointment base. The choice of a base depends upon the clinical indication for the ointment.

Characteristics of an Ideal Ointment

1. It should be chemically and physically stable.
2. It should be smooth and free from grittiness.
3. It should melt or soften at body temperature and be easily applied.
4. The base should be non-irritant and should have no therapeutic action.
5. The medicament should be finely divided and uniformly distributed throughout the base.

Classification of Ointments

Ointment can be classified into three types according to their therapeutic properties based on penetration of skin as given in Table 3.3. Ointment can also be classified according to its therapeutic uses as given in Table 3.4.

Table 3.3: Classification of ointment based on penetration of skin	
a. Epidermic ointments	• These ointments are intended to produce their action on the surface of the skin and produce local effect. • They are not absorbed. • They act as protective, antiseptic and parasiticide.
b. Endodermic ointments	• These ointments are intended to release the medicaments that penetrate into the skin. • They are partially absorbed and acts as emollients, stimulants and local irritants.
c. Diadermic ointments	• These ointments are intended to release the medicaments that pass through the skin and produce systemic effects.

Table 3.4: Classification of ointment according to its therapeutic uses

Ointment classification	Use	Example of drugs
Antiacne	Acne treatment	Resorcinol, sulfur
Antibiotics	Used to kill microorganisms	Bacitracin, chlortetracycline, neomycin
Antieczematous	Used to stop oozing and exudation from vesicles on the skin	Hydrocortisone, coal tar, ichthamol, salicylic acid
Antifungal	Used to inhibit or kill the fungi	Benzoic acid, salicylic acid, nystatin, clotrimazole
Anti-inflammatory	Used to relieve inflammatory, allergic and pruritic conditions of the skin	Betamethasone valerate, hydrocortisone, triamcinolone acetonide
Antipruritic	Used to relieve itching	Benzocaine, coal tar.
Antiseptic	Used to stop sepsis	Ammoniated mercury, zinc oxide
Astringent	Reduces the secretion of glands or discharge from skin surface	Calamine, zinc oxide, aluminium acetate and subacetate, acetic acid and tannic acid
Counter-irritant	These are applied locally to irritate the intact skin, thus reducing or relieving another irritation or deep seated pain	Capsicum oleoresin, iodine (Iodex), methyl salicylate
Anti-dandruff	Dandruff treatment	Salicylic acid and cetrimide (cetyl trimethyl ammonium bromide)
Emollient	Used to soften the skin (for example, in the dry season).	Soft paraffin
Keratolytic	Used to remove or soften the horny layer of the skin	Resorcinol, salicylic acid and sulfur
Keratoplastic	Tends to increase the thickness of horny layer	coal tar
Parasiticide	These ointments destroy or inhibit living infestations such as lice and ticks	Benzyl benzoate, gamma-benzene hexachloride (GBH), sulfur
Protective	Protects the skin from moisture, air, sun rays or other substances such as soaps or chemicals.	Silicones, titanium dioxide, calamine, zinc oxide, petrolatum

FORMULATION OF SEMISOLID DOSAGE FORMS

Inert pharmaceutical ingredients are used in combination with drugs to formulate the product. However, many times topical bases are used for therapy, e.g. cold cream.

Ingredients Used in Preparation of Semisolids

Ingredients used for formulating semisolids include API, bases, antimicrobial preservative, chelating agents, humectants, fragrances.

1. Active Pharmaceutical Ingredients

Active pharmaceutical ingredients are described in Table 3.5.

Table 3.5: Medicaments prescribed for semisolids

Disease treated	API
Keratolytic	Salicylic acid
Acne	Sulfur, resorcinol
Antipruritic	Benzocaine, menthol, camphor
Emollient	Lanolin
Anti-inflammatory	Corticosteroid
Antifungal	Benzoic acid, salicylic acid

2. Bases

A large number of drugs for external use are presented as semi-solid formulations, e.g. ointments, suppositories, creams and pastes. While ointments are considered as semisolids, suppositories are regarded as molded solid dosage forms. Ointment and suppository bases do not merely act as the carriers of the medicaments, but they also control the extent of absorption of medicaments incorporated in them.

An ointment base should be compatible with skin, stable, smooth and pliable, non-irritating, non-sensitizing, inert, capable of absorbing water or other liquid preparations, and of releasing the incorporated medicament, readily. A base for ophthalmic ointments must be non-irritating to the eye, should permit the diffusion of the drug through the secretions batting the eye, and should retain the activity of the medicament for a reasonable period often under proper storage conditions. It should also be sterilizable conveniently.

Selection of ointment base depends on following:

1. Desired release rate of the drug substance from the ointment base.
2. Rate and extent of topical or percutaneous drug absorption.
3. Desirability of occlusion of moisture from skin.
4. Stability of the drug in the ointment base.
5. Effect of drug on the consistency of base.
6. Easy removal of base on washing.
7. Characteristic of the surface to which it is applied.

Ointment bases may be classified in several ways but the following classifications based on composition are generally used which are as follows:

1. Oleaginous bases.
2. Absorption bases.
3. Emulsion bases.
4. Water-soluble bases.
5. Water removable bases.

Oleaginous bases: These generally consist of a combination of more than one oleaginous material such as water-insoluble hydrophobic oils and fats. Most of the early ointment bases used to be exclusively oleaginous in nature but nowadays the materials obtained from plant, animal, mineral as well as synthetic origin are employed as oleaginous ointment bases. Combinations of these materials can produce a wide range of melting points and viscosities.

Absorption (emulsifiable) bases: These are essentially anhydrous systems composed of hydrophobic ingredients already discussed under oleaginous bases. They are called as emulsifiable bases because they initially contain no water but are capable of taking it up to yield w/o and o/w emulsions. Absorption bases are w/o type emulsions and have capacity to absorb considerable quantities of water or aqueous solution without marked changes in consistency. Absorption bases are mostly mixtures of animal sterols with petrolatum. Combinations of cholesterol and/or other suitable lanolin fractions with white petrolatum are available under different commercial names, e.g. Eucerin and Aquaphor.

Emulsion bases: According to the type of emulsion, these bases are classified as either w/o or o/w. All w/o emulsions are not water-washable as the oil is in the external phase and o/w emulsions are used in dermatological preparations and cosmetic creams. Some of the popular creams include cold creams, vanishing creams, skin creams, emollient creams, foundation creams, hand creams, etc. Fundamentally, creams can be divided into cold and vanishing types.

Types of creams depending on formulation are as follow:

1. *Sterol creams:* They are water in oil emulsions where emulgent is wool fat or wool alcohol. Classical example is lanolin.

2. *Soap creams:* Triethanolamine creams are neutral soaps, produces o/w emulsion with oleic acid and triethanolamine (good emulgents for liquid paraffin).

3. *Anionic emulsifying wax creams:* These emulsifiers produce oil in water type.

4. *Cationic emulsifying wax creams:* These emulsifiers produce water in oil type.

5. *Creams emulsified with non-ionic surfactants:* Cream bases prepared with self-emulsifying monostearin, a sorbitan ester, a macrogol ester, a non-emulsifying wax containing a macrogol ether, etc.

6. *Divalent creams:* Classical example is lime creams which is of water in oil type. Emulgent in these is oleic acid and calcium hydroxide.

7. *Vanishing creams:* They are oil in water type creams which when rubbed on to the skin and disappear with little or no trace of their former presence.

Water-soluble bases: These include both anhydrous and hydrous dermatological non-emulsion bases which are water-soluble and contain no oil phase. These are generally based on either polyethylene glycols or one or more of the other hydrocolloids.

Polyethylene glycols (carbowaxes) are water-soluble, non-volatile, unctuous compounds. They do not hydrolyse or deteriorate and do not support mold growth. They have low irritancy and dermal/oral toxicities. Carbowaxes also allow easy diffusion of medicaments to the body tissues but the degree of their absorption is low. Different grade of cabowaxes are available which are designated by a number roughly representing their average molecular weights, e.g. 200–300,

400, 600, 1000, 1540, 4000 and 6000. At room temperature, carbowaxes 200 to 400 are clear liquids whereas carbowaxes 1000 to 60000 are white, waxy solids.

A variety of water-washable ointment bases with consistencies ranging from semisolid to solid can be obtained by blending different polyethylene glycols. Polyethylene glycol ointment USP is a blend of carbowaxes 4000 and 400. Medicaments containing acidic hydrogen may interact with high molecular weight polyethylene glycols forming molecular complexes.

An example of formulation containing plastibase official in BPC is triamcinolone dental paste which contains an anti-inflammatory agent triamcinolone acetonide in adhesive, sodium CMC, pectin and gelatin.

Water removable bases: Popular example of this includes vanishing cream.

Note: Mineral oils are added to petrolatum to lower its fusion point, however, by doing so problem of phase separation on storage is seen. This separation can be prevented by the addition of small quantities of natural waxes like ozokerite, ceresine or microcrystalline wax.

Semisolid ophthalmic vehicles contain soft petrolatum, a bland absorbing base or a water-soluble base.

3. Antimicrobial Preservatives

Some bases, although, resist microbial attack but because of their high water content, they require an antimicrobial preservative. Commonly used preservatives include methylhydroxyl-benzoate, propylhydroxybenzoate, chlorocresol, benzoic acid, phenyl mercuric nitrate, benzalkonium chloride, chlorhexidine acetate, benzyl alcohol and mercurial.

4. Antioxidants

An antioxidant is a molecule that inhibits the oxidation of other molecules. Oxidation is a chemical reaction that transfers electrons or hydrogen from a substance to an oxidizing agent. Oxidation reactions can produce free radicals. In turn, these radicals can start chain reactions. Antioxidants terminate these chain reactions by removing free radical intermediates, and inhibit other oxidation reactions. They do this by being oxidized themselves, so antioxidants are often reducing. Examples of commonly used antioxidants include butylated hydroxy anisole, and butylated hydroxy toluene.

5. Chelating Agents

Chelating agents are chemical substances that contain molecules capable of bonding securely to minute particles of metal called ions. Examples of commonly used chelating agents include citric acid, maleic acid.

6. Humectants

A substance, especially a skin lotion used to reduce the loss of moisture. Examples of commonly used humectants include polyethylene glycol, glycerol or sorbitol.

7. Fragrances

To ipmport fragrance to the formulation. Examples of widely used fragrances are lavender oil, rose oil, lemon oil, almond oil, etc.

8. Ideal Emulsifier (Table 3.6)

Ideal properties of emulsifier includes:
  a. Must reduce surface tension for proper emulsification.
  b. Prevents coalescence should quickly absorb around the dispersed phase.

Table 3.6: Emulsifiers

Anionic	Cationic	Non-ionic
Alkyl sulfates	Quaternary ammonium compounds	Polyoxyethylene alkyl-aryl ethers
Soaps	Alkoxyalkylamines	Polyoxyethylene fatty acid ester
Dodecyl benzene sulfonate		Polyoxyethylene sorbitan esters
Lactylates		Sorbitan fatty acid esters
Sulfosuccinates		Glyceryl fatty acid esters
Monoglyceride sulfonates		Sucrose fatty acid esters
Phosphate ester		Polyoxyethylene
Silicones		Polyoxypropylene block
Taurates		Polymers

c. Ability to increase the viscosity at low concentration.

d. Effective at low concentration.

Table 3.7: HLB system

HLB range	Application
4–6	w/o emulsifier
7–9	Wetting agent
8–18	o/w emulsifier
13–15	Detergent
10–18	Solubilizers

9. Gelling Agents

These are organic hydrocolloids or hydrophilic inorganic substances. They are tragacanth, sodium alginate, pectin, starch, gelatin, cellulose derivatives, carbomer, and poly vinyl alcohol, clays.

There are numerous gelling agents varying in gelling ability. Commonly used gelling agents are listed in Table 3.8.

Table 3.8: Gelling agents

Material	%	Brookfield viscosity 'CPS'
Carbomer 941 resin NF	0.15	2900
Carbomer 941 resin NF	0.25	6300
Carbomer 941 resin NF	0.50	44000
Carbomer 941 resin NF	1.00	81000
Sodium carboxymethyl cellulose	1.50	5000
Guar gum	1.50	8040
Methylcellulose	2.00	5200
Locust bean gum	2.50	22800
Sodium alginate	2.50	10400

10. Permeability Enhancer

Skin can act as a barrier and prevent deep penetration of drug molecules. With the introduction of various penetration enhancers, however, systemic drug delivery through the transdermal route has gained major footing (Table 3.9).

Penetration enhancer works by:

a. Reversibly disordering the lamellar packing of stratum corneum.

Table 3.9: Penetration enhancer used with drugs for topical semisolids

Sr. no	Permeation enhancer	Drugs used
1.	Menthol, carvacrol, linalol	Propranolol hydrochloride
2.	Limonene	Indomethacin, ketoprofen
3.	Geraniol, nerolidol	Diclofenac sodium
4.	Oleic acid	Piroxicam
5.	Lecithin	Hydrocortisone acetate, heparin
6.	Propylene-glycol-dipelargonate	Heparin
7.	Cyclodextrins	Hydrocortisone

b. Increasing the thermodynamic activity of the drug.

c. Increasing the amount of drug in solubilized form at the skin surface.

In addition to the use of penetration enhancers alone, their combination with cosolvents that deliver a drug in solubilized form has led to the achievement of higher drug permeability (Tables 3.10 and 3.11).

Table 3.10: Combination of penetration enhancer and cosolvent for topical semisolids

Sr. no	Permeation enhancer	Cosolvent	Drugs used
1.	Isopropyl myristate	Propylene glycol	Diclofenac sodium
2.	Cineole	Ethanol	TRH analogue p-Glu-3-methyl-His-Pro amide
3.	Ethanol	Propylene glycol	Aspirin

Table 3.11: Compilation of constituents of semisolid dosage form

Function	Sample ingredients	
Polymeric thickeners	Gums	Acrylic acids
	Acacia	Carbomers
	Alginates	Polycarbophil
	Carageenan	Colloidal solids
	Chitosan	Silica
	Collagen	Clays
	Tragacanth	Microcystalline cellulose
	Xanthan	Hydrogels
	Celluloses	Polyvinyl alcohol

(Contd...)

Table 3.11: Compilation of constituents of semisolid dosage form *(Contd.)*

Function	*Sample ingredients*	
	Sodium carboxymethyl	Polyvinylpyrrolidone
	Hydroxyethyl	Them reversible polymers
	Hydroxypropyl	Poloxamers
	Hydroxypropylmethyl	
Oil phase	Mineral oil	Isopropyl myristate
	White soft paraffin	Isopropyl palmitate
	Yellow soft paraffin	Castor oil
	Beeswax	Canola oil
	Stearyl alcohol	Cottonseed oil
	Cetyl alcohol	Jojoba oil
	Cetostearyl alcohol	Arachis (Peanut) oil
	Stearic acid	Lanolin (and derivatives)
	Oleic acid	Silicone oils
Surfactants	**Non-ionic**	**Anionic**
	Sorbitan esters	Sodium dodecyl sulfate
	Polysorbates	Cationic
	Polyoxyethylene alkyl ethers	Cetrimide
	Polyoxyethylene alkyl esters	Benzalkonium chloride
	Polyoxyethylene alkyl ethers	Polyethylene glycols
	Glycerol esters	Propylene carbonate
	Cholesterol	Triacetin
Solvents	**Polar**	**Non-polar**
	Water	Isopropyl alcohol
	Propylene glycol	Medium chain triglycerides
	Glycerol	
	Sorbitol	
	Ethanol	
	Industrial methylated spirit	
Preservatives	**Antimicrobial**	**Antioxidants**
	Benzalkonium chloride	α-tocopherol
	Benzoic acid	Ascorbic acid
	Benzyl alcohol	Ascorbyl palmitate
	Bronopol	Butylated hydroxyanisole
	Chlorhexidine	Butylated hydroxytoluene
	Chlorocresol	Sodium ascorbate

(Contd...)

Table 3.11: Compilation of constituents of semisolid dosage form *(Contd.)*

Function	Sample ingredients	
	Imidazolidinyl urea	Sodium metabisulfite
	Paraben esters	Chelating agents
	Phenol	Citric acid
	Phenoxyethanol	Edetic acid
	Potassium sorbate	
	Sorbic acid	
pH adjusters	Diethanolamine	Sodium hydroxide
	Lactic acid	Sodium phosphate
	Monoethanolamine	Triethanolamine

Methods of Preparation

Before discussing method of preparation of ointment, we must understand the characteristics of well-made ointment.

A well-made ointment is:

a. Uniform throughout, i.e. it contains no lumps of separated high melting point ingredients of the base, there is no tendency for liquid constituents to separate and insoluble powders are evenly dispersed.

b. Free from grittiness, i.e. insoluble powders are finely subdivided and large lumps of particles are absent. Methods of preparation must satisfy these criteria.

Two mixing techniques are frequently used in making ointments:

1. Fusion, in which ingredients are melted together and stirred to ensure homogeneity.

2. Trituration, in which finely-subdivided insoluble medicaments are evenly distributed by grinding with a small amount of the base or one of its ingredients followed by dilution with gradually increasing amounts of the base.

1. Ointments Prepared by Fusion Method

When an ointment base contains a number of solid ingredients such as white beeswax, cetyl alcohol, stearyl alcohol, stearic acid, hard paraffin, etc. as components of the base, it is required to melt them. The melting can be done in two methods:

Method-I

The components are melted in the decreasing order of their melting point, i.e. the higher melting point substance should be melted first, the substances with next melting point and so on. The medicament is added slowly in the melted ingredients and stirred thoroughly until the mass cools down and homogeneous product is formed.

Advantages

This will avoid over-heating of substances having low melting point.

Method-II

All the components are taken in subdivided state and melted together.

Advantages

The maximum temperature reached is lower than method-I, and less time was taken possibly due to the solvent action of the lower melting point substances on the rest of the ingredients.

Precautions to be taken while Preparing Ointment

i. Melting time is shortened by grating waxy components (i.e. beeswax, wool alcohols, hard-paraffin, higher fatty alcohols and emulsifying waxes) by stirring during melting and by lowering the dish as far as possible into the water bath so that the maximum surface area is heated.

ii. The surface of some ingredients discolors due to oxidation, e.g. wool fats and wool alcohols and this discolored layers should be removed before use.

iii. After melting, the ingredients should be stirred until the ointment is cool, taking care not to cause localized cooling, e.g. by using a cold spatula or stirrer, placing the dish on a cold surface (e.g. a plastic bench top) or transferring to a cold container before the ointment has fully set. If these precautions are ignored, hard lumps may separate.

iv. Vigorous-stirring, after the ointment has begun to thicken, causes excessive aeration and should be avoided.

v. Because of their greasy nature, many constituents of ointment bases pickup dirt during storage, which can be seen after melting. This is removed from the melt by allowing it to sediment and decanting the supernatant, or by passage through muslin supported by a warm strainer. In both instances, the clarified liquid is collected in another hot basin.

vi. If the product is granular after cooling, due to separation of high melting point constituents, it should be remelted, using the minimum of heat, and again stirred and cooled.

Examples

i. Simple ointment BP contains

- Wool fat—50 g
- Hard paraffin—50 g
- Cetostearyl alcohol—50 g
- White soft paraffin—850 g

Type of preparation: Absorption ointment base

Procedure:

Hard paraffin and cetostearyl alcohol are mixed and heated on water-bath. Wool fat and white soft paraffin are mixed and stirred until all the ingredients are melted.

If required decanted or strained and stirred until cold and packed in suitable container.

ii. Paraffin ointment base

Type of preparation: Hydrocarbon ointment base

iii. Wool alcohols ointment BP

Type of preparation: Absorption base

iv. Emulsifying ointment BP

Type of preparation: Water-miscible ointment base.

v. Macrogol ointment BPC

Type of preparation: Water-soluble ointment base

Formula: Macrogol 4000

Liquid Macrogol 300

Method: Macrogol 4000 is melted and previously warmed liquid macrogol 300 is added. It is stirred until cool.

2. Ointment Prepared by Trituration

This method is applicable in the base or a liquid present in small amount.

i. Solids that are finely powdered are passed through a sieve (#250, #180, #125).

ii. The powder is taken on an ointment-slab and triturated with a small amount of the base. A steel spatula with long, broad blade is used. To this, additional quantities of the base are incorporated and triturated until the medicament is mixed with the base.

iii. Finally, liquid ingredients are incorporated. To avoid loss from splashing, a small volume of liquid is poured into a depression in the ointment and thoroughly incorporated before more is added in the same way. Splashing is more easily controlled in a mortar than on a tile.

Example

Whitfield ointment (compound benzoic acid ointment BPC.)

Formula:

Benzoic acid, in fine powder—6 gm

Salicylic acid, in fine powder—3 gm

Emulsifying ointment—91 gm

Method: Benzoic acid and salicylic acid are sieved through no. 180 sieves. They are mixed on the tile with small amount of base and levigated until smooth and dilute gradually.

ii. Salicylic acid sulfur ointment BPC.

3. Ointment Preparation by Chemical Reaction

Chemical reactions were involved in the preparation of several famous ointments of the past, e.g. strong mercuric nitrate ointment, both of the 1959 BPC.

a. *Ointment containing free iodine:* Iodine is only slightly soluble in most fats and oils but readily soluble in concentrated solution of potassium iodide due to the formation of molecular complexes $KI.I_2$, $KI.2I_2$, $KI.3I_2$, etc. These solutions may be incorporated in absorption-type ointment bases, e.g. strong iodine ointment B.Vet.C (British

Veterinary Pharmacopoeia) is used to treat ringworm in cattle. It contains free iodine. At one time, this type of ointments was used as counter-irritants in the treatment of human rheumatic diseases but they were not popular because:

i. They stain the skin a deep red color.

ii. Due to improper storage, the, water dries up and the iodine crystals irritate the skin, hence glycerol was some times to dissolve the iodine-potassium iodide complex instead of water.

Example: Strong Iodine Ointment B. Vet.C., iodine, woolfat, yellow soft paraffin, potassium iodide, water.

Procedure

i. KI is dissolved in water. I_2 is dissolved in it.

ii. Woolfat and yellow soft paraffin are melted together over water bath. Melted mass is cooled to about 40°C.

iii. I_2 solution is added to the melted mass in small quantities at a time with continuous stirring until a uniform mass is obtained.

iv. It is cooled to room temperature and packed.

Use: Ringworm in cattle.

b. *Ointment containing combined iodine:* Fixed oils and many vegetable and animal fats absorb iodine which combines with the double bonds of the unsaturated constituents, e.g. $CH_3.(CH_2)_2.CH = CH.(CH_2)_7.COOH + I_2 \Rightarrow CH_3.(CH_2)_2.CHI$ $CHI.(CH_2)_7.COOH$ (oleic acid di-iodostearic acid).

Example: Non-staining Iodine Ointment BPC. 1968, iodine arachis oil, yellow soft paraffin.

Method

a. Iodine is finely powdered in a glass mortar and required amount is added to the oil in a glass-stoppered conical flask and stirred well.

b. The oil is heated at 50°C in a water-bath and stirred continually. Heating is continued until the brown color is changed to greenish-black; this may take several hours.

c. From 0.1 g of the preparation the amount of iodine is determined by BPC method and the amount of soft paraffin base is calculated to give the product the required strength.

d. Soft paraffin is warmed to 40°C. The iodized oil is added and mixed well. No more heat is applied because this causes deposition of a resinous substance.

e. The preparation is packed in a warm, wide-mouthed, amber color, glass bottle. It is allowed to cool without further stirring.

4. Preparation of Ointments by Emulsification

An emulsion system contains an oil phase, an aqueous phase and an emulsifying agent. For o/w emulsion systems, the following emulsifying agents are used:

i. Water-soluble soap

ii. Cetyl alcohol

iii. Glyceryl monostearate

iv. Combination of emulsifiers: Triethanolamine stearate + cetyl alcohol

v. Non-ionic emulsifiers: Glyceryl monostearate, glyceryl mono-oleate, propylene glycol stearate. For w/o emulsion creams, the following emulsifiers are used:

- Polyvalent ions, e.g. magnesium, calcium and aluminum are used.

- Combination of emulsifiers: beeswax + divalent calcium ion. The viscosity of this type of creams prevents coalescence of the emulsified phases and helps in stabilizing the emulsion.

Example: Cold Cream

Procedure:

i. Water immiscible components, e.g. oils, fats, waxes are melted together over water bath (70°C).

ii. Aqueous solution of all heat-stable, water-soluble components is heated (70°C).

iii. Aqueous solution is slowly added to the melted bases with continuous stirring until the product cools down and a semisolid mass is obtained.

Note: The aqueous phase is heated otherwise high melting point fats and waxes will immediately solidify on addition of cold aqueous solution.

Stability of Ointments

The ointments should remain stable from the time of preparation to the time when the whole of it is consumed by the user.

i. To stop microbial growth, preservatives are added. Preservatives for ointment includes: p-hydroxybenzoates, phenol, benzoic acid, sorbic acid, methylparaben, propylparaben, quaternary ammonium compounds, mercury compounds, etc.

ii. The preservatives should not react with any of the components of the formulation. Plastic containers may absorb the preservative and thereby decreasing the concentration of preservative available for killing the bacteria.

iii. Some ingredients like wool fat and wool alcohols are susceptible to oxidation. Therefore, a suitable antioxidant may be incorporated to protect the active ingredients from oxidation.

iv. Incompatible drugs, emulsifying agents and preservatives must be avoided. The drugs which are likely to hydrolyze must be dispensed in an anhydrous base.

v. Humectants such as, glycerin, propylene glycol and sorbitol may be added to prevent the loss of moisture from the preparation.

vi. Ointment must be stored at an optimum temperature otherwise separation of phases may take place in the emulsified products which may be very difficult to remix to get a uniform product.

Paste

Pastes are basically ointments into which a high percentage of insoluble solid has been added. The extraordinary amount of particulate matter stiffens the system through direct interactions of the dispersed particulates and by adsorbing the liquid hydrocarbon fraction the vehicle on the particle surface.

Pastes are usually prepared by incorporating solids directly into a congealed system by levigation with a portion of the base to form a paste-like mass. The remainders of the base are added with continue levigation until the solids are uniformly dispersed in the vehicle.

Properties of Paste

- Pastes are less penetrating and less macerating and less heating than ointment.
- Pastes make particularly good protective barrier when placed on the skin for, in addition to forming an unbroken film, the solid they contain can absorb and thereby neutralize certain noxious chemicals before they ever reach the skin.
- Like ointments, pastes form an unbroken relatively water impermeable film unlike ointments the film is opaque and, therefore, an effective sun block accordingly. Skiers apply paste around the nose and lips to gain a dual protection.
- Pastes are less greasy because of the absorption of the fluid hydrocarbon fraction to the particulates.

There are two types of paste:

a. Fatty pastes (e.g. zinc paste)
b. Non-greasy pastes (e.g. bassorin paste is also named tragacanth jellies since hydrophilic component of tragacanth gels in water).

Differences Between Pastes and Ointments

i. Pastes generally contain a large amount (50%) of finely powdered solids. So they are often stiffer than ointments.
ii. When applied to the skin, pastes adhere well, forming a thick coating that protects and soothes inflamed and raw surfaces and minimizes the damage done by scratching in itchy conditions such as chronic eczema. It is comparatively easy to confine pastes to the diseased areas whereas ointments, which are usually less viscous, tend to spread on to healthy skin, and this may result in sensitivity reactions, if the preparations contain a powerful medicament such as dithranol.

iii. Because of the powder contents, pastes are porous; hence, perspiration can escape. Since the powder absorbs exudate, pastes with hydrocarbon base are less macerating than ointments with a similar base.

iv. They are less greasy than ointments but since their efficacy depends on maintaining a thick surface layer they are far from attractive cosmetically.

v. Most of the pastes are unsuitable for treating scalp conditions because they are difficult to remove from the hair.

BASES OF PASTES

1. *Hydrocarbon base:* Soft paraffin and liquid paraffin are commonly used bases for the preparation of paste (Table 3.12).
2. Water miscible base (Table 3.13).
3. *Water-soluble bases:* Water-soluble bases are prepared from mixtures of high and low molecular weight polyethylene glycols (or macrogols) (Table 3.14).

METHODS OF PREPARATION

Like ointment, pastes are prepared by trituration and fusion methods. Trituration method is used when the base is liquid

Table 3.12: Examples of hydrocarbon base pastes			
Name of the preparation	*Active ingredients*	*Base*	*Use*
1. Compound zinc paste BP	Zinc oxide	Soft paraffin	Eczema, psoriasis
2. Compound zinc and salicylic acid paste BP (Lassar's paste)	Zinc oxide and salicylic acid	Soft paraffin	Eczema, psoriasis
3. Coal tar paste	Coal tar	Soft paraffin	Eczema
4. Dithranol paste compound	Dithranol	Soft paraffin	Ring worm or psoriasis
5. Aluminum paste BPC (Baltimore paste)	Aluminum oxide	Liquid paraffin	Protectant

or semisolid. Fusion method is used when the base is semisolid and/or solid in nature.

Table 3.13: Examples of water miscible pastes

Name of the preparation	Base	Use
1. Resorcinol and sulfur paste BPC	Emulsifying ointment	Anti-dandruff
2. Zinc and coal tar paste	Emulsifying wax	Eczema
3. Magnesium sulfate paste BPC	Magnesium sulfate-45%	
(Morison's paste)	Phenol in glycerol	Treat boils, because of their powerful osmotic effect of the salt and the glycerol
4. Titanium dioxide BPC	Suspension of TiO_2, ZnO, light kaolin and paste red Fe_2O_3 in glycerol + water	Absorbs exudates from weeping skin conditions

Table 3.14: Examples of water-soluble base pastes

Name of the preparation	Base	Use
1. Water-soluble dental pastes	Neomycin sulfate	Sterilizing infected root canal
2. Triamcinolone dental paste BPC	Triamcinolone acetonidein an adhesive paste (NaCMC, pectin and gelatin)	Anti-inflammatory

Preparation 1

Name: Compound zinc paste

Formula:

- Zinc oxide, finely sifted—25 g
- Starch, finely sifted—25 g
- White soft paraffin—50 g

Type of preparation: Paste with semisolid base prepared by fusion and trituration.

Procedure

a. Zinc oxide and starch powder are passed through no. 180 sieve.
b. Soft paraffin is melted on a water bath.
c. The required amount of powder is taken in a warm mortar, triturated with little melted base until smooth. Gradually rest of the base is added and mixed until cold.

Preparation 2

Name: Zinc and coal tar paste BPC.
Formula:

- Zinc oxide, finely sifted
- Coal tar emulsifying wax
- Starch
- Yellow soft paraffin.

Type of preparation: Paste with semisolid base prepared by fusion.

Procedure

Method-I:

a. Emulsifying wax is melted in a tared dish (70°C).
b. The coal tar is weighed in the dish and stirred to mix. Soft paraffin is melted in a separate dish (70°C) and about half is added to the tar-wax mixture; stirred well. Remainder is added; stirred again until homogeneous. Allowed to cool at about (30°C) and zinc oxide (previously passed through 180 mesh) and starch, in small amount with constant stirring. It is stirred until cold.

Method-II: Wax and paraffin melted together, mixed well and stirred until just setting. Powders are mixed on a slightly warm tile and the tar is incorporated. This method eliminates the risk of overheating.

Gels (Jellies)

Gels are semisolid system in which a liquid phase is constrained within a 3-D polymeric matrix (consisting of natural or synthetic gum) having a high degree of physical or chemical cross-linking or in other words gels are semisolid systems that consist of either suspensions of small inorganic particles or large organic molecules interpenetrated by a liquid. Gels can be either water based (aqueous gels) or organic solvent based (organogels).

Jellies are transparent or translucent non-greasy semisolid gels. Some are as transparent as water itself, an aesthetically pleasing state, other are turbid, as the polymer is present in colloidal aggregates that disperse light. They are used for medication, lubrication and some miscellaneous applications like carrier for spermicidal agents to be used intravaginally with diaphragms as an adjunctive means of contraception.

Types of Jellies

1. Medicated Jellies

i. Water-soluble drugs like local anesthetics, spermicides and antiseptics are suitable for incorporation in the jellies.

ii. They are easy to apply and evaporation of the water content produces a pleasant cooling effect. The medicinal film usually adheres well and gives protection but is easily removed by washing when the treatment is complete.

Examples:

a. Ephedrine sulfate jelly—used to arrest bleeding from nose.

b. Pramoxine HCl, a local anesthetic—relieves discomfort of pruritis and haemorrhoids.

c. Phenylmercuric nitrate—as spermicidal contraceptive.

2. Lubricant Jellies

i. Catheters, items of eletrodiagnostic equipment, such as cystoscopies, and rubber gloves or finger stalls used for rectal and other examinations require lubrication before use.

ii. The lubricants must be sterile for articles inserted into sterile regions of the body, such as urinary bladder.

iii. For painful investigations, a local anesthetic may be included as in Lignocaine Gel BPC.

3. Miscellaneous Jellies

The following are more specialized jellies:

a. *Patch testing:* Here the jelly is the vehicle for allergens applied to the skin to detect sensitivity. Several allergens may be applied on one person. The viscosity of the jelly and it leaves on drying help to keep the particles separate.

b. *Electrocardiography:* To reduce electrical resistance between the patient's skin and electrodes of the cardiograph, an electrode jelly may be applied. This contains NaCl to provide good conductivity and often pumice powder which, when applied on to the skin, removes part of the horny layer of the epidermis, the main layer of electrical resistance.

FORMULATION

Pharmaceutical jellies are usually prepared by adding a thickening agent such as tragacanth or carboxy methylcellulose (CMC) to an aqueous solution in which drug has been dissolved. The mass is triturated in a mortar until a uniform product is obtained. For the preparation of jellies, whole gum is preferred rather than powdered gum because the former gives a clear preparation of uniform consistency.

The following gelling agents are used for the preparation of jellies.

1. Tragacanth

The main hydrophilic component of tragacanth that gels in water has been named bassorin—hence, tragacanth jellies are sometimes called bassorin paste.

The amount of gum required for a preparation varies with its use:

a. For lubricating jelly, 2 to 3%.

b. For dermatological vehicles, about 5%.

c. For incorporation of ichthamol, resorcinol, salicylic acid and other medicaments, about 5% is generally used. All formulations contain alcohol and/or glycerol and/or a volatile oil to disperse the gum and prevent lumpiness when water is added.

d. They vary in viscosity, due to the natural origin of the gum and variations in milling and storage.

e. The film left on the skin tends to flake.

f. Viscosity is rapidly lost outside the pH range of 4.5 to 7.0; for example, if benzoic acid is used as the preservative.

g. They are susceptible to microbial growth.

Example

Formula:

- Ichthamol—1.0 g
- Tragacanth—2.5 g
- Alcohol 90%—5.0 g
- Glycerin—1.0 g
- Purified water—q.s. up to 50 g

Procedure

i. Alcohol is taken in a 100 ml, wide-mouthed jar; and then tragacanth is added to it. (The reverse order may lead to lump formation). Mixed well.

ii. Water is added as quickly as possible and mixed.

iii. Separately, ichthamol, glycerin and 10 ml water are mixed. Final weight is adjusted by adding more of water.

2. Sodium Alginate

Uses: As lubricant—1.5 to 2 % is used. As dermatological vehicle— 5 to 10 % is used.

A trace of Ca-salt ($CaCl_2$) may be added to increase the viscosity and most formulations contain glycerol as a dispersing agent.

Advantage: Sodium alginate has an advantage over tragacanth that is available in several grade or standardized viscosity.

3. Pectin

Pectin is a very good gelling agent and is used in the preparation of many types of jellies including edible jellies.

Glycerin is used as a dispersing agent and humectant in dermatological jellies.

Jellies must be packed in well-closed containers because they lose water rapidly by evaporation and this is increased by the susceptibility of pectin gels to syneresis (i.e. exudation of the aqueous phase as a result of contraction of the gel).

4. Starch

Starch in combination with gelatin and glycerin is commonly used for preparations of jellies. Glycerin in 50% may act as preservative. Medicaments are incorporated in the cold jelly by trituration.

5. Gelatin

Insoluble in cold water but swells and softens in it. It is soluble in hot water. Hot solution contains 2% gelatin forms a jelly on cooling. Very stiff (15%) jellies are melted before used and after cooling to desired temperature are applied with a brush to the affected area. The area is covered with bandage and the dressing may be left in place for several weeks.

Zinc-gelatin jelly (Unna's paste) is such an example.

Formula

- Zinc oxide—15 g
- Gelatin—15 g
- Glycerin—35 g
- Water—35 g

Procedure

i. Gelatin soaked in water until softened.
ii. Glycerin is added and heated over bath until the glycerin is dissolved.
iii. Adjust the weight to 85 g, if necessary by adding more amount of water.
iv. ZnO is passed through sieve (#120). Required amount is added in small amounts to the molten base with gentle stirring. Stirring is continued until a viscous product is obtained.
v. The product so obtained is poured in a tray to a depth of about 1 cm with continuous trituration throughout the operation. When the mass is set, carefully the mass is cut into pieces of about 1.5 cm^2 with a blade or sharp knife.

6. Cellulose Derivative

Methylcellulose and sodium carboxymethylcellulose are generally used. They produce neutral jellies of stable viscosity. They have good resistance against microbial growth and clear due to freedom from insoluble impurities. It produces strong film after drying on the skin.

Use: Sodium carboxymethylcellulose can be used to prepare lubricating jellies and sterile jellies, e.g. lignocine gel—because it can withstand autoclaving temperature.

N.B: Other cellulose derivatives are hydroxypropyl methyl-cellulose (hypermellose), carbomer polyvinyl alcohols.

7. Clays

Gels containing 7 to 20% of bentonite can be used as dermatological bases.

Disadvantages

1. They are opalescent and lack attractiveness.
2. Their pH is about 9.0, i.e. not suitable for application on the skin.
3. Residue on the skin is powdery and rather silky.

Preservation of jellies: Although some bases like clays and cellulose derivative(s) resist microbial contamination but since all the jellies contain large amount of water, therefore, must be suitably preserved, e.g. methylparaben 0.1 to 0.2 % is commonly used. Loss of water can quickly lead to skin formation on jellies and to prevent the hygroscopic substances, e.g. glycerol, propylene glycol or sorbitol solution may be added. Bases and medicaments sensitive to heavy metals are sometimes protected by a chelating agent, e.g. ethylene diamine tetra-acetic acid (EDTA).

Poultices

They are soft, viscous, pasty preparations for external use. They are applied to skin while they are hot. Poultices must retain heat for a considerable time because they are intended to supply warmth to inflamed parts of body, e.g. Kaolin poultice (BPC).

Uses

i. Glycerol, because of its hygroscopic nature, is believed to draw infected materials from the tissues when the poultice is used for boils and similar infections.

ii. Methyl salicylate (an antirheumatic drug), thymol (a powerful bactericide), boric acid (a weak antimicrobial agent), and peppermint oil (which contributes to the smell) are used for different purposes.

Method of Applying the Poultice

i. For use, the poultice is heated, with occasional stirring, until it can only be tolerated on the back of the hand.

ii. Then it is spread thickly on lint or other dressing and applied to the affected area which is sometimes first covered with muslin to facilitate removal after use.

iii. A thick layer of cotton wool is applied to retain the heat and a covering of oiled silk may be added to protect clothing.

Example: The only example given in the pharmacopoeia is Kaolin Poultice BPC.

Formula:

- Heavy kaolin, finely sifted and dried at 100°C—52.7 g
- Boric acid, finely sifted—4.5 g
- Methyl salicylate—0.2 ml
- Thymol—50 mg
- Peppermint oil—0.05 ml
- Glycerin—42.5 g

Procedure

a. Kaolin is spread in a suitable quantity of kaolin in a thin layer, e.g. on a tray of aluminum foil, and dried at 100°C until the weight is constant. Allowed to cool down and then passed through no. 180 sieve.

b. Boric acid and kaolin are mixed in a mortar. Gradually the mixed powder is triturated with glycerol to form a smooth paste.

c. The paste is transferred to a heat-resistant glass-jar, protected either with a paper or aluminum foil and heated at 120°C for 1 hour in a hot-air oven, with occasional stirring. The antimicrobial effects of the heat and glycerol destroy the sporing pathogens that may be in the kaolin. (Above 120°C glycerin may degrade).

d. After cooling, a mixture of thymol, methyl salicylate and peppermint oil is mixed (eutectic mixture).

e. Kaolin poultice is stored in well-closed containers to prevent loss of volatile ingredients and absorption of moisture from the atmosphere by glycerin.

Machines used in Manufacturing of Semisolid Dosage Form

Size Reduction Apparatus

1. Mortar and pestle
2. Hammer mill
3. Ball mill
4. Colloid mill

Mixing Equipments

1. Agitator mixers: Sigma mixers and planetary.
2. Shear mixers: Triple roller mill and colloidal mill.

Centrifugation Apparatus

1. Conical disc centrifuge or De laval clarifier
2. Supercentrifuge

Evaluation of Semisolid Dosage Form

Most semisolids are heated to high temperature, processed and packaged in a hot or warm liquid state. There is a considerable lapse time until they achieve their final physical state. At this point they should be tested for conformity with final specifications. Test to be perform are as follows:

A. Microbial Test

With exception of ophthalmic ointments, topical preparations are not require being sterile. They must meet acceptable standards for microbial contents and preparations that are prone to microbial growth must contain antimicrobial preservatives.

Microbial limits are stated in USP. For example, betamethasone valerate ointment USP, must meet the requirements of the tests for absence of *Staphylococcus aureus* and *Pseudomonas aeruginosa*.

In the USP chapter titled "Microbial Attributes of Non-sterile Pharmaceutical Products", emphasis is placed on strict adherence to environmental control and application of GMP to minimize both type and the number of microorganisms in unsterilized pharmaceutical product.

The USP states that dermatological products of such type should be examined for *Pseudomonas aeruginosa* and *Staphylococcus aureus* and those intended for rectal or urethral or vaginal use should be tested for yeasts and molds, common offenders at these sites of application.

B. Physical Tests

Viscosity measurement: It is done with the help of Brookfield viscometer, cone and plate viscometer and pen etrometer for consistency measurement (Fig. 3.2).

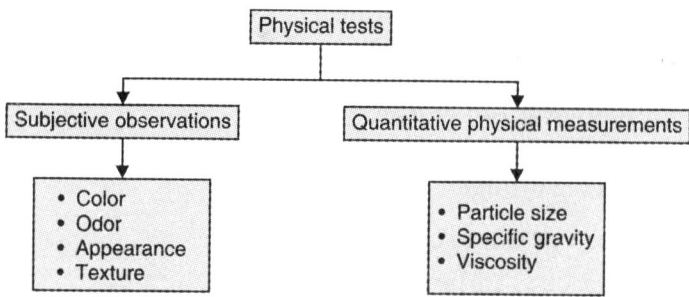

Fig. 3.2: Physical tests

Texture analysis: Stable micro-systems have launched a new Q.C. device–texture analyzer which is used to detect:

a. Ointment flow characteristic

b. Ointment consistency

Gel strength: Gels have gained wide acceptance as semisolid dosage forms. It has been postulated that the strength rather than the viscosity of a gel layer plays a major role in determining the amount of drug release from hydrophilic matrices. Recent advances have occurred in the development of an optimal apparatus to characterize gel strength. One proposed apparatus consists of a sample holder placed on an electronic microbalance connected to a computer. A probe is lowered into the sample by means of a motor equipped with a speed transformer, and the force required to penetrate the gel is measured. The increase in force with time is a function of the mechanical resistance of the sample to the penetration of the probe. Because the lowering speed is known, the displacement covered by the probe as a function of time is calculated and used to compute the gel-strength parameter or mechanical resistance of the gel system.

Flavor release: A theory of flavor release from gelatin-sucrose gels has been developed based on combined interfacial mass and heat transport. The driving force for flavor release is shown to depend on the bulk melting temperature of the gel, which depends on the gelatin and sucrose concentrations. For gels possessing melting points below the mouth temperature, the driving force for flavor release is the rate at which heat can diffuse into the gels matrix and initiate melting. For harder gels with melting points above mouth temperature, the diffusion of sucrose from the surface of the gel into the adjacent saliva phase is the rate limiting step for flavor release, because this lowers the melting temperature of the surface layer. The theoretical model gives good agreement with *in vitro* release experiments using gelatin gels containing sucrose and dye.

Sachet or Tube extrusion force measurement: Stable micro-systems have launched a new Q.C. device that quantifies the force required to extrude the contents from either tube or sachet style packaging. This device allows manufacturers to tests the force required to extrude the content of a sachet or tube at regular intervals over a long period of time, throughout its shelf life and adopt formulation accordingly.

C. Chemical Tests

Chemical tests to be performed include:
a. Chemical potency test
b. Content uniformity test–API should be distributed uniformly.
c. pH measurement

In vitro Release Profile Test

The principal *in vitro* technique for studying skin penetration involves use of some variety of a diffusion cell like Franz cell and Flow through cell in which animal or human skin is fastened to a holder and the passage of compounds from the epidermal surface to a fluid bath is measured.

Hairless rats were sacrificed by an overdose of halothane anesthesia. The skin from the dorsal surface was excised, and the adherent fat and subcutaneous tissue were removed. The skin was mounted on Franz diffusion cells with the epidermis facing the donor compartment. The skin permeation studies were performed by the procedure as described under "release studies."

For the skin retention studies, the donor cell was removed, and the excess formulation was removed from the surface of the skin using a cotton swab. The skin was then washed with 50% ethanol: water and blotted dry with lint-free absorbent wipes. The entire dosing area (0.636 cm²) was collected with a biopsy punch. The epidermis was separated from the dermis, and the tissues were minced using a dissection blade. Where applicable, the stratum corneum (SC) was stripped 20 times using breathable medical tape and the stripped skin was used to conduct permeation and skin retention experiments. Active drug content of epidermis and dermis was extracted using a previously reported method. Briefly, the samples were homogenized and boiled for 10 minutes in solvent (xM). The samples were then centrifuged and the supernatant was collected for analysis of drug by HPLC. The experiments were repeated at least 3 times using the skins from different rats.

Modified USP Type II Dissolution Apparatus

A USP Type II dissolution apparatus was modified for studying the *in vitro* release of phenol from ointment. It comprised a 200 ml vessel, 2.5 × 1.5 cm paddle, and an enhancer diffusion cell (VanKel, Cary, NC). The cell contained an adjustable-capacity sample reservoir, a washer for controlling the exposure of the surface area, and an open screw-on cap to secure the washer and membrane over the sample reservoir. The water bath was maintained at 37°C. Filled cells were placed in the bottom of the vessels, and the paddles were lowered to 1 cm above the sample surface. 50 ml of high-performance liquid chromatography–grade filtered water, degassed and prewarmed to 37°C, was used as the dissolution medium. The system was found to yield reproducible results with good reliability in the data generated.

Analysis of Gel using FT-NIR Transmission Spectroscopy

The objective of this study was to demonstrate the use of transmission Fourier transform near-infrared (FT-NIR) spectroscopy for quantitative analysis of an active ingredient in a translucent gel formulation. Gels were prepared using Carbopol 980 with 0%, 1%, 2%, 4%, 6%, and 8% ketoprofen and analyzed with an FT-NIR spectrophotometer operated in the transmission mode. The correlation coefficient of the calibration was 0.9996, and the root mean squared error of calibration was 0.0775%. The percent relative standard deviation for multiple measurements was 0.10%. The results prove that FT-NIR can be a good alternative to other more time-consuming means of analysis for these types of formulations.

Topical formulations, such as gels, creams, and ointments, represent a small but significant overall fraction of marketed pharmaceutical products. Most of these formulations present analytical challenges to those who must develop methods to test them. Typically, test procedures for these products require tedious extractions and difficult sample preparation procedures.

Fourier transform near-infrared (FT-NIR) spectroscopy is an analytical technique that has gained popularity in recent years for analyzing raw materials, intermediate products, and finished dosage forms. Among the finished products that have been most often analyzed using NIR spectroscopy are tablets, capsules, and lyophilized materials.

The major strengths of FT-NIR include fast and easy equipment operation, good accuracy and precision, and the potential to perform non-destructive analyses. However, the most attractive advantage of FT-NIR with respect to the analysis of topical formulations is that samples do not typically have to be manipulated before analysis. A literature review showed that FT-NIR has not often been used for routine analysis of topical formulations such as gels, creams, and ointments; hence, in this study, quantitative analysis of a clear topical gel formulation containing ketoprofen as the active ingredient was performed using transmission FT-NIR. Carbopol 980 gel was selected for this study because of its wide use as a topical gel in commercial formulations.

PACKAGING OF SEMISOLIDS

Most semisolid products are manufacture by heating and are filled into the container while cooling still in the liquid state. It is important to establish optimum pour point, the best temperature for filling and set or congealing point, the temperature at which the product become immobile in the container.

Topical dermatological products are packed in either jar or tubes whereas ophthalmic, nasal, vaginal and rectal semisolid products are almost always packed in tubes.

The specific FDA regulation pertaining to drug products state that,

"Container closures and other component part of drug packages, to be suitable for that intended use must not be reactive, additive or absorptive to the extent that identity, strength, quality or purity of drug will be affected."

All drug product containers and closures must be approved by stability testing of product in the final container in which it is marketed. This includes stability testing of filled container at room temperature, e.g. 20°C as well as under accelerated stability testing condition, e.g. 40–50°C.

Ointment jars are made up of clear or opaque glass or plastic. Some are colored green, amber or blue. Opaque jars are used for light sensitive products, are porcelain white, dark green or amber. Commercially available empty ointment jars vary in size from about 0.5 ounce to 1 pound. In commercial manufacture and packaging of topical products, the jars and tubes are first tested for compatibility and stability for the intended product. This includes stability testing of filled containers. Tubes use to package topical pharmaceutical products are gaining popularity since they are light in weight, relatively inexpensive, convenient for use, compatible with most formulative components and provide protection against external contamination

Ointment tubes are made of aluminum or plastic. When the ointments are used for ophthalmic, rectal, vaginal or nasal application, they are packed with special applicator tips.

The multiple dose tube used for pharmaceutical has conventional continuous thread closure. Single dose tube may be prepared with a teraway tip. Meter dose, temper evident and child resistant closures are also available. Standard size of empty tubes has capacity of 1.5, 2, 3.5, 5, 15, 30, 45, 60 and 120 gm.

Ointment, creams and gels are most frequently packed in 5, 15 and 30 gm tubes. Ophthalmic ointments typically are packed in small aluminum or collapsible plastic tubes holding 3.5 gm of ointment.

RECENT DEVELOPMENT IN SEMISOLID DOSAGE FORMS

Submicron Emulsion Vehicle System (SMEVS)

Conventional creams have a mean droplet size ranging from 10 to 100 μm. Such formulations have demonstrated poor penetration of drug-loaded oil droplets into deep skin layers. It has been reported that microparticles with diameters penetrate follicular ducts, whereas particles 10 μm remain on the skin surface, and those 3 μm are distributed randomly into hair follicles and stratum corneum. Taking these constraints into consideration, researchers have developed the submicron emulsion vehicle system (SMEVS) for improving drug permeation. The submicron lipid particles of an SMEVS penetrate the layers of the stratum corneum, increasing its fluidity and leading to the disruption of barrier continuity. Significant hydration of the stratum corneum, assisted by gap formation, permits the penetration of submicron emulsion particles by forming a drug depot in the skin. The result is slow, continuous, and controlled systemic delivery of the drug. An SMEVS can be formulated by processing a medium-chain triglyceride emulsion with a high pressure homogenizer. In addition, the presence of lecithin, an efficient dispersing agent, causes a drastic reduction in droplet size, usually to between 100 and 300 nm.

Oleo-hydrogel Systems

Oleo-hydrogel systems for localized skin have been explored successfully. It was examined that transdermal permeation using various vehicle systems to avoid systemic side effects and gastrointestinal irritation from ketoprofen upon oral administration. The researchers examined an oleo-hydrogel system that consisted of ketoprofen incorporated into an emulsion of oil and carbomer hydrogel mixture, with N-methylpyrrolidone as a permeation enhancer. The greater bioavailability of ketoprofen in the oleo-hydrogel system was ascribed to good drug release properties, higher emulsion droplet stability of the carbomer gel, and the penetration-enhancing effect of N-methylpyrrolidone. The formulation of ketoprofen oleo-hydrogel that showed maximum percutaneous absorption was one that contained 3% ketoprofen, 1% carbomer, 10% N-methylpyrrolidone, 10% oils, 8% surfactant, and water adjusted to pH 4.6 using triethanolamine.

Volatile Vehicle–Antinucleant Polymer Systems

Studies have investigated various techniques to enhance the transdermal permeation of topically applied drug molecules. Increasing the thermodynamic activity of drug molecules was found to be the most efficient approach. This increase can be achieved by the volatile vehicle–antinucleant polymer system. Enhanced permeation of sodium nonivamide acetate (an antinociceptive agent) was observed with ethanol–buffer solutions (pH 4.2) containing antinucleant polymers. The system used supersaturation (achieved by evaporation of the vehicle) for penetration enhancement. In supersaturated solutions, the drug is in a high state of activity and has a great leaving tendency, resulting in increased flux.

Lecithin Microemulsion Gel

Lecithin microemulsion gel is a promising matrix system for transdermal drug delivery. Microemulsion gels are obtained by dispersing soybean lecithin (a mixture of phosphatidyl-cholines) in a non-polar organic solvent, thereby forming an entangled network of long and flexible multimolecular aggregates. Fatty-acid esters such as isopropyl palmitate are preferred organic solvents because of their relatively high viscosity and complete optical transparency.

Cream Containing Lipid Nanoparticles

For enhanced penetration of topical drugs, occlusion of skin is the prime criterion. This requirement can be achieved easily by the incorporation of large quantities of fats and oils, especially liquid and semisolid paraffin. However, such formulations have the limitations of poor cosmetic properties characterized by a greasy feel and glossy appearance. The development of a water-in-oil cream wherein the aqueous phase was divided into small droplets solved this problem.

Solid Lipid Nanoparticles (SLNs)

Solid lipid nanoparticles of glyceryl behenate have been investigated as efficient carrier systems for topical use. They provide both burst and sustained drug release. Burst release improves the penetration of drug into the skin. Solid lipid nanoparticles possess the advantages of better drug penetration because the small particle size of their drug-carrier system ensures close contact to the stratum corneum and increases the amount of encapsulated drug penetrating the skin.

Liposomes as Drug Carriers

Liposomes have shown great potential as novel drug carriers for dermal and transdermal systems. Liposomes are micro-scopic vesicles composed of membrane-like lipid layers surrounding an aqueous compartment they also serve as a reservoir for the prolonged release of drugs within various skin layers, thereby reducing the rapid elimination of drug into the blood or lymphatic circulation.

Advantages of Novel Approaches

1. Carriers like liposomes delivers drug into the dermal and transdermal systems and retained for providing the prolonged release of drugs.
2. SLNs provide sustained drug release also better penetration of drugs because the small particle size of their drug-carrier system ensures close contact to the stratum corneum and increases the amount of encapsulated drug penetrating the skin.
3. Microemulsion gels are used for systemic drug delivery, i.e. lecithin microemulsion gels.

4. Ethosomes, cubosomes are used for cosmetics due to their better penetration in the stratum corneum.

5. Iontophoresis, electroporation and phonosoresis are used to deliver ionic drugs, in systemic circulation.

6. Oleo-hydrogel used for local action to avoid systemic side effects.

Disadvantages

1. Their production cost is high.
2. Not available easily.
3. Generally low efficacy.

Summary

Semisolids constitute a significant proportion of pharmaceutical dosage forms. It has their peculiar Rheological behavior; semisolids can adhere to the application surface for sufficiently long periods before they are washed off. The novel approaches discussed were applicable for transdermal delivery of pharmaceuticals.

ISOLATED KEY POINTS

- **Semisolid dosage** forms are dermatological preparations intended to apply externally on the skin to produce local or systemic effect.
- *Physical properties:* (a) Smooth texture, (b) elegant in appearance, (c) non-dehydrating, (d) non-gritty, (e) non-greasy and non-staining, (f) non-hygroscopic.
- *Physiological properties:* (a) Non-irritating, (b) Do not alter membrane/skin functioning, (c) miscible with skin secretion, (d) have low sensitization effect.
- *Application properties:* (a) Easily applicable with efficient drug release, (b) high aqueous washability.
- **Ointments** are semisolid preparations meant for external application to the skin or mucous membrane. They usually contain a medicament or medicaments dissolved, suspended or emulsified in the base.
- **Creams** are viscous emulsions of semisolid consistency intended for application to the skin or mucous membrane; two types—o/w type and w/o type.

- **Pastes** are the preparations contain a large amount of finely powdered solids such as starch and zinc oxide. These are generally very thick and stiff.
- **Jellies** are thin transparent or translucent, non-greasy preparations. They are similar to mucilages because they are prepared by using gums but they differ from mucilages in having jelly like consistency.
- **Gels** are jelly-like semisolid dispersions of drug meant to be applied on the skin.
- **Suppositories** are meant for insertion into the body cavities other than mouth. They may be inserted into rectum, vagina or urethra.
- **Poultices** are also known as cataplasams. They are soft viscous wet masses of solid substances.
- **Plasters** are semisolid masses applied to the skin to enable prolonged contact of drug with the skin. Or substances intended for external application, made of such materials and consistency as to adhere to the skin and thereby attach as dressing.
- The skin is the largest organ of the body. Human skin is, on average, 0.5 mm thick (ranging from 0.05 mm in eye lid to 2 mm).
- Classification of skin based on the epidermis alone especially the surface layer (stratum corneum): Thick: palms of hand, soles of feet. Thin: rest of the body. Although the skin is one of the major sites for non-invasive delivery of therapeutic agents into the body, this task can be relatively challenging owing to the impermeability of the skin.
- *Skin structure:* The skin consists of three major layers: epidermis dermis and subcutaneous tissues
- *Percutaneous absorption:* It involves passive diffusion of substance through skin. Transepidermal penetration: Intracellular penetration, intercellular penetration and transappendegeal penetration.
- **Bases:** There are four classes or types of bases which are differentiated on the basis of their physical composition. These are: (1) Oleaginous bases; (2) Absorption bases; (3) Emulsifying base (Water in oil emulsion bases and oil

in water emulsion bases) (4) Water-soluble bases. Semi-solid bases.

- *Oleaginous base + w/o surfactant:* These bases are generally anhydrous substances which have the property of absorbing (emulsifying) considerable quantities of water but still retaining their ointment-like consistency.

- *The absorption bases are of two types:* (i) Non-emulsified bases, and (ii) water in oil emulsion. Absorption bases. The non-emulsified bases absorb water and aqueous solution producing w/o emulsion. Examples: Wool fat, wool alcohol, beeswax and cholesterol.

- *Water in oil emulsion bases:* These are anhydrous, hydrophilic, absorb water and non-water removable, with low thermal conductivity and occlusive. They have the same properties as the absorption bases. They are used as emollients, cleansing creams, vehicles for solid, liquid, or non-hydrolyzable drugs. Examples: Cold cream type, Hydrous Lanolin, Rose Water Ointment, Hydrocream™, Eucerin®, Nivea®, emulsifying base.

- *Oil in water emulsion bases:* These bases are anhydrous, water-soluble, absorb water and water-washable. They are either carbowaxes polyethylene glycols (PEGs) or hydrated gums (bentonite, gelatin, cellulose derivatives). They are used as drug vehicles. Examples: PEG ointment, Polybase™.

- *Water-soluble bases:* Water-soluble bases do not contain oily and are called greaseless base and are completely soluble in water. Example: (A) polyethylene glycol (PEGs), polyoxyl 40 stearate and polysorbates. (B) Macrogols: They are mixture of water and polycondensation products of ethylene oxide. They are of three types: (i) Solid macrogols (ii) Liquid macrogols; (iii) Semisolid macrogols.

- The water-soluble bases have the advantages of being: Water-soluble and washable, non-greasy, non-staining, non/less occlusive, lipid free, relatively inert, does not support mold growth, little hydrolysis, stable. Disadvantages: May dehydrate skin and hinder percutaneous absorption.

- Requirement for percutaneous or topical absorption. After of the drug on the consistency and other properties of the base. Physicochemical properties like solubility and stability of a drug in the base. Required rate of drug release from the base. Compatibility of the base with the drug and additives. Types of skin lesion at the affected site. Need for preventing the loss of moisture from the skin. Quantity of the liquids to be incorporated in the formulation

- *Selection of semisolid base:* Selection of the appropriate base based on: 1. Dermatological factors and 2. Pharmaceutical factors.

- *Dermatological factors:* (a) Absorption and penetration: 'Penetration' means passage of the drug across the skin, i.e. cutaneous penetration, and 'absorption' means passage of the drug into bloodstream. Medicaments which are both soluble in oil and water are most readily absorbed though the skin, whereas animal and vegetable fats and oils normally penetrate the skin. Animals fats, e.g. lard and wool fat when combined with water, penetrates the skin. o/w emulsion bases release the medicament more readily than greasy bases or w/o emulsion bases. (b) Effect on the skin: Greasy bases interfere with normal skin functions, i.e. heat radiation and sweating. They are irritant to the skin. o/w emulsion bases and other water miscible bases produce a cooling effect due to the evaporation of water. (c) Miscibility with skin secretion and serum: Skin secretions are more readily miscible with emulsion bases than with greasy bases. Due to this, the drug is more rapidly and completely released to the skin. (d) Compatibility with skin secretions: The bases used should be compatible with skin secretions and should have pH about 5.5 because the average skin pH is around 5.5. Generally neutral ointment bases are preferred. (e) Non-irritant: All bases should be highly pure and bases specially for eye ointments should be non-irritant and free from foreign particle. (f) Emollient properties: Dryness and brittleness of the skin causes discomfort to the skin, therefore, the bases should keep the skin moist. For this purpose, water and humectants such as glycerin, propylene glycol are used. Ointments should prevent rapid loss of moisture from the skin. (g) Ease of application and removal: The ointment bases should be easily applicable as well as easily removable from the skin by simple washing with water. Stiff and sticky ointment bases require much force to spread on the skin and during rubbing newly formed tissues on the skin may be damaged.

2. Pharmaceutical factors: (a) Stability: Fats and oils obtained from animal and plant sources are prone to oxidation unless they are suitably preserved. Due to oxidation, odor comes out. This type of reactions is called rancidification. Lard, from animal origin, rancidifies rapidly. Soft paraffin, simple ointment and paraffin ointment are inert and stable. Liquid paraffin is also stable but after prolonged storage it gets oxidized. Therefore, an antioxidant like tocopherol (vit. E) may be incorporated. Other antioxidants those may be used are butylated hydroxytoluene (BHT) or butylated hydroxy anisole (BHA). (b) Solvent properties: Most of the medicaments used in the preparation of ointments are insoluble in the ointment bases, therefore, they are finely powdered and are distributed uniformly throughout the base. (c) Emulsifying properties: Hydrocarbon bases absorb very small amount of water. Wool fat can take about 50% of water and when mixed with other fats can take up several times its own weight of aqueous solution. Emulsifying ointment, cetrimide emulsifying ointment and cetomacrogol emulsifying ointment are capable of absorbing considerable amount of water, forming w/o creams. (d) Consistency: The ointments produced should be of suitable consistency. They should neither be hard nor too soft. They should withstand climatic conditions. Thus in summer, they should not become too soft and in winter not too hard to be difficult to remove from the container and spread on the skin. The consistency of an ointment base can be controlled by varying the ratio of hard and liquid paraffin.

- **Methods of preparation of semisolids:** (1) Trituration method, (2) fusion method, (3) emulsification method: (a) Preparation of oil and aqueous phases; (b) mixing of the phases; (c) cooling the emulsion; (d) homogenization; (4) chemical reaction method.

1. Trituration method: It is most commonly used for the preparation of semisolid. When base contains soft fats and oils, or medicament is insoluble or liquid, then this method is used with spatula or motar and pestle.

2. *Fusion method:* The ingredients of the base are melted together and properly mixed to obtain a uniform product. On small scale, fusion method is carried out in a porcelain dish, which is placed in a waterbath. Initially, the ingredient of high melting point is melted. Then remaining ingredients of the base are added in the decreasing order of their melting points and melted with constant stirring. The above mixture is removed from the water bath and stirred in order to cool it. If the drug is soluble in the base, then its powdered form is added to the molten base. Liquid or semisolid are added at a temperature of 40°C. Insoluble additives are added in small quantities with proper stirring, when the thickening of the base starts. Localized cooling of the molten base and vigorous stirring should be avoided to prevent aeration of the ointment.

3 *Emulsification method:* Preparation of oil and aqueous phases Place the ingredients of the oil phase into the stainless steel steam-jacketed kettle and melt them while mixing. Filter the oil phase through several layers of cheese cloth to remove any foreign matter. Heat the emulsion mixing kettle to the temperature of the oil phase. This avoids congealing of higher melting component. Transfer the oil phase into the emulsion mixing kettle. Dissolve the ingredient of the aqueous phase in purified water and filter the solution. A soluble drug which is thermostable may be added to the aqueous phase in this step.

- The phases are usually mixed at a temperature of 70 to 72°C, because at this temperature intimate mixing of the liquid phases can occur. The properties of some emulsions depend on the temperature at which the phases are mixed. The initial mixing temperature must be raised above 70 to 72 degrees.

- *Mixing of the phases:* Three ways of mixing the phases: 1. Simultaneous blending of the phases; 2. Addition of the discontinuous phase to the continuous phase and 3. Addition of the continuous phase to the discontinuous phase.

- *Equipment used for mixing of phases:* Agitator mixers: Sigma mixer and planetary mixer. Shear mixers: Triple roller mill and colloidal mill.
- The rate of cooling is generally slow to allow for adequate mixing while the emulsion is still liquid. The temperature of the cooling medium in the equipment should be decreased gradually and at a rate consistent with the mixing of the emulsion and scrapping of the kettle walls to prevent formation of congealed masses of the ointment or cream. Cooling the emulsion perfume should be added at 43 to 45°C to avoid chilling the emulsion in case of oil in water type emulsion. Perfume should be added at room temperature in water in oil type emulsion. If the drug is not added in the aqueous phase, then it should be added in solution form or in the form of crystals.
- *Yield value:* It is a measure of the force required to extrude the material from the deformable bottle tube. It can be determined by the use of an instrument called the Penetrometer. Penetrometer consists of a metal needle that pierces through the system and the distance of penetration of the needle is measured, from which the yield value may be calculated.
- *Spreadability:* The spreadability test is performed to determine the extent of spreadability of gels based on their rheological properties.
- *Stability:* This test is known as the shipping test and is performed to determine the extent of stability of gels at varying temperature, which the product may experience while exporting to other countries.
- *Safety:* The safety of the product on use should be determined in order to check the effect of the product by evaluating the physiological properties of the raw materials.
- The term "*disperse system*" refers to a system in which one substance (the dispersed phase) is distributed, in discrete units, throughout a second substance (the continuous Phase or vehicle). Each phase can exist in solid, liquid, or gaseous state.
- The phase which is dispersed in a medium is known as an internal phase or dispersed phase. The medium is known as external phase, continuous phase, or dispersion medium

- *Suspension:* A pharmaceutical suspension is a coarse dispersion in which internal phase is dispersed uniformly throughout the external phase. The internal phase consisting of insoluble solid particles having a specific range of size which is maintained uniformly throughout the suspending vehicle with aid of single or combination of suspending agent. The external phase (suspending medium) is generally aqueous in some instance, may be an organic or oily liquid for non-oral use.

- *Classification of suspensions:*

1. Based on general classes oral suspension, e.g. antacid, antibiotic. Externally applied suspension, e.g. lotion, parenteral suspension, ophthalmic suspension

2. Based on proportion of solid particles: Dilute suspension (2 to 10% w/v solid) Concentrated suspension (50% w/v solid).

3. Based on electrokinetic nature of solid particles: Flocculated suspension, deflocculated suspension.

- Structured vehicles are aqueous solutions of natural and synthetic gums. These are used to increase the viscosity of the suspension. It is applicable only to deflocculated suspensions, e.g. methylcellulose, sodium carboxymethyl cellulose, acacia, gelatin and tragacanth. These are non-toxic, pharmacologically inert, and compatible with a wide range of active and inactive ingredients.

- *Wetting agents:* These are the substances which reduce the interfacial tension between the solid particles and liquid medium, thus producing a suspension of required quality. This may achieved by adding a suitable wetting agent which is absorbed at the solid/liquid interface in such a way that the affinity of the particles for the surrounding medium is increased and interparticular forces are decrease. Example: Alcohol in tragacanth mucilage, glycerin in sodium alginate or bentonite dispersion, polysorbate in oral and parenteral suspension.

- *Flocculating agents:* Electrolytes, surfactants, polymers. Flocculating agents are used to obtain and promote controlled flocculation. Example of flocculating agents: NaCl, sulfate, citrates, phosphates salts. Reduce or decrease the zeta potential (energy of potential) between the solid particles. This leads to decrease in repulsion potential and makes the particles come together to from loosely arranged structure (floccules). The flocculating power increases with the valency of the ions. As for example, calcium ions are more powerful than sodium ions because the valency of calcium is two whereas sodium has valency of one. Electrolytes, e.g. bismuth subnitrate with KH_2PO_4.

- Both ionic and non-ionic surfactants can be used to bring about flocculation of suspended particles. (I) Ionic surfactants: They cause neutralization of the charge on each particle. The particles are then attracted towards each other by van der Waals forces and forms loose agglomerates. (II) Non-ionic surfactant: They are adsorbed on to more than one particle thus forming a loose flocculated structure.

- *Properties of flocculated and deflocculated suspension particles:* (A) Flocculated: 1. Particles form loose aggregates and form a network like structure. 2. Rate of sedimentation is high. 3. Sediment is rapidly formed. 4. Sediment is loosely packed and doesn't form a hard cake. 5. Sediment is easy to redisperse. 6. Suspension is not pleasing in appearance. 7. The floccules stick to the sides of the bottle. (B) Deflocculated: 1. Particles exist as separate entities. 2. Rate of sedimentation is slow. 3. Sediment is slowly formed. 4. Sediment is very closely packed and a hard cake is formed. 5. Sediment is difficult to redisperse. 6. Suspension is pleasing in appearance. 7. It does not stick to the sides of the bottle.

- Suspensions can be evaluated by using parameter of sedimentation and official method. 1. Parameter: These are two parameters, i.e. (a) sedimentation volume (F) and (b) degree of flocculation. 2. Official method: (a) Sedimentation method, (b) electrokinetic method, (c) rheological method and (d) micromeritic method.

- Emulsion may be defined as a biphasic system consisting of two immiscible liquids usually water and oil, one of which is finely subdivided and uniformly dispersed as droplets throughout the other. Since such a system is thermodynamically, unstable emulsifying agent is required to stabilize the system. To stabilize these droplets, emulsifying agent should be added.

- The phase which makes globules or droplets is known as internal phase or disperse phase and other is external or continuous phase. Oil can be present as internal and external phase and water also as internal or external phase. Emulsion is normally opaque. It can be used orally, topically and parenterally. Microemulsion: Droplets size range 0.01 to 0.1 mm. Macroemulsion: Droplets size range approximately 5 mm. Oil in water (o/w) emulsions and 2. Water in oil (w/o) emulsions.

- Formulation of emulsion involves following components: Emulsifying agents. Other additives: (I) Antioxidant, (II) Preservative, (III) Flavors.

- *Antioxidant:* During storage of emulsions, the fats (obtained from vegetable and animal sources) and emulsifying agents (such as wool fat, wool alcohol) undergo oxidation by atmospheric oxygen. This can be avoided by using antioxidant, such as, tocopherol, gallic acid, propyl gallate and ascorbic acid. Some times oxidation occurs due to enzymes produced by microorganism. Such problems should be prevented by adding a suitable antimicrobial preservative.

- The following are some of the qualities of an ideal antioxidant: 1. It should be readily soluble or dispersible in the medium. 2. It should be non-toxic. 3. It should be non-irritant. 4. It should be colorless, odorless and tasteless.

- *Flavors:* Vanillin is a good flavoring agent for liquid paraffin emulsion. Benzaldehyde is generally used as a flavoring and sweetening agent provides greater palatability to emulsion.

- *Preservatives:* Emulsion which are prepared by using emulsifying agent, such as carbohydrates, proteins, sterol, and non-ionic surfactants may lead to the growth of bacteria, fungi and molds in the presence of water. The contamination of emulsions by these microorganisms may cause unpleasant odor, taste and discoloration. Due to breakdown of emulsifying agent, changes occur in the consistency of an emulsion which may lead to cracking of emulsion.

- The contamination of an emulsion may occur due to any one of the following reasons: 1. The equipment used in the preparation of emulsion are carelessly cleaned. 2. By using contaminated natural emulsifying agents such as gums, starches and clays. 3. The ratio of oil and water is not proper. 4. By using not properly stored deionized and purified water. 5. pH of the preparation.

- *Preparation:* The following methods are commonly used for the preparation of emulsion on a small scale: Dry gum method, wet gum method, bottle method, other methods.

- 1. *Dry gum method:* Measure the required quantity of oil in a dry measure and transfer it into a dry mortar. Add calculated quantity of gum acacia into it and triturate rapidly so as to form a uniform mixer. Add required quantity of water and triturate vigorously till a clicking sound is produced and the product becomes white or nearly white due to the total internal reflection of light. This emulsion produced at this stage is known as primary emulsion. Add more of water to produce required volume.

- 2. *Wet gum method:* In this method, the proportion of oil: water: gum for preparing the primary emulsion. Calculate the quantity of oil, water and gum required for preparing the primary emulsion. Powder the gum acacia in a mortar. Add water and triturate it with gum so as to form a mucilage. Add the required quantity of oil in small portions with rapid trituration until a clicking sound is produced and the product becomes white or nearly white. At this stage, the emulsion is known as primary emulsion. Add more of water in small portions to the primary emulsion with trituration to produced the required volume. Stirr thoroughly so as to form a uniform emulsion. Transfer the emulsion to a bottle, cork, label and dispense.

- 3. *Bottle method:* It is used for preparation of emulsions of volatile and other non-viscous oils. The proportion of oil: water: gum is 2:2:1. Measured the required quantity of the oil and transfer into a large bottle. Add the required quantity of powdered gum acacia. Shake the bottle vigorously, until the oil and gum are mixed thoroughly. Add the calculated amount of water all at once. Shake the mixture vigorously to form a primary emulsion. Add more of water in small portion with constant agitation to produce the required volume.

- 4. *Other methods:* Various blenders and homogenizers are used for preparing emulsion. Hand homogenizer, silversion mixer homogenizer and colloidal mill are some of the homogenizers which are used for preparation of extemporaneous emulsion.

- *Factors affecting the stability of an emulsion:* Particle size: Increased particle size of the internal phase causes the decreased stability of an emulsion. Smaller size of the particles of internal phase is always preferable. Particle-particle interaction: Deflocculated particles are always preferable because the less the particle-particle interaction the more the stability of an emulsion. Particle density: The less the particle density the more the stability of an emulsion. Bulk phase/external phase density: The more the bulk phase density the more the stability of an emulsion. Bulk phase viscosity: Generally the more the viscosity of bulk phases, the more the stability of emulsion.

Stability testing of Emulsion:

- *Flocculation:* Flocculation is the joining together of globules to form large clumps or floccules within the emulsion. In flocculation, the interfacial film and the individual droplets remain intact; the globules do not coalesce and may be redispersed by shaking.

- *Creaming:* It is a concentration of the floccules of the internal phase formed upward or downward layer according to the density of internal phase.

- *Cracking:* When an emulsion cracks during preparation, i.e. the primary emulsion does not become white but acquires an oily translucent appearance. Cracking of emulsion can be due to: 1. Addition of an incompatible emulsifying agent, e.g. monovalent soap + divalent soap, e.g. anionic + cationic emulsifying agent. 2. Chemical or microbial decomposition of emulsifying agent, e.g. alkali soaps decomposed by acids. 3. Exposure to increased or reduced temperature. 4. Addition of common solvent, e.g. addition of a solvent in which the two phases are soluble (alcohol).

- *Phase inversion:* In phase inversion, o/w type emulsion changes into w/o type and vice versa. It is a physical instability. It may be brought about by: 1. The addition of an electrolyte, e.g. addition of $CaCl_2$ into o/w emulsion formed by sodium stearate can be inverted to w/o. 2. By changing the phase volume ratio. 3. By temperature changes. Phase inversion can be minimized by: 1. Using the proper emulsifying agent in adequate concentration. 2. Keeping the concentration of dispersed phase between 30 and 60%. 3. Storing the emulsion in a cool place.

LONG ANSWER TYPE QUESTIONS

Q 1. What are semisolid dosage forms? Discuss in brief various types of semisolid dosage form along with their properties.

Q 2. Discuss in brief ideal properties of semisolid dosage form.

Q 3. What are the various factors affecting drug penetration and route of absorption of semisolid dosage form?

Q 4. Give mechanism of drug absorption in detail. How various types of skin structure govern mechanism of absorption?

Q 5. What are ointments? Give classification and discuss in brief ideal characteristics of an ointment.

Q 6. What are the various ingredients used in the preparation of semisolid dosage form? Give suitable examples.

Q 7. Write short notes on:
   a. Bases
   b. Preservatives
   c. Antioxidant
   d. Chelating agent
   e. Humectants
   f. Surfactants

Q 8. What are the various types of permeability enhancer? Give their mechanism of action.

Q 9. Give various methods of preparation of ointments with suitable example.

Q 10. What are pastes? Give properties of an ideal paste.

Q 11. Compare and contrast between paste and ointment.

Q 12. Discuss in detail the various bases used in the preparation of pastes. Give methods of preparation of pastes.

Q 13. Write short notes on

    a. Gels

    b. Types of jellies

    c. Poultices

    d. Packaging of semisolid dosage forms.

Q 14. What are the various evaluation methods used for evaluation of semisolid dosage form?

Q 15. Write in brief about recent development in semisolid dosage form. What are the advantages and disadvantages of novel approach?

SHORT ANSWER TYPE QUESTIONS

1. Semisolid dosage forms are dermatological preparations intended to apply........................ on the skin to produce local or systemic effect.

2. .... also known as cataplasms and are soft viscous wet masses of solid substances.

3. The skin consists of three major layers ....

4. The phase which is dispersed in a medium is known as an ....

5. A pharmaceutical ....is a coarse dispersion in which internal phase is dispersed uniformly throughout the external phase.

6. .... are the substances which reduce the interfacial tension between the solid particles and liquid medium.

7. Emulsion may be defined as a .... system consisting of two .... liquids usually water and oil, one of which is finely subdivided and uniformly dispersed as droplets throughout the other.

8. .... is used for preparation of emulsions of volatile and other non-viscous oils.

9. .... is the joining together of globules to form large clumps or floccules within the emulsion.

10. Creaming can be .... depending upon the density of internal phase.

11. When the primary emulsion does not become white but acquires an oily translucent appearance, it is called ....

12. In phase inversion, o/w type emulsion changes into .... type and vice versa.

ANSWERS

1. Externally
2. Poultices
3. Epidermis, dermis, subcutaneous tissues
4. Internal phase or dispersed phase
5. Suspension
6. Wetting agents
7. Biphasic, immiscible
8. Bottle method
9. Flocculation
10. Upward or downward
11. Cracking
12. w/o

4

Suppositories

INTRODUCTION

Suppositories are solid unit dosage forms suitably shaped for insertion into the rectum. The bases used either melt when warmed to body temperature, or dissolve or disperse when in contact with mucous secretions. Suppositories may contain medicaments, which are intended to exert a systemic effect, either dissolved or dispersed in the base. Suppositories are prepared by incorporating any medicaments in the base, which may then be shaped by cold compression into molds. The molten mass is poured at a suitable temperature into molds and allowed to cool until set.

Pessaries are solid unit dosage forms suitably shaped for insertion into the vagina, and containing medicaments intended to exert a local action. They may be prepared by molding as described above or may be compressed as suitably shaped tablets.

The ideal suppository base should be non-toxic, non-irritating, inert, compatible with medicaments, and easily formed by compression or molding. It should also dissolve or disintegrate in the presence of mucous secretions or melt at body temperature to allow for the release of the medication. The suppository base composition plays an important role in rate and extent of release of medications.

The shapes of suppositories are generally tapering at one end and depending upon the need various sizes are prepared (Fig. 4.1).

- Number 0 is for children, and can also be used for the ear or nose.

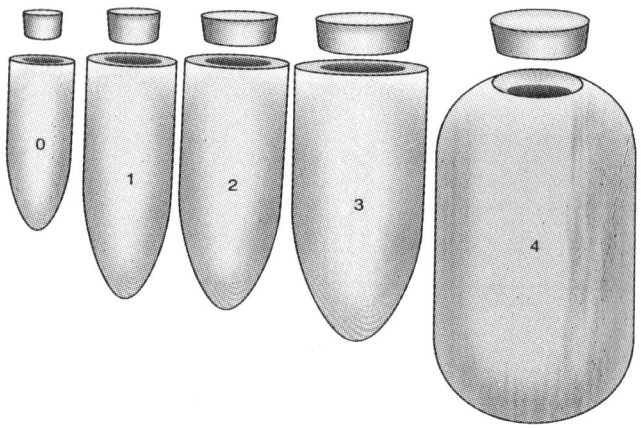

Fig 4.1: Various types of suppositories

- Number 1, 2, and 3 are for the rectum.
- Number 4 is a pessary.

Advantages of Suppositories

1. Suppositories are dosage forms containing accurate quantities of medicament(s).
2. When the oral administration is not suitable, as in unconscious patients and infants, suppositories are used for systemic effect.
3. Suppositories allow administration of some medicaments, which are sensitive to the gastric pH and gastric enzymes and are not tolerated orally.
4. Suppositories permit administration of medicaments that interrupt the functionality of the gastrointestinal tract, e.g. drugs irritating to the stomach. Also suitable in case of nausea and vomiting.
5. Drugs destroyed by first past metabolism in portal circulation may bypass the liver circulation, where many drugs are subject to metabolic changes (first pass effect).
6. Suppositories are suitable when local effect is wanted as in the treatment of rectal, vaginal and urethral diseases.
7. Suppositories have shown faster onset of action than found after oral administration as the drug is directly absorbed from the mucosa into the venous circulation.

Disadvantages of Suppositories

1. Poor patient acceptability.
2. Suppositories are not suitable for patients suffering from diarrhea.
3. Incomplete absorption may be obtained because suppository usually promotes evacuation of the bowel.

Indications

The use of suppositories is indicated under the following circumstances:

1. To empty the bowel before certain types of surgery.
2. To empty the bowel to relieve acute constipation or when other treatments for constipation have failed.
3. To empty the bowel before endoscopic examination.
4. To introduce medication into the system.
5. To soothe and treat hemorrhoids or anal pruritus.

Dosage of Suppositories

a. Rectal suppositories for adults weigh 2 gm and are torpedo shape. Children's suppositories weigh about 1 gm.
b. Vaginal suppositories or pessaries weigh about 3–5 gm and are molded in globular or oviform shape or compressed on a tablet press into conical shapes.
c. Urethral suppositories called bougies are pencil shape. Those intended for males weigh 4 gm each and are 100–150 mm long while those for females are 2 gm each and 60–75 mm in length.

Contraindications

The use of suppositories is contraindicated when one or more of the following pertain:

1. Chronic constipation, which would require repetitive use.
2. Paralytic ileus.
3. Colonic obstruction.
4. Following gastrointestinal or gynecological operations, unless on the specific instructions of the doctor.

Routes of Administration that Utilize Suppositories

They are made in a variety of shapes and sizes because they are used in many different routes of administration (body cavities).

Rectal

Rectal route is used for local effect or to achieve a systemic effect. Local effects may include the soothing of inflamed hemorrhoidal tissues, promoting laxation, and enemas. Using rectal administration to achieve systemic activity is preferred when the drug is destroyed in the GI tract, if oral administration is not possible because of vomiting, or the patient is unconscious or incapable of swallowing oral formulations. Rectal administration has been used to treat a variety of conditions such as asthma, nausea, motion sickness, anxiety, and bacterial infections.

The most common rectal formulations are suppositories, solutions, and ointments. Suppositories are manufactured in a variety of shapes. Rectal suppositories for adults are tapered at one end and usually weigh about 2 grams. Infant rectal suppositories usually weight about 1 gram or about half that of adult suppositories.

The major disadvantages of rectal suppositories are:

1. Poor patient acceptability; they are inconvenient.
2. Rectal absorption of most drugs is frequently erratic and unpredictable.
3. Some suppositories "leak" or are expelled after insertion.

Vaginal

Vaginal administration has many advantages:

1. Generally, there is less drug degradation via this route of administration compared to oral administration
2. The dose can be retrieved, if necessary
3. There is the potential of long-term drug absorption with various intrauterine devices (IUDs).

Vaginal administration does lead to variable absorption since the vagina is a physiologically and anatomically dynamic organ that causes pH and membrane permeability to change over time. There is also a tendency of some dosage forms to be expelled after insertion into the vagina.

Vaginal formulations include solutions, powders for solutions, ointments, creams, aerosol foams, suppositories, and tablets. Vaginal suppositories are employed as contraceptives, feminine hygiene antiseptics, bacterial antibiotics, or to restore the vaginal mucosa. Vaginal suppositories are inserted high in the vaginal tract with the aid of a special applicator. The suppositories are usually globular, oviform, or cone-shaped and weigh between 3–5 grams. Patients should be instructed to quickly dip the suppository in water before insertion. Because suppositories are generally used at bedtime and can be messy, if the formulation is an oleaginous base, patients should wear a sanitary napkin to protect nightwear and bed linens.

Urethral

Urethral suppositories are cylindrical in shape (3–6 mm in diameter) and vary in length according to gender. Female urethral suppositories can be 25–70 mm in length while male urethral suppositories can be about 50–125 mm in length. The one commercially available urethral suppository is actually marketed as a "pellet" and is 1.4 mm in diameter and 3 or 6 mm in length depending on strength. Urethral suppositories are unusual and may not be encountered in a compounding practice.

Inserting Suppositories

Inserting Rectal Suppositories (Fig. 4.2)

1. If possible, go to the toilet and empty bowels.
2. Wash hands carefully with soap and warm water.
3. Remove any foil or plastic wrapping from the suppository.
4. Lubricate the tapered end of the suppository with a small amount of jelly. If the jelly is not available, moisten the suppository with a small amount of water.
5. Either stand with one leg on a chair, or lay on one side with one leg straight and the other leg bent toward your stomach.
6. Separate buttocks to expose the rectal area.

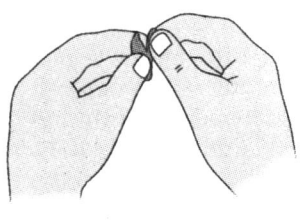

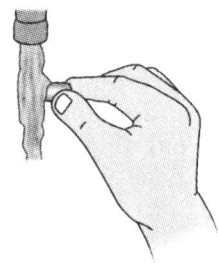

1. Remove foil wrapper.

2. Moisten the suppository with water or water-based lubricating jelly

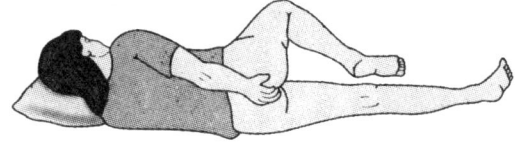

3. Lie on your left side and bend your right knee up toward your chest. Gently push the suppository into your rectum

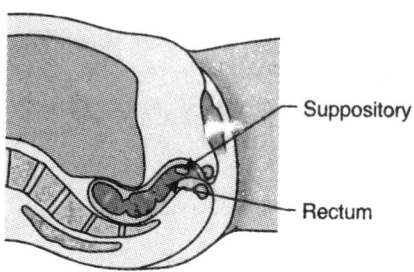

Suppository

Rectum

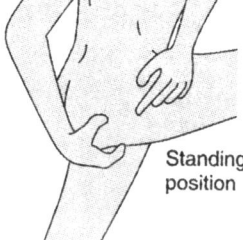

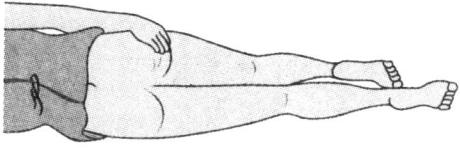

Standing position

Laying Position

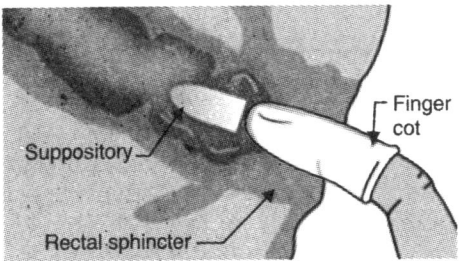

Fig. 4.2: Method of inserting rectal suppository

7. Gently but firmly push the suppository into the rectum until it passes the sphincter (about 1/2 to 1 inch in infants, and 1 inch in adults).

8. Close your legs and sit (or lay) still for about 15 minutes. Avoid emptying bowels for at least one hour (unless the suppository is a laxative). Avoid excessive movement or exercise for at least one hour.

9. Wash hands again with soap and warm water immediately after inserting the suppository.

Inserting Vaginal Suppositories (Fig. 4.3)

1. Wash your hands carefully with soap and warm water.

2. Remove any foil or plastic wrapping from suppository.

3. Place suppository in applicator.

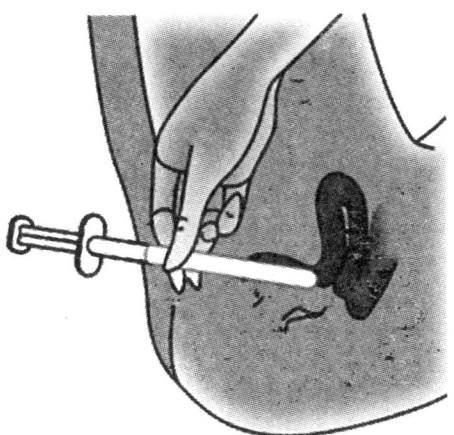

Fig. 4.3: Insertion of vaginal suppository

4. Hold the applicator by the opposite end.

5. Either lay on your back with your knees bent, or stand with your feet spread a few inches apart and your knees bent.

6. Gently insert the applicator into the vagina as far as it will go comfortably. Once you are ready, push the inside of the applicator in and place the suppository as far back in the vagina as possible.

7. Remove the applicator from the vagina.

8. Wash your hands again with soap and warm water.

Factors Affecting the Rectal Absorption

1. *Physiologic factors:* Among the physiologic factors affecting drug absorption from the rectum are the colonic contents, circulation route, and the pH and lack of buffering capacity of the rectal fluids.

    a. *Colonic content:* When systemic effects are desired from the administration of a medicated suppository, greater absorption may be expected from a rectum that is void than from one that is distended with fecal matter. This is because the drug will obviously have greater opportunity to make contact with the absorbing surface of the rectum and colon in the absence of fecal matter. Other conditions such as diarrhea, colonic obstruction due to tumor growths and tissue dehydration can all influence the rate and degree of drug absorption from the rectal site.

    b. *Circulation route:* Drugs absorbed rectally, bypass the portal circulation during their first pass into the general circulation, thereby enabling drugs to exert systemic effects. The lower hemorrhoidal veins surrounding the colon receive the absorbed drug and initiate its circulation throughout the body, bypassing the liver.

    c. *pH and lack of buffering capacity of the rectal fluids:* Because rectal fluids are essentially neutral in pH (7–8) and have no effective buffer capacity, the form in which the drug is administered will not generally be chemically changed by the rectal environment. For systemic drug action, it is preferable to incorporate the ionized rather than the unionized form of a drug in order to maximize bioavailability.

2. *Physicochemical factors of the drug and the base:*

a. *Lipid-water solubility:* The lipid-water partition coefficient of a drug is an important consideration in the selection of the suppository base. A lipophilic drug that is distributed in a fatty suppository base in low concentration has less tendency to escape to the surrounding aqueous fluids. Water-soluble bases, for example, polyethylene glycol, which dissolve in the anorectal fluids, release for absorption both water-soluble and oil-soluble drugs.

b. *Particle size:* For drugs present in the suppository in the undissolved state, the size of the drug particle will influence its rate of dissolution and its availability for absorption. The smaller the particle size, the more readily the dissolution of the particle and the greater the chance for rapid absorption.

c. *Nature of the base:* As indicated earlier, the base must be capable of melting, softening, or dissolving to release its drug components for absorption. If the base interacts with the drug inhibiting its release, drug absorption will be impaired or even prevented. Also, if the base is irritating to the mucous membranes of the rectum, it may initiate a colonic response and prompt a bowel movement, thereby inhibiting the drug release and absorption.

Suppository Bases

Suppository bases may be conveniently classified as according to their composition and physical properties:

- Oleaginous (fatty) bases
- Water-soluble or miscible bases

Oleaginous Bases

Oleaginous bases include theobroma oil and synthetic triglyceride mixtures.

1. Theobroma Oil

Theobroma oil or cocoa butter is used as a suppository base because, in large measure, it fulfills the requirements of an ideal base. At ordinary room temperatures of 15° to 25°C (59° to 77°F), it is a hard, amorphous solid, but at 30° to 35°C (86° to 95°F), i.e. at body temperature, it melts to a bland, non-irritating oil. In warm climates, theobroma oil suppositories should be refrigerated.

While preparing suppositories with cocoa butter base, two things should be kept in mind. Firstly, this base must not be heated above 35°C (95°F) because cocoa butter is a polymorphic compound and if overheated will convert to a metastable structure that melts in the 25° to 30°C (77° to 86°F) range. The second factor is the change in melting point caused by adding certain drugs to cocoa butter suppositories. For example, chloral hydrate and phenol tend to lower the melting point. It may be necessary to add spermaceti or beeswax to raise the melting point of finished suppositories back to the desired range.

2. Synthetic Triglycerides

The synthetic triglycerides consist of hydrogenated vegetable oils. Their advantage over cocoa butter is that they do not exhibit polymorphism, but they are more expensive. Some of the bases are single entity formulations. Some of the names may denote a series of bases. In a series, the bases are varied to give a range of melting points. For example, Fattibase® is a single entity base that consists of triglycerides from palm, palm kernel, and coconut oils. Wecobee® is a series of bases. Wecobee FS, M, R, and S are all made from triglycerides of coconut oil. But FS has a melting point range of 39.4 to 40.5°C, M has a range of 33.3 to 36.0°C, R has a range of 33.9 to 35.0°C, and S has a range of 38.0 to 40.5°C. Other triglyceride type bases include Dehydag®, Hydrokote®, Suppocire®, and Witepsol®.

Water-soluble/Water-miscible Bases

Water soluble/water miscible bases are those containing glycerinated gelatin or the polyethylene glycol (PEG) polymers.

1. Glycerinated Gelatin

It is useful especially for vaginal suppositories. It is suitable for use with a wide range of medicaments including alkaloids, boric acid, and zinc oxide. Glycerinated gelatin suppositories are translucent, resilient, gelatinous solids that tend to dissolve or disperse slowly in mucous secretions to provide prolonged release of active ingredients. Suppositories made with glycerinated gelatin must be kept in well-closed containers in a cool place since they will absorb and dissolve in atmospheric moisture. For extended shelf-life a preservative is added, such as methylparaben or propylparaben, or a suitable combination of the two. To facilitate administration, glycerinated gelatin suppositories should be dipped in water just before use.

2. Polyethylene Glycol Polymers

They are chemically stable, non-irritating, miscible with water and mucous secretions, and can be formulated, either by molding or compression, in a wide range of hardness and melting point. Like glycerinated gelatin, they do not melt at body temperature, but dissolve to provide a more prolonged release than theobroma oil. Certain polyethylene glycol polymers may be used singly as suppository bases but, more commonly two or more molecular weights substances mixed in various proportions are needed to yield a finished product of satisfactory hardness and dissolution time. Since the water-miscible suppositories dissolve in body fluids and need not be formulated to melt at body temperature, they can be formulated with much higher melting points and thus may be safely stored at room temperature.

Characteristics of Ideal Suppositories

An ideal suppository should:

1. Melts at rectal temperature 37.5°C.
2. Completely non-toxic and non-irritating to sensitive and inflamed tissues.
3. Compatible with a broad variety of drugs.
4. Not show polymorphism.
5. Shrinks sufficiently on cooling to release itself from the mold without the need for mold lubricants.
6. Have small interval between "melting point" and "solidification point".
7. Has wetting and emulsifying properties.

8. Have high "water number". So, a high percentage of water can be incorporated in it.
9. Stable on storage, dose not change color, odor, and drug release pattern.
10. Can be manufactured by molding either by hand, machine compression, or extrusion.
11. Have "acid value" below 0.2.
12. "Saponification value" ranges from 200 to 245.
13. "Iodine value" less than 7.

Functions of Suppository Bases

1. Dilute the drug to non-irritating level.
2. Control the rate of drug release.
3. Represent the drug in an acceptable usable form.

Types of Suppository Bases

Four main types of bases are available:

1. Oily bases.
2. Hydrophilic bases.
3. Water dispersible bases.
4. Emulsifying bases.

1. Oily or Oleaginous or Fatty Bases

a. Cocoa Butter (Theobroma Oil)

One of the most widely used suppository base, used in compounding prescription when no base is specified. Cocoa butter is defined as the fat obtained from roasted seed of *Theobroma cacao*. Chemically, it is a triglyceride with the predominant glyceride chains being oleopalmitostearin and oleodistearin. It is a yellowish-white, solid, brittle fat, which smells and tastes like chocolate. Because cocoa butter can easily melt and rancidify, it must be stored in cool, dry place, and protected from light.

Advantages

1. Has a melting point range of 34–38°C. (i.e. solid at normal room temperature but melts at body temperature).
2. Readily melts on warming, rapid sets on cooling.

3. Easily miscible with other ingredients.
4. Bland, innocuous, non-reactive and non-irritating.

Disadvantages

1. *Gets adhere to the mold:* Sticking is a problem which may be overcome by adequate lubrication.
2. Softening point too low for hot climate.
3. Melting point reduced by soluble ingredients, Additives such as beeswax may be incorporated to raise the melting point sufficiently to counteract the effects of medicaments and/or climate.
4. Rancid on storage due to oxidation of unsaturated glycerides.
5. Poor water absorbing ability. Improved by the addition of emulsifying agents.
6. Leakage from the body. Sometimes melted base escapes from the rectum or vagina, for this reason, oil of theobroma is rarely used as a pessary base.
7. It is costly.
8. Shows polymorphism.

b. Emulsified Theobroma oil

In order to increase the diffusion and absorption, several agents have been used to form emulsified theobroma oil suppositories. The addition of an emulsifying agent to cocoa butter also prevents unnecessary melting because the suppository will swell and disintegrate in the presence of moisture. Thus, the melting point may be raised without fear of interfering with disintegration. Also, more aqueous solution may be incorporated in such emulsified suppositories.

Examples: The addition of 5% glyceryl monostearate has been recommended for preparing emulsified cocoa butter suppositories. These products are said to have a melting point above 35°C and may be made by either the hot or the cold method.

The incorporation of 2 to 3% cetyl alcohol with theobroma oil also makes a satisfactory emulsified base. A suppository mass containing 2% lecithin and 98% theobroma oil forms an oil-in-water emulsified base. A water-in-oil emulsion is formed by the inclusion of 2% cholesterol with theobroma oil.

c. Synthetic Hard Fat (Hydrogenated Oils)

Synthetic hard fat bases are prepared by first hydrolyzing the vegetable oil, then hydrogenating the resulting fatty acids and finally reemulsifying the acids by heating with glycerol, e.g. hydrogenated palm kernel oil is used in tropical countries as a base for suppositories.

Advantages of these Bases Over Theobroma Oil

1. Their solidifying points are unaffected by overheating.
2. They have good resistance to oxidation because their unsaturated fatty acids have been reduced.
3. The difference between melting and setting points is small, generally only 1.5–2°C and seldom over 3°C. When the setting point of a base is well below the melting point, the suppository soften quickly when handled and become too slippery to administer.
4. They usually contain a proportion of partial glycerides some of which, e.g. glyceryl monostearate, are w/o emulsifying agents and, therefore, their water-absorbing capacities are good.
5. No mold lubricant is necessary because they contract significantly on cooling.
6. They produce suppositories that are white and almost odorless and have an attractive, clean, polished appearance.

Disadvantages

1. Low viscosity when melted allows sedimentation of suspended ingredients at the melted stage. This problem can be avoided by the use of thickeners.
2. Brittle, if cooled rapidly.

2. Hydrophilic Bases

a. Glycerinated Gelatin

This substance has many properties that make it a desirable base for suppositories. Suppositories made with glycerinated gelatin slowly dissolve in the aqueous secretions and provide a slow, continuous release of medication. Glycerinated gelatin may be used to prepare all types of suppositories and it is particularly useful in vaginal suppositories. It is well adapted for the incorporation of solid extracts such as belladonna. It may also be used for suppositories containing boric acid; bromides, chloral hydrate, iodide, iodoform and other drugs. Care should be taken in the selection of the type of gelatin used in suppositories. There are two major types of gelatin, each of which has its specific applications.

Type A (also called pharmagel A) is derived from an acid-treated precursor and has a pH between 3.8 and 4.5. This gelatin has an isoelectric point between pH 7 and 9. In solution, type A gelatin carries a strong positive charge and behaves as a cationic agent. It has the customary incompatibilities of both a weak acid and chlorides.

Type B (also called as pharmagel B). It is made from an alkali treated precursor and has a pH between 5 and 7. Since this pH is above its isoelectric point (pH 4.7 to 5), it carries a negative charge and behaves as an anionic agent, unless its pH is lowered below 4.7, when it becomes cationic.

The type of gelatin selected must be based upon the properties of the medicament to be incorporated. It was found that ichthammol suppositories made with type A gelatin were granular. Mild silver protein suppositories made with type A gelatin shrink because they contain protein that is anionic in relation to the cationic properties of type A gelatin. Glycerinated gelatin is also the best and most reliable vehicle for the effective use of antiseptics such as hexyl resorcinol, nitromersol, and phemerol in suppository form. Many formulae have been recommended for glycerinated gelatin, differing in the proportion of glycerin, gelatin, and water.

Advantages

1. The base does not melt at body temperature, but rather dissolve in the secretions of the cavity in which they are inserted.

2. Solution time is regulated by the proportion of gelatin: glycerin: water used, the nature of gelatin used, and the chemical reaction of the drug with gelatin.

3. The consistency of a 20% gelatin formula was found inadequate for rectal use. The gelatin content is sometimes increased to as high as 30%.

Disadvantages

1. Glycerol suppositories have laxative action.
2. Unpredictable solution time. This varies with the batch of gelatin and the age of the base.
3. The base requires protection from heat and moisture and also has a dehydrating effect on the rectal or vaginal mucosa leading to irritation.
4. The base may require preservatives leading to problems of incompatibility.
5. The base is more time consuming to prepare than fatty bases and may be difficult to remove from the mold.
6. Lubrication of the mold is essential.

b. The Polyethylene Glycols (Macrogols)

Polyethylene glycols are polymers of ethylene oxide and water, prepared to various chain length, molecular weights, and physical states. Polyglycols exist as liquids when their average molecular weight ranges from 200 to 600, and as wax-like solids with molecular weights about 1000. Their water solubility, hygroscopicity and vapor pressure decrease with increasing average molecular weights.

The polyethylene glycol suppositories can be prepared by both moldings and cold compression methods.

Several combinations of polyethylene glycols have been prepared for suppository bases having desired consistency and different physical characteristics.

Advantages

1. No laxative effect.
2. Microbial contamination less likely.
3. The base contracts slightly on cooling and no lubricant is necessary.
4. Melting point generally above body temperature. Cool storage is, therefore, not so critical; they are suitable for hot climates and less likely to melt on handling. The high melting point also means that the bases do not melt in the body but dissolve and disperse the medication slowly, providing a sustained effect.

5. Produce high viscosity solution. This means that after dispersing in the body, leakage is less likely.

6. Good solvent properties.

7. Give product with clean smooth appearance.

Disadvantages

1. Hygroscopic. Like glycerogelatin base, polyethylene glycol bases may cause irritation to the mucosa. This can partly overcome by incorporation of 20% water in the mass or by instructing the patient to dip the preparation in water prior to insertion.

2. Poor bioavailability of medicaments. The good solvent properties may result in retention of the drug in the liquefied base with consequence reduction in therapeutic effect.

3. Incompatibilities. Polyethylene glycol bases are incompatible with some medicaments, e.g. bismuth salts, ichthamol, benzocaine and phenol, and reduces the activity of quaternary ammonium compounds and hydroxy-benzoate. They also interact with some plastics which limits the choice of container.

4. Brittleness. Polyethylene glycol suppositories may be brittle unless poured at as low temperature as possible. The addition of surface active agents or plasticizer may reduce brittleness. Products sometimes fracture on storage, particularly if they contain water. One cause is the high solubility of the macrogols, which can lead to a super-saturated solution in the water and subsequent crystallization. This in turn makes the mass granular and brittle.

5. Crystal growth of certain medicaments may occur, particularly if they are partly in solution or suspension in the base.

c. Soap Glycerin

Stearin soap (i.e. curd soap, sodium stearate) is used as a suppository base. The soap used in this base is formed in glycerin solution by interaction between stearic acid and sodium carbonate.

It has certain *advantages* over gelatin for making glycerin sufficiently hard for suppositories:

1. A larger quantity of glycerin can be incorporated actually up to 95% of the mass.
2. Soap assists the action of glycerin, whereas gelatin does not.

The *disadvantage* is that soap glycerin suppositories are very hygroscopic, and require to be wrapped in waxed paper or pure tin foil, and protected from the atmosphere.

3. Water Dispersible Bases

Several non-ionic surfactants can be used for formulating both water-soluble and oil-soluble drugs. The water dispersible bases offer the additional advantages of storage and handling at elevated temperatures having broad drug compatibility, non-support of microbial growth, non-toxicity, and non-sensitivity. The surfactants most commonly used in suppository formulations are the Tween, Myrj, Span and Ariacel. These surfactants may be used alone, blended or in combination with other suppository vehicle materials to yield a wide range of melting points and consistencies.

4. Emulsifying Bases

a. Massa Estrinum (Adeps Solidus)

This is a mixture of the monoglycerides, diglycerides, and triglycerides of the saturated fatty acids having the formula $C_{11}H_{23}COOH$ to $C_{17}H_{35}COOH$.

Several grades are available to suit climate changes such as Massa estrinum A, AB, AS, B, BB, BC, BD and C. They possess a melting range of 33 to 38°C.

b. Massupol

This consists of glyceryl esters, mainly of lauric acid, to which a very small amount of glyceryl monostearate has been added. They exhibit a melting range of 34–37°C, and are suitable for mass production.

c. Witepsols

They consist of hydrogenated triglycerides of lauric acid with added monoglycerides. Nine grades are available of which

Witepsol H_{12}, H_{15}, W_{35}, S_{55}, E_{75} and E_{55} are in common uses. The fatty acids, of which the trigycerides in Witepsol are composed, are derived from natural saturated fatty acid of C_{12}–C_{18} with predominance of lauric acid. They are formerly marketed under the trade name of Imhausen bases. They are suitable for formulation of eutectic mixtures and tropical suppositories, e.g. Witepsol H_{15} disintegrates almost as fast in the rectum as cocoa butter. The melting times were 4 minutes for cocoa butter, 6 minutes for Witepsol.

Differences between witepsol and cocoa butter suppository

1. Witepsol enables the suppository to ascend more in the rectum before disintegration, while a cocoa butter suppository, melting more rapidly at a lower temperature and more likely to cause leakage.

2. Witepsols do not undergo structural changes at temperatures above their melting points.

3. They absorb water, due to the presence of glycerol mono and diesters as emulsifiers. The interval between softening and melting is small and the masses congeal just one or two degrees below their softening points.

4. Witepsols solidify rapidly after being poured at their melting temperature into the mold and chilling of the mold is unnecessary.

5. Witepsols contract more upon solidification than cacao butter, thus eliminating the need for lubricating the mold. Combinations of Witepsol H_{15} and E_{85} cover a wide melting point range.

d. Wecobee Bases

They are triglycerides of higher melting fractions of coconut oil and palm kernel oil and may contain 0.25% of lecithin. The incorporation of glyceryl monostearate and propylene glycol monostearate makes them emulsifiable. Wecobee W, R, S, M and FS are presented in commerce.

e. Dehydag Bases

Three grades are manufactured and marketed as suppository base I, II and G. Base I and II are composed of hardened fatty alcohols and fats, but base G is formed from a saturated fatty alcohols known as Guerbet alcohols. Waxes or high-melting alcohol may be added to raise the melting point of base I and base II.

None of the Dehydag exhibits polymorphism. They may be heated above their melting points without lowering their congealing temperatures. Waxes or high melting alcohols may be added to raise the m.p. of these bases.

f. Emulsified Propylene Glycol Derivatives

Propylene glycol α-monostearate (monolene) was developed as a suppository base. This base melts within body temperature and is self-emulsifying in water, forming soft bulky non-irritant emulsion, suitable for rectal treatment. Its properties permit diffusion of the medicament and absorption of water-soluble drug irrespective of melting range, while insoluble substances are emulsified and kept in intimate contact with mucosal tissue.

Advantages of emulsifying bases

1. The physical properties do not change by overheating.
2. They do not stick to the mold.
3. They solidify rapidly.
4. As they all contain an emulsifying agent, they can absorb fairly high percentages of aqueous liquids.
5. The emulsifying agents are monoglycerides which form water-in-oil emulsions and this would seem more rational than the use of oil-in-water emulsifying agents.

Methods of Preparation

Suppositories can be extemporaneously prepared by one of three methods.

1. Hand Mold Suppositories (Fig. 4.4)

This is the oldest and simplest method of preparing suppositories. A skilled person is required for the preparation of suppositories. General process for preparation of suppositories is as follows:

   a. Mix measured quantity of medicinal substances with sufficient quantity of theobroma oil.

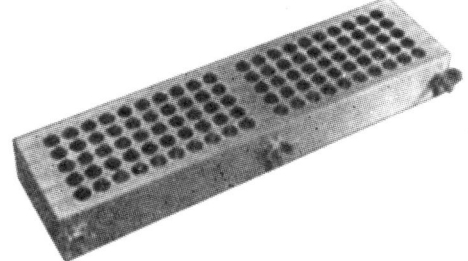

Fig. 4.4: Suppository hand mold

b. Triturate and, if required, soften with diluted alcohol and rub until a smooth paste is formed.

c. Add remaining quantity of theobroma oil and add wool fat for consistency.

d. When the mass becomes plastic by vigorous kneading of the pestle quickly remove from the mortar with a spatula.

e. Transfer with spatula to a piece of filter paper and keep in hands during the kneading and rolling procedure.

f. Roll the mass by quick rotating movements of the hands and immediately place on a pill tile.

g. Rolling the mass on the tile with a flat board forms a cylindrical suppository.

h. Cut in pieces by spatula.

i. Give the shape by rolling one end on the tile with a spatula.

j. Pack in butter paper or in proper container and store in cool place (Fig. 4.5).

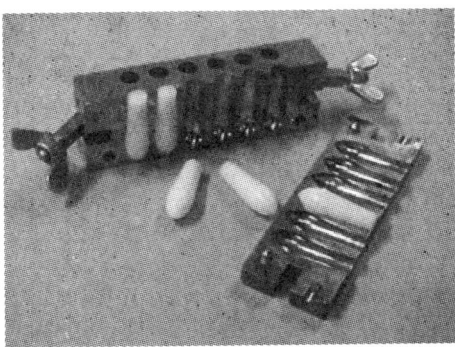

Fig. 4.5: Hand mold (open) showing prepared suppository

2. Compression Mold Suppositories (Cold Compression)

a. Mix theobroma oil and drug.
b. Mixture is forced into a mold under pressure, using a wheel-operated press.
c. Mold is removed, opened and replaced.
d. On large-scale, cold-compression machines are hydraulically operated by water-jacketed cooling and screw fed.

3. Fusion or Melt Mold Suppositories

a. Drug is dispersed or dissolved in a melted suppository base.
b. Pour the mixture into suppository molds and allow cooling in ice bath.
c. Finished suppositories are removed by opening the mold.
d. Various types and sizes of molds are available for preparation of suppositories. Molds are made of aluminum alloys, brass or plastic and are available with from six to several hundred cavities.

4. Automatic Mold Machine

All filling, ejection, and mold cleaning operations are fully automatic. The output of a typical rotary machine ranges from 3500 to 6000 suppositories per hour. The suppository mold is lubricated by brushing or spraying and then filled to a slight excess. Excess material is removed after the mass gets solidified and collected for re-use. All heating and cooling systems are fully automatic.

When the density factor is not known

When bases other than cocoa butter are used, or when the density factor for a drug in cocoa butter is not known, then the density factor can be estimated by calculation or experimentally determined by the double casting technique.

The weight of the blank suppository is easily determined. A portion of the suppository base is melted, poured into the suppository mold and allowed to congeal. The suppositories are removed from the mold, and the total weight of the suppositories is determined. The average weight of the blank suppository is determined by dividing the total weight by the number of suppositories.

Estimation by Calculation

One method to determine the density factor of a drug in a base other than cocoa butter requires the use of the ratio of a blank suppository of the non-cocoa butter base to a blank suppository of the cocoa butter base. This information is generally obtained by calibrating the mold first with one base and then the other base.

As an example of the method, a mold was calibrated with the PEG base and the average blank suppository weighed 2.24 grams. The same mold was calibrated with cocoa butter and those blank suppositories weighed 1.87 grams on average. Therefore, the ratio of the two weights was:

$$\frac{\text{Weight of PEG suppositories}}{\text{Weight of cocoa butter suppositories}} = \frac{2.24 \text{ g}}{1.87 \text{ g}} = 1.20$$

If 200 mg of aspirin is to be incorporated into each PEG suppository, it is necessary to determine how much PEG base will be displaced by the aspirin. That displacement amount can be calculated as follows:

- Density factor of aspirin in cocoa butter = 1.3 (from reference sources)
- Density of PEG base relative to cocoa butter = 1.20 (the ratio obtained from the calibrations)
- 0.2 g of aspirin will displace $\dfrac{0.2 \text{ g}}{1.3} \times 1.20 = 0.18 \text{ g}$ of PEG base

For each PEG suppository to be formulated, 0.2 g of aspirin and 2.06 g (2.24 g − 0.18 g = 2.06 g) of the PEG base will be needed.

Double Casting Technique (Fig. 4.6)

The total quantity of drug is mixed with an amount of base which is inadequate to fill the number of cavities. The mixture is poured into the mold, partially filling each cavity, and the remaining portion of the cavities are filled with the melted blank base. The cooled suppositories are then removed, remelted, mixed, and recast to evenly distribute the active ingredient. By recording the necessary information, the pharmacist can determine the weight of base displaced by the drug and then calculate the density factor.

Note: A portion of the formula will be lost during this process, so you should always prepare for 2 extra suppositories to ensure that you have enough mixture for the desired number of suppositories.

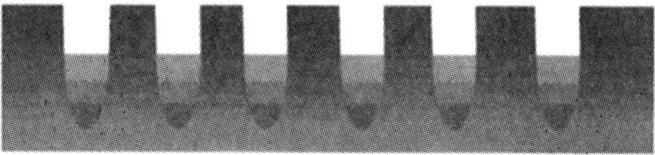

1. Mix all of the drug with a portion of the base and use the mixture to partially fill each of the suppository mold cavities.

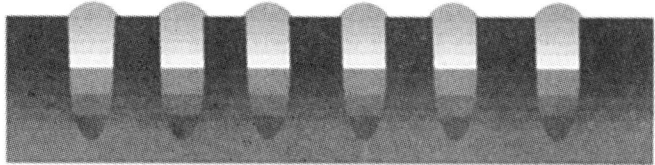

2. Use plain base to overfill each cavity.

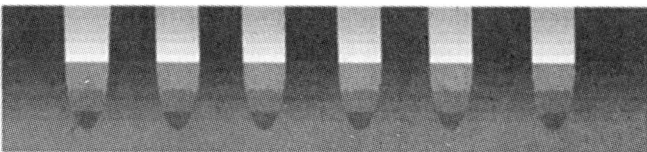

3. Let cool, then remove excess base from top of mold. Remove suppositories, remelt, and recast to evenly distribute the drug.

Fig. 4.6: Double casting method of suppository preparation

Suppositories are usually formulated on weight basis. The medicament replaces the portion of base having same density as that of theobroma oil. If the drug substance is heavier, it will replace a proportionally smaller amount of theobroma oil.

Example 1

Prepare six suppositories containing 0.1 g tannic acid in each suppository.

Density of tannic acid is 1.6 as compared with cocoa butter.

Weight of blank suppositories = 2.0 g

Cocoa butter replaced by drug = 0.1/1.6 = 0.062 g

Cocoa butter required for one suppository = 2.000 – 0.062 =1.938 g

Actual weight of one suppository = 1.938 + 0.10 = 2.038 g

Weight of cocoa butter for 8 suppositories (take excess weigh of 2 suppositories as required) = 1.938 × 8 = 15.504 g

Weight of tannic acid for 8 suppositories (take excess weigh of 2 suppositories as required) = 0.10 × 8 = 0.80 g

Total weight of all suppositories = 15.504 + 0.80 = 16.304 g

Example 2

Prepare 0.1 g tannic acid 6 suppositories using polyethylene glycol as base. Density factor of cocoa butter is 1.6 and density factor of polyethylene glycol is 1.25.

Weight of polyethylene glycol suppository = 1.75

Cocoa butter replaced by drug = (0.1/1.6) x 1.25 = 0.078 g

Polyethylene glycol required for one suppository = 1.750 – 0.078 = 1.672 g

Actual weight of one suppository = 1.672 + 0.10 = 1.772 g

Weight of polyethylene glycol for 8 suppositories (take excess weigh of 2 suppositories as required) = 1.672 × 8 = 13.376 g

Weight of tannic acid for 8 suppositories (take excess weigh of 2 suppositories as required) = 0.10 × 8 = 0.80 g

Total weight = 13.376 + 0.80 = 14.176 g

Displacement Value of Medicaments

The amount of base displaced will depend on the "densities" of the ingredient and the base. The amount displaced may be calculated from the displacement value of the medicament. The *displacement value* of an ingredient is defined as the number of *parts by weight of the ingredient which displace one part by weight of theobroma oil.* The displacement values for other fatty bases (e.g. Witepsol W) are taken to be the same as those quoted for theobroma oil. For glycerol suppository base, the displacement values will be 1/1.2 of those values for theobroma oil.

Determination of Displacement Value

Weight of six suppositories of theobroma oil or any other base = a g

Weight of six suppositories containing, say 40% of drug(s) = b g

Calculate weight of theobroma oil = $60/100 \times b = c$ g

Calculate drug(s) = $40/100 \times b = d$ g

$(a - c)$ g = the weight of theobroma oil displaced by d g of drug substances

Displacement value of the medicament = $d/(a - c)$

Example 1: Calculate the quantities required to make 10 theobroma oil suppositories (2 g mold) each containing 400 mg of zinc oxide (Displacement value = 4.7)

Calculation

1. Calculate the total weight of zinc oxide required.
2. Calculate what weight of base would be required to prepare 10 unmedicated suppositories.
3. Determine what weight of base would be displaced by the medicament.
4. Calculate, therefore, the weight of base required to prepare the medicated suppositories.

Total weight of zinc oxide required = 400 mg × 10 = 4 g.

Weight of base required for unmedicated suppositories = 2 g × 10 = 20 g.

As the displacement value of zinc oxide = 4.7.

This means that 4.7 g of zinc oxide would displace 1 g of theobroma oil.

1 g of zinc oxide would displace 1 ÷ 4.7 g of theobroma oil. So, 4 g of zinc oxide will displace (4 × 1) ÷ 4.7 g of theobroma oil = 0.85 g.

Therefore, the weight of base required to make medicated suppositories = 20 − 0.85 g = 19.15 g.

Answer: 19.15 g

Example 2: Calculate the quantities required to make six glycerogelatin suppositories (4 g mold), each containing 100 mg aminophylline (Displacement value = 1.3).

Calculation

1. Calculate the total weight of aminophylline required.
2. Calculate what weight of glycerogelatin base would be required to prepare 10 unmedicated suppositories.
3. Determine what weight of base would be displaced by the medicament.
4. Calculate, therefore, the weight of base required to prepare the medicated suppositories.

Total weight of aminophylline required = 100 mg × 6 = 600 mg or 0.6 g.

Weight of base required for unmedicated suppositories = 4 g × 6 × 1.2 (to take account of the greater density of this base) = 28.8 g.

As the displacement value of aminophylline = 1.3

This means that 1.3 g of aminophylline displaces 1 g of theobroma oil.

So, 1 g of aminophylline displaces 1 ÷ 1.3 g of theobroma oil. 0.6 g of aminophylline displace (1 × 0.6) ÷ 1.3 g of theobroma oil = 0.46 g of theobroma oil.

This means that the aminophylline would displace 0.46 g × 1.2 of the glycerogelatin base = 0.55 g.

Therefore, the weight of base required to make medicated suppositories = 28.8 g – 0.55 g = 28.25 g

Answer: 28.25 g

Example 3: What quantities are required to prepare eight theobroma oil suppositories, in a 4 g mold, containing 1% w/w lignocaine hydrochloride?

Calculation

1. Calculate the total weight of the medicated suppositories.
2. Calculate, therefore, the weight of the drug required (1% of the total weight).
3. Subtract the weight of the drug from the total weight of the suppositories to find the weight of the base required.

Total weight of the suppositories = 32 g

Weight of drug required (1% w/w) = (32 × 1) ÷ 100 g = 0.32 g

Therefore, weight of base required = 32 g – 0.32 g = 31.68 g

Answer: 31.68 g

Example 4: Prepare 12 glycerogelatin suppositories, containing 0.5% w/w cinchocaine hydrochloride. Use a 2 g mold.

Calculation:

1. Calculate the total weight of the medicated suppositories, allowing for the greater density of the glycerogelatin base.
2. Calculate the weight of the drug required.
3. Subtract the weight of the drug from the total weight of the suppositories to determine the weight of the base required.

Total weight of the suppositories = 12×2 g $\times 1.2 = 28.8$ g

Weight of drug required = $(28.8$ g $\times 0.5) \div 100 = 0.144$ g (or 144 mg)

Therefore, weight of base required = 28.8 g $- 0.144$ g $= 28.66$ g

Answer: 28.66 g

Quality Control of Suppositories

1. Appearance

This includes odor, color, surface condition and shape. Suppositories are elongated, smooth and have a uniform texture and appearance. They may also consist of several layers. Evidence of physical and/or chemical instability is demonstrated by noticeable changes in:

— Surface texture or form; and

— Color and odor.

2. Uniformity of Weight (Weight Variation) (BP 1980)

a. *Weigh* 20 suppositories *individually.* $w_1, w_2, w_3, ..., w_{20}$

b. *Weigh all* the suppositories together = W.

c. Calculate the *average weight* = W/20.

d. *Limit:* not more than 2 suppositories differ from the average weight by more than 5%, and no suppository differs from the average weight by more than 10%.

$\because$ Upper limit = average weight $+ \dfrac{5 * avg.wt.}{100}$

$\because$ Lower limit = average weight $- \dfrac{5 * avg.wt.}{100}$

Not more than two of the suppositories differ from the average weight by more than the % *error* listed. If more than two suppositories are different from the average weight by 5%, calculate double the percent error as follows:

$$\text{Upper limit} = \text{average weight} + \frac{10 * avg.wt.}{100}$$

$$\text{Upper limit} = \text{average weight} - \frac{10 * avg.wt.}{100}$$

Note: No suppository differs by more than double that percentage.

3. Hardness of Suppositories (Breaking Test)

a. The suppository is placed in the instrument.
b. Add 600 g; leave it for one min (use a stop watch).
c. If not broken, add 200 g every one min. until the suppository is broken.

Calculations: The hardness of the suppository is calculated by adding the weights together. But if the suppository is broken before the end of the last min, the last weight is canceled.

Results

- Using polyethylene suppositories → H = 1.7 kg
- Using indocid suppositories → H = 4 kg
- Using glycerin suppositories → H = 1.4 kg

4. Melting Range Test

a. This test is also called the macromelting range test and is a measure of the time it takes for the entire suppository to melt when immersed in a constant-temperature (37°C) water bath.
b. The apparatus commonly used for measuring the melting range of the entire suppository is the USP Tablet Disintegration Apparatus.

Procedure: The suppository is completely immersed in the constant temperature water bath, and the time for the entire suppository to melt or disperse in the surrounding water is measured.

The suppository is considered disintegrated when:

a. It is completely dissolved or

b. Dispersed into its component part.

c. Become soft "change in shape" with formation of core which is not resistant to pressure with glass rod.

5. Liquefaction Time or Softening Time Test

a. In this test, a U tube is partially immersed in a constant temperature bath and is maintained at a temperature between 35 to 37°C. There is a constriction in the tube in which the suppository is kept and above the suppository, a glass rod is kept. The time taken for the glass rod to go through the suppository and reach the constriction is known as the liquefaction time or softening time.

b. Another apparatus is there for finding "softening time" which mimics *in vivo* conditions. It uses a cellophane tube, and the temperature is maintained by water circulation. Time taken for the suppository to melt is noted.

6. Disintegration

Suppositories should comply with the "disintegration test for suppositories" unless intended for modified release. Unless otherwise stated in the individual monograph, for each of the three suppositories, examine the state of the sample after 30 minutes for fat-based suppositories and rectal capsules, and after 60 minutes for water-soluble based suppositories.

7. Uniformity of Mass

Not more than two of the individual masses should deviate from the average mass by more than 5%, and none by more than 10%.

8. Dissolution Test

By using different types of apparatus such as wire mesh basket, or dialysis tubing is used to test for *in vitro* release from suppositories.

9. Stability Testing

a. Cocoa butter suppositories on storage, "bloom", i.e. they form a white powdery deposit on the surface. This can be avoided by storing the suppositories at uniform cool temperatures and by wrapping them in foils.

b. Fat-based suppositories harden on storage, i.e. there is an upward shift in melting range due to slow crystallization to the more stable polymorphic forms of the base.

c. The softening time test and differential scanning calorimetry can be used as stability indicating test methods.

d. If we store the suppositories at an elevated temperature, just below its melting range, immediately after manufacture, the aging process is speeded up.

Labeling

The preparation must comply with the labeling requirements established by good manufacturing practices.

The label on the immediate container should include:

1. The name of the pharmaceutical product.
2. The name(s) of the active ingredient(s); International Nonproprietary Names (INN) should be used wherever possible.
3. The amount of the active ingredient(s) in each suppository and the number of suppositories in the container.
4. The batch (lot) number assigned by the manufacturer.
5. The expiry date and, when required, the date of manufacture.
6. Any special storage conditions or handling precautions that may be necessary.
7. Directions for use, warnings and precautions that may be necessary.
8. The name and address of the manufacturer or the person responsible for placing the product on the market.
9. If applicable, the names and concentrations of the antimicrobial agents and/or antioxidants incorporated in the preparation.

Packaging and Storage

1. Suppositories are usually packed in tin or aluminum, paper or plastic.
2. Poorly packed suppositories may give rise to staining, breakage or deformation by melting.

3. Both cocoa butter and glycerinated gelatin suppositories stored preferably in a refrigerator.

4. Polyethylene glycol suppositories stored at usual room temperature without the requirement of refrigeration.

ISOLATED KEY POINTS

- Suppositories are medicated solid dosage forms of various shapes and sizes meant for insertion into body cavities like rectum, vagina, urethra, ear and nose.

- Suppositories are medicated, solid bodies of various sizes and shapes suitable for introduction into body cavities for local or systemic effect. The medicament is incorporated into a base such as cocoa butter which melts at body temperature, or into one such as glycerinated gelatin or PEG which slowly dissolves in the mucous secretions.

- Suppositories are suited particularly for producing local action, but may also be used to produce a systemic effect or to exert a mechanical effect to facilitate emptying the lower bowel.

- *Suppository base* 1. Oleaginous (fatty) bases: Cocoa butter or theobroma oil. 2. Water-soluble or miscible bases: Glycerinated gelatin, polyethylene glycol.

- *Suppositories—method of preparation:* Hand rolling: It is the oldest and simplest method of suppository preparation and may be used when only a few suppositories are to be prepared in a cocoa butter base. It has the advantage of avoiding the necessity of heating the cocoa butter. A plastic-like mass is prepared by triturating grated cocoa butter and active ingredients in a mortar.

- *Compression molding:* Compression molding is a method of preparing suppositories from a mixed mass of grated suppository base and medicaments which is forced into a special compression mold using suppository making machines. The suppository base and the other ingredients are combined by thorough mixing. The friction of the process causing the base to soften into a past-like consistency.

- On a small scale, a mortar and pestle may be used (preheated mortar facilitate softening of the base). On large scale, mechanically operated kneading mixers and a warmed mixing vessel may be applied. In the compression machine, the suppository mass is placed into a cylinder which is then closed. Pressure is applied from one end to release the mass from the other end into the suppository mold or die.

- When the die is filled with the mass, a movable end plate at the back of the die is removed and when additional pressure is applied to the mass in the cylinder, the formed suppositories are ejected. The end plate is returned, and the process is repeated until all of the suppository mass has been used. The method requires that the capacity of the molds first be determined by compressing a small amount of the base into the dies and weighing the finished suppositories. When active ingredients are added, it is necessary to omit a portion of the suppository base, based on the density factors of the active ingredients.

- Fusion molding involves: 1. Melting the suppository base. 2. Dispersing or dissolving the drug in the melted base. 3. The mixture is removed from the heat and poured into a suppository mold. 4. Allowing the melt to congeal. 5. Removing the formed suppositories from the mold. The fusion method can be used with all types of suppositories and must be used with most of them.

- *Suppository molds:* Small scale molds are capable of producing 6 or 12 suppositories in a single operation. Industrial molds produce thousands of suppositories per hour from a single molding.

- *Packaging:* Suppositories must be packed in such a manner that they do not touch each other. Staining, breaking or deformation by melting caused by adhesion can result from poorly wrapped and packaged suppositories. Suppositories usually are foiled in tin or aluminum, paper or plastic strips. Overwrapping is done with hand or machine. Hand packing yields a nonuniform product. Machines overcome this problem and can wrap 8000 suppositories per hour.

- *Storage:* Suppositories should be protected from heat, preferably by storing in the refrigerator. Polyethylene glycol suppositories and suppositories enclosed in a solid shell are less prone to distortion to temperature slightly above body temperature. Store in a cool place or refrigerator for external use only.

- *Testing/evaluation of suppositories:* Finished suppositories are routinely inspected for: Appearance. Content uniformity, melting range test, breaking test, drug release test, disintegration test, dissolution testing, liquefaction or softening time.

- *Breaking test (hardness):* To measure the brittleness of suppository, double wall chamber in which the test suppository is placed. Water at 37°C is pumped through the double wall. The suppository supports a disc to which rod is attached. The other end of the rod consist of another disc to which weights are applied.

- The test was conducted by placing the suppository to support the axis of 600 g weight. At one minute intervals, 200 gm weights are added. The weight at which the suppository collapses is the breaking point. When the breaking point reached in the first 20 sec, the added weight was not calculated. When the breaking point reached in the second 20 sec, half the added weight was calculated. When the breaking point reached in the third 20 sec, all the added weight was calculated.

- *Melting range test:* Macromelting range is a measure of the time it takes for the entire suppository to melt when immersed in a constant-temperature (37°C) water bath. The apparatus commonly used for measuring the melting range of the entire suppositories is a USP tablet disintegration apparatus.

- *In vitro drug release: In vitro* drug release pattern is measured by using the same melting rang apparatus. Aliquots of the release medium were taken at different time intervals within the melting period. The drug content in the aliquots was determined. The drug release pattern was plotted (time versus drug release curve).

LONG ANSWER TYPE QUESTIONS

1. What are 'suppositories'? Classify different suppository bases used in the preparation of suppositories. Describe briefly each base.

2. Define the term 'suppositories'. What are the advantages and disadvantages of suppositories.

3. What do you mean by 'suppositories'? Describe in brief the various types of suppositories.

4. Discuss in brief, the various methods of preparation of suppositories.

5. Write short notes on the following:
   a. Theobroma oil
   b. Displacement value
   c. Pessaries
   d. Fusion method of preparation of suppositories
   e. Prior to insertion
   f. Compounding suppositories using the fusion method
   g. Your mold has been calibrated and the average weight per suppository is 2 g.

6. What is an advantage of the oleaginous bases with regards to membrane tissues?

7. Describe the procedure used for melting cocoa butter.

8. What release characteristics would one expect to be associated with hydrophobic drugs and oleaginous suppository bases?

9. What do PEG suppository bases do when inserted into the body?

10. List three advantages and disadvantages of PEG suppository bases.

11. Enumerate various factors to consider when selecting a suppository base.

12. What is the rationale for recommending that patients moisten PEG suppositories?

13. What type of base is preferred when an emollient effect is desired?

14. What are the two methods used for compounding suppositories?

15. Why are density calculations and mold calibration so important?

16. Define the term density displacement factor.

17. Perform the calculations for preparing 10 suppositories each containing 180 mg of phenobarbital as the sole active ingredient and using cocoa butter as your base.

SHORT ANSWER TYPE QUESTIONS

1. Define the term 'suppository'.

2. Explain the term 'displacement value'.

3. Name the different types of suppositories which are available in the market.

4. Write the various types of lubricants used to lubricate the suppository mold.

5. Why cocoa butter is not used in the preparation of suppositories?

6. Mention different methods of preparation of suppositories.

7. What is the importance of calibration of the mold?

8. Write the advantages and disadvantages of suppositories.

9. Mention the qualities of an ideal suppository base.

10. Write in brief, the advantages and disadvantages of theobroma oil as suppository base.

11. What are the advantages and disadvantages of hydrogenated oil as suppository base?

OBJECTIVE TYPE QUESTIONS

1. Suppositories are .... dosage form of drugs.

2. Suppositories are used to produce ...., ...
and .... action.

3. Cocoa butter is a mixture of .... of stearic, palmitic, oleic and other fatty acids.

4. In suppositories, the drug is released either due to .... of base or .... its contents in .... fluid.

5. Compression method is suitable for the preparation of suppositories containing .... and .... drugs.

6. Cocoa butter is not a suitable base for .... and .... suppositories.

ANSWERS

1. Unit
2. Local, systemic mechanical
3. Glyceryl esters
4. Melting, dissolving, body cavity
5. Thermolabile, insoluble
6. Pessaries, nasal

Aerosols

DEFINITION

Pharmaceutical aerosols are defined as the products containing therapeutically active ingredients dissolved, suspended or emulsified in a propellant or a mixture of solvent and propellant and intended for oral or topical administration into body cavities. The packaging of an aerosol product consists of self-pressurized non-returnable dispenser, constructed of metal, glass or plastic which contains a fluid product and which is fitted with a valve to dispense the product in the form of a spray, liquid, paste, foam or powder.

Advantages

- The medication can be delivered directly to the affected area in a desired form, such as spray, steam, quick breaking foam or stable foam.
- Product can be maintained free of contamination. Substances that get spoiled by oxygen or moisture can be maintained.
- Irritation produced by the mechanical application of topical medication is reduced or eliminated.
- Ease of convenience of application.
- Application of medication in thin layer.

Disadvantages

- Aerosol packs must not be subjected to heat since high pressures in most aerosol can cause explosion.
- Toxicity of propellants.

- Catalytic oxidation of drugs such as ascorbic acid and epinephrine has been caused by traces of metal from valve parts of container.

Components of Aerosol Product (Fig. 5.1)

An aerosol product consists of the following component parts:

1. *Propellant:* Propellant includes one propellant or a mixture of propellants. Mixture of propellants is used to get the desired vapor pressure.
2. *Product concentrate:* Product concentrate includes drug, surfactants, solvents, antioxidants, etc.
3. Containers
4. Valves and actuator

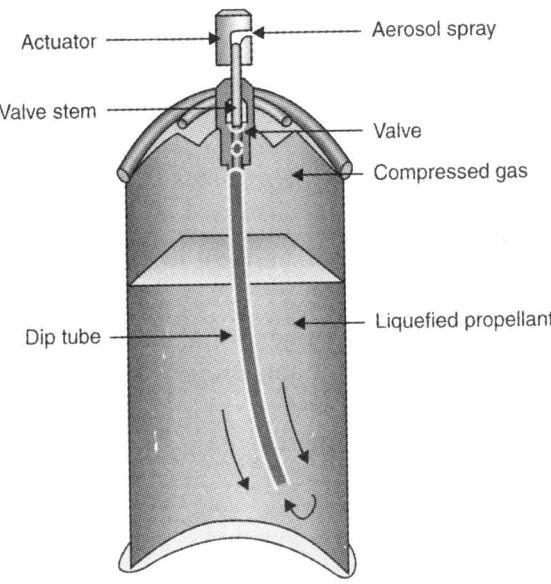

Fig. 5.1: Components of aerosol

Propellants

A propellant is a chemical with a vapor pressure greater than atmospheric pressure at 40°C. The propellant is the driving force (or you could say, the 'engine'), behind the aerosol. An propellant is a material that is used to move ('Propel') an object.

The material is usually expelled by gas pressure through a nozzle. The pressure may be from a compressed gas, or a gas produced by a chemical reaction. The exhaust material may be a gas, liquid, plasma, or before the chemical reaction, a solid, liquid or gel. The propellant supplies the necessary pressure within an aerosol system to expel material from the container and, in combination with other components, to convert the material into the desired physical form.

The contents of the aerosol are made up of two components:

1. The product, in the form of a liquid, emulsion or suspension.
2. The propellant, which can be a liquefied gas, or even a compressed gas.

The propellants produce the necessary pressure within the aerosol system to expel the material from the container and convert the material into desired physical form in combination with other components. A good propellant system should have the proper vapor characteristics compatible with the other aerosol components. The mixture of propellants is frequently used to obtain the desirable pressure, delivery and spray characteristics.

Desired Characteristics of Aerosol Propellant

- It should be non-toxic.
- Inert and unreactive in the formulation.
- Chemically should be stable under a range of conditions.
- It should be of high purity.
- Acceptable taste and odor.

Types of Propellants

Types of propellants commonly used in pharmaceutical aerosols include:

1. Chlorofluorocarbons
2. Hydrochlorofluorocarbons and hydrofluorocarbons
3. Hydrocarbons
4. Compressed gases.

1. Chlorofluorocarbon (CFC) Propellants

For many years, the chlorofluorocarbon (CFC) propellants P-11, P-12, and P-114 were used in aerosol products. Their use has been severely curtailed due to their role in depleting the ozone layer of the atmosphere. Since January 1996, worldwide production of these CFCs has been reduced to only the amount needed for aerosols used in the treatment of asthma and chronic obstructive pulmonary disease. Alternatives to P-12 (i.e. P-134a and P-227) have now been developed and are being incorporated in aerosol formulations. Currently, there are not alternatives for P-11 and P-114. Small amounts of P-11 are required in most aerosol suspensions to make a slurry of the active drug and other ingredients. It also is used to dissolve surfactants in some formulations.

P-11, P-12, and P-114 are the CFCs of choice for oral, nasal, and inhalation aerosols. These particular chlorofluorocarbon propellants are well accepted due to their relatively low toxicity and inflammability. The chlorofluorocarbons as a class are inert but P-11 is subject to hydrolysis and will form hydrochloric acid in the presence of water. The acid increases the corrosion of the container and may be irritating when applied to membranes. If water is present, P-12 or a mixture of P-12 and P-114 is used (Fig. 5.2).

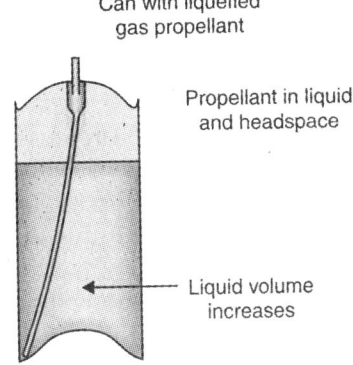

Can with liquefied
gas propellant

Propellant in liquid
and headspace

Liquid volume
increases

Fig. 5.2: Propellants in a container

The CFCs are gases at room temperature that can be liquefied by cooling them below their boiling point or by compressing them at room temperature. For example, dichlorodifluoromethane (P-12) will form a liquid when cooled to –21.6°F or when compressed to 84.9 psia at 70°F (psia = pounds per square inch absolute). These liquefied gases also have a very large expansion ratio compared to the compressed gases (e.g. nitrogen, carbon dioxide). The usual expansion ratio for liquefied gases is about 240 which means that 1 ml, of liquefied gas will occupy a volume of approximately 240 ml, if allowed to vaporize. Compressed gases have an expansion ratio of about 3–10 (Table 5.1).

Table 5.1: Properties of chlorofluorocarbon propellants

Name	Formula	No	VP @ 70°F (psia)[a]	BP °F (1 atm)	Liquid density @ 70°F (g/ml)
Trichloromonofluoromethane	CCl_3F	11	13.4	74.7	1.485
Dichlorodifluoromethane	CCl_2F_2	12	84.9	-21.6	1.325
Dichlorotetrafluoroethane	$CClF_2ClF_2$	114	27.6	39.4	1.468

[a] psia (pounds per square inch absolute) = psig (pounds per square inch gauge + 14.7)

The numerical designations for fluorinated hydrocarbon propellants have been designed so the chemical structure of the compound can be determined from the number. The system consists of three digits.

- The digit at the extreme right refers to the number of fluorine atoms in the molecule.
- The second digit from the right represent one greater in the number of hydrogen atoms in the molecule.
- The third digit from the right is one less the number of carbon atoms in the molecule; if this third digit is 0, it is omitted and a two digit number is used.
- The capital letter "C" is used before a number to indicate the cyclic nature of a compound.
- The small letters following a number are used to indicate decreasing symmetry of isomeric compounds. The most symmetrical compound is given the designated number, and all other isomers are assigned a letter (i.e. a, b, etc.) in descending order of symmetry.
- The number of chlorine atoms in a molecule may be determined by subtracting the total number of hydrogen and fluorine atoms from the total number of atoms required to saturate the compound.

When a liquefied gas propellant or propellant mixture is sealed in an aerosol container with the product concentrate, an equilibrium is establish between the propellant which remains liquefied and a portion that vaporizes and occupies the upper portion of the container. The pressure at this equilibrium is referred to as the vapor pressure (expressed as psia) and is a characteristic of each propellant at a given temperature. Since the vapor pressure is exerted equally in all directions and is independent of the quantity of liquefied phase present, the pressure forces the liquid phase up the dip tube and out of the container when the valve is actuated. As the propellant reaches the air, it evaporates due to the drop in pressure and leaves the product concentrate as airborne liquid droplets or dry particles. As the liquid is removed from the container through the dip tube, the equilibrium between the propellant's liquefied phase and vapor phase is rapidly re-established. Thus, the pressure within the container remains virtually constant and the product may be continuously released at an even rate and with the same propulsion.

In the case when there is no dip tube in the container, the container is used in the inverted position so that the liquid phase will be in direct contact with the valve. When the valve is actuated, the liquid phase is emitted and immediately reverts to the vapor phase in the atmosphere.

2. Hydrochlorofluorocarbons (HCFC) and Hydrofluoro-carbons (HFC)

The hydrochlorofluorocarbons (HCFC) and hydrofluoro-carbons (HFC) differ from CFCs in that they may not contain chlorine and have one or more hydrogen atoms. These compounds break down in the atmosphere at a faster rate than the CFCs resulting in a lower ozone depleting effect (Table 5.2).

P-22, 142b, and 152a are used in topical pharmaceuticals. These three propellants have a greater miscibility with water and, therefore, are more useful as solvents compared to the other propellants. They are also slightly more flammable than the other propellants but this is not perceived as a disadvantage.

Table 5.2: Properties of hydrochlorofluorocarbon and hydrofluorocarbon propellants

Name	Formula	No. @70°F (psia)	BP °F (1 ATM)	VP	Liquid density @70°F (g/ml)
Chlorodifluoromethane	$CHClF_2$	22	−135.7	−41.4	1.21
Trifluoromonofluoroethane	CF_3CH_2F	134a	85.8	−15.0	1.21
Chlorodifluoroethane	CH_3CClF_2	142b	43.8	14.4	1.12
Difluoroethane	CH_3CHF_2	152a	76.4	−12.5	0.91
Heptafluoropropane	CF_3CHFCF_3	227	57.7	2.3	1.41

3. Hydrocarbons

The hydrocarbons are used in topical pharmaceutical aerosols because of their environmental acceptance and their low toxicity and non-reactivity. They are also useful in making three phase (two layer) aerosols because of their density being less than 1 and their immiscibility with water. The hydrocarbons remain on top of the aqueous layer and provide the force to push the contents out of the container. However, they are flammable and can explode. They contain no halogens and, therefore, hydrolysis does not occur making these good propellants for water based aerosols (Table 5.3).

Table 5.3: Properties of hydrocarbon propellants

Name	Formula	No @70°F (psia)	BP °F (1 ATM)	VP	Liquid density @68°F (g/ml)
Propane	C_3H_8	A-108	124.7	−43.7	0.50
Isobutane	C_4H_{10}	A-31	45.1	10.9	0.56
Butane	C_4H_{10}	A-17	31.2	31.1	0.58

Propane, butane, and isobutane are the most commonly used hydrocarbons. They are used alone or as mixtures or mixed with other liquefied gases to obtain the desired vapor pressure, density, and degree of flammability. The flammability hazard has been substantially reduced by using mixtures of propellants and with the development of newer types of dispensing valves (i.e. valve with vapor tap).

4 Compressed Gases

Gases such as nitrogen, nitrous oxide, and carbon dioxide have been used as aerosol propellants for products dispensed as fine mists, foams, or semisolids. But due to their low expansion ratio, the sprays are fairly wet and the foams are not as stable as produced by liquefied gas propellants. However, using a compressed gas that is insoluble in the product concentrate (e.g. nitrogen) will emit the product concentrate in essentially the same form as it was placed in the container (Fig. 5.3).

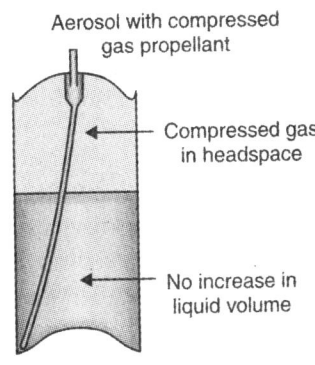

Aerosol with compressed gas propellant

Compressed gas in headspace

No increase in liquid volume

Fig. 5.3: Compressed gas propellant

The pressure of the compressed gas contained in the headspace of the aerosol container forces the product concentrate out of the container. But unlike aerosols prepared with liquefied gas propellants, there is no propellant reservoir. So higher gas pressures are required in these aerosols and the pressure diminishes as the product is used. These gases have been used for the most part to dispense food products, dental creams, hair preparations, and ointments (Table 5.4).

Table 5.4: Properties of compressed gases				
Name	Formula	VP @70°F (psia)	BP °F (1 ATM)	Gas density @70°F (g/ml)
Nitrogen	N_2	492	– 320	0.97
Nitrous oxide	N_2O	735	– 127	1.53
Carbon dioxide	CO_2	852	– 109	1.53

OTHER TYPICAL PROPELLANTS

Liquefied Petroleum Gas (LPG)

The LPG grade aerosol propellant consists of high purity hydrocarbons derived directly from oil wells, and as a by-product from the petroleum industry. They consist of a mixture of propane, isobutane and n-butane. These propellants are used in most aerosols today, and have been used for many years in household aerosol products.

Dimethyl Ether (DME)

This is an alternative liquefied propellant, and is more common in personal care products, and some air fresheners.

Chlorofluorocarbons (CFCs)

These liquefied propellant gases used to be very common prior to the discovery that they were affecting the ozone layer. They are no longer used in consumer aerosols in the western world. They are, however, permitted in inhalation aerosols, as used in the treatment of asthma.

An aerosol formulation consists of two components, the product concentrate and the propellant. The product concentrate is the active drug combined with additional ingredients or cosolvents required to make a stable and efficacious product. The concentrate can be a solution, suspension, emulsion, semisolid, or powder. The propellant provides the force that expels the product concentrate from the container and additionally is responsible for the delivery of the formulation in the proper form (i.e. spray, foam, semisolid). When the propellant is a liquefied gas or a mixture of liquefied gases, it can also serve as the solvent or vehicle for the product concentrate. If the product characteristics are to change on dispensing, additional energy in the form of a mechanical breakup system may be required.

Product Concentrates

Solution aerosols are two-phase system consisting of the product concentrate in a propellant, a mixture of propellants, or a mixture of propellant and solvent. Solvents may also be added to the formulation to retard the evaporation of the propellant. Solution aerosols can be difficult to formulate because many propellants or propellant-solvent mixtures are non-polar and are poor solvents for the product concentrate. Also, there is a limited number of solvents that can be used. Ethyl alcohol is the most commonly used solvent but propylene glycol, dipropylene glycol, ethyl acetate, hexylene glycol, and acetone have also been used.

Aerosol solutions have been used to make foot preparations, local anesthetics, spray on protective films, anti-inflammatory preparations, and aerosols for oral and nasal applications. They contain 50 to 90% propellant for topical aerosols and up to 99.5% propellant for oral and nasal aerosols. As the percentage of propellant increases, so does the degree of dispersion and the finest of the spray. As the percentage of propellant decreases, the wetness of the spray will increase. The particle sizes of the sprays can vary from 5 to 10 mm in inhalation aerosols and 50 to 100 mm for topical sprays (Fig. 5.4).

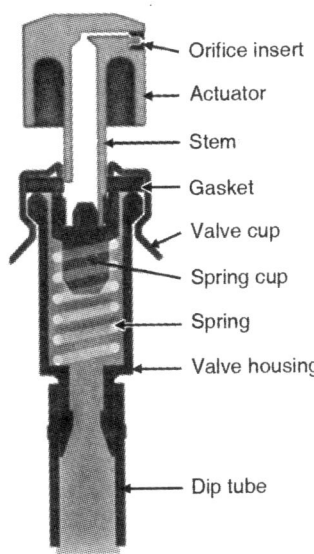

Fig. 5.4: Various parts of aerosol

Suspensions aerosols can be made when the product concentrate is insoluble in the propellant or mixture of propellant and solvent, or when a cosolvent is not desirable.

Antiasthmatic drugs, steroids, and antibiotics are delivered as suspension aerosols. When the valve is actuated, the suspension formulation is emitted as an aerosol and the propellant rapidly vaporizes and leaves a fine dispersion of the product concentrate (Fig. 5.5).

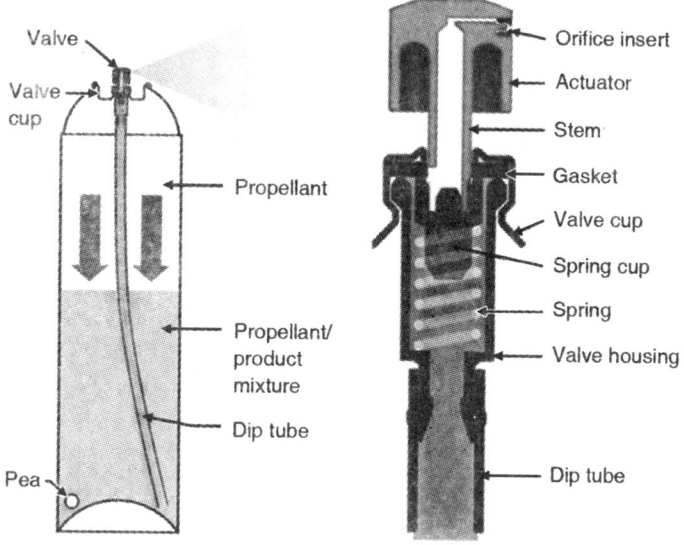

Fig. 5.5: Diagram showing functioning of various parts of aerosol

Formulation considerations for suspension aerosols that are not necessary with solution aerosols include agglomeration, particle size growth, valve clogging, moisture content, and particle size of the dispersed aerosolized particles. Lubricants such as isopropyl myristate and light mineral oil, and surfactants such as sorbitan trioleate, oleic acid, and lecithin have been used to overcome the difficulties of particle size agglomeration and growth which are directly related to the clogging problems. The moisture content of the entire formulation should be kept below 200 to 300 ppm so all of the ingredients need to be the anhydrous form of the chemical or be capable of becoming anhydrous after a drying process. The particle size of the insoluble product concentrate ingredients should be in the 1 to 10 μm range for inhalation aerosols and between 40 to 50 μm for topical aerosols.

The product concentrate in an emulsion aerosol will consist of the active ingredient, aqueous and/or non-aqueous vehicles, and a surfactant. Depending on the components, the emitted product can be a stable foam (shaving cream type) or a quick breaking foam. A quick breaking foam creates a foam when emitted from the container but the foam collapses in a relatively short time. This type of foam is used to apply the product concentrate to a large area without having to manually rub or spread the product. Also, the active drug is more rapidly available because the foam quickly collapses.

Foams are produced when the product concentrate is dispersed throughout the propellant and the propellant is in the internal phase; i.e. the emulsion behaves like o/w emulsion. When the propellant is in the external phase (i.e. like a w/o emulsion), foams are not created but sprays or wet streams result. Stable foams are produced when surfactants are used that have limited solubility in both the organic and aqueous phases. Surfactants concentrate at the interface between the propellant and the aqueous phase forming a thin film referred to as the "lamellae." It is the specific composition of this lamellae that dictates the structural strength and general characteristics of the foam. Thick and tightly layered lamellae produce very structured foams which are capable of supporting their own weight.

Surfactants used in emulsion aerosols have included fatty acids saponified with triethanolamine, anionic surfactants, and more recently non-ionic surfactants such as the polyoxyethylene fatty esters, polyoxyethylene sorbitan esters, alkyl phenoxy ethanols, and alkanolamides. The non-ionic surfactants are present fewer compatibility problems because they charge no electronic charge.

When liquefied gases (CFC, HCFC, HFC, hydrocarbons) are used as propellants, one of two systems can be formulated. The two-phase system is the simplest system. Here the product concentrate is dissolved or dispersed in liquefied propellant and solvents creating a homogenous system. The propellants exist in both the liquefied phase and the vapor phase. When the aerosol valve is actuated, some liquefied propellant and solvent containing the product concentrate is emitted from the container. These aerosols are designed to produce a fine mist or wet spray by taking advantage of the large expansion of the propellant when it enters room temperature and atmospheric pressure. The two-phase system is commonly used to formulate aerosols for inhalation or nasal application.

A three-phase system (i.e. a heterogeneous system) is made up of a layer of water immiscible liquid propellant, a layer of propellant immiscible liquid (usually water) which contains the product concentrate, and the vapor phase. This type of system is used when the formulation requires the presence of a liquid phase that is not propellant miscible. When the aerosol valve is actuated, the pressure of the vapor phase causes the liquid phase to rise in the dip tube and be expelled from the container. If the product is to maintain the liquefied gas reservoir, the dip tube must not extend beyond the aqueous phase. Sometimes it is desirable to have some liquefied propellant mixed with the aqueous phase to facilitate in the dispersion of the spray or to create a foam. In this case, the container should be shaken immediately prior to use.

If CFCs, HCFCs, and HFCs are used as the propellants, they will reside on the bottom of the container since their density is greater than water. The dip tube will then need to end somewhere in the middle of the container. If hydrocarbons are used as the propellants, they will reside on the aqueous layer since their density is less than water. In this case, the dip tube can be extended through the liquid propellant all the way down to the bottom of the container. Thus an important characteristic of any aerosol is the density of the propellant, propellants, or blend of propellants.

Foam aerosols are a three-phase system in which the liquid propellant is emulsified with the product concentrate. When the valve is actuated, the emulsion is forced through the nozzle and the entrapped propellant reverts to the vapor phase and whips the emulsion into a foam when it reaches the atmosphere. To facilitate the formulation of a foam, some aerosols are shaken prior to use to disperse some of the propellant throughout the product concentrate. If a dip tube is present, the container is used while being held upright. If there is no dip tube, the container must be inverted prior to use.

Foam products operate at a pressure of about 40 to 50 psig at 70°F and contain about 4 to 7% propellant. Generally, a blend of propane and isobutane is used for foam aerosols. Contraceptive foam aerosols use A-31 as the propellant. Other foams use P-152a since it will produce a more stable foam and is less flammable than hydrocarbons. Other propellants that have been used include the compressed gases—nitrous oxide and carbon dioxide. Typical products include whipped creams and toppings and several pharmaceutical and veterinary products.

Aerosols using compressed gases as the propellant operate essentially as a pressure package. The pressure of the gas forces the product concentrate out of the container in essentially the same form as it was placed in the container. Only the product concentrate is expelled; the compressed gas remains in the container occupying the headspace. The pressure drops in the container as the product concentrate is removed and the gas expands to occupy the newly vacated space. The pressure will continue to drop as the product concentrate is expelled. Therefore, the initial pressure in these containers is higher than used in liquefied gas aerosols and is usually 90 to 100 psig at 70°F. The amount of product left in the container after the pressure is exhausted varies with the viscosity of the product and loss of pressure due to gas seepage.

Depending on the nature of the formulation and the type of compressed gas used, the product may be dispensed as a semisolid (solid stream) foam or spray. Semisolid aerosols are used to dispense more viscous concentrates such as dental creams, hair dressings, ointments, creams, cosmetic creams, and foods.

In barrier pack systems, the propellant is physically separated from the product concentrate. The propellant pressure on the outside of the barrier serves only to push the contents from the container. In the piston type system, a polyethylene piston is fitted into the container. The product concentrate is placed into the upper portion of the container and a compressed gas or hydrocarbon gas is placed on the other side of the piston. The gas pushes against the piston and pushes the product concentrate out of the container when the valve is actuated. As the rises in the container, it scrapes against the side of the container which helps dispense most of the product concentrate.

This system is used to dispense cheese spreads, cake decorating icings, and ointments. Since these product concentrates are semisolid and viscous, they emit from the container as a lazy stream rather than a foam or spray. The piston type system is limited to viscous materials since liquids tend to pass around the edges of the piston into the gas compartment.

A collapsible plastic bag fitted into a container is another type of barrier pack system. In some systems, the bag is a thin-walled aluminum pouch. The product concentrate is placed in the bag and the propellant surrounds the bag. The bag is accordion pleaded to prevent the gas from pinching it closed. These types of systems are used to dispense liquids as fine mists or streams, and semisolids as streams. These systems can also be used for topical creams, ointments, or gels.

Gels that foam after being dispensed are placed in both the piston type and collapsible plastic bag type of systems. The dispensed gel contains a low boiling liquid such as isopentane or pentane in it. The liquid will vaporized when the gel is placed in the warmth of the hands and this will produce the foaming gel.

The Valve Assembly

The effectiveness of a pharmaceutical aerosol depends on achieving the proper combination of product concentrate formulation, container, and valve assembly. The valve mechanism is the part of the product package through which the contents of the container are emitted. The valve must withstand the pressure required by the product concentrate and the container, be corrosive resistant, and must contribute to the form of the emitted product concentrate.

The primary purpose of the valve is to regulate the flow of product concentrate from the container. But the valve must also be multifunctional and regulate the amount of emitted material (metered valves), be capable of delivering the product concentrate in the desired form, and be easy to turn on and off. Among the materials used in the manufacture of the various valve parts are plastic, rubber, aluminum, and stainless steel (Fig. 5.6).

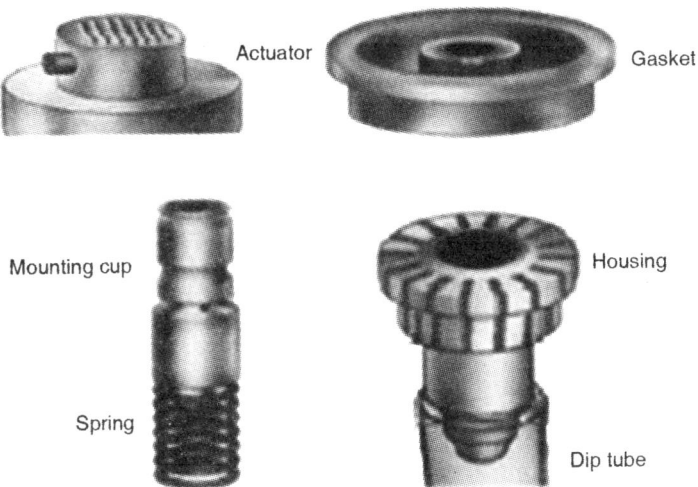

Fig. 5.6: Various parts of valve assembly of an aerosol

The basic parts of a valve assembly can be described as:

1. **Actuator:** The actuator is the button which the user presses to activate the valve assembly and provides an easy mechanism of turning the valve on and off. In some actuators, mechanical breakup devices are also included. It is the combination of the type and quantity of propellant used and the actuator design and dimensions that determine the physical form of the emitted product concentrate.

2. **Stem:** The stem supports the actuator and delivers the formulation in the proper form to the chamber of the actuator.

3. **Gasket:** The gasket, placed snugly with the stem, serves to prevent leakage of the formulation of the valve is in the closed position.

4. **Spring:** The spring holds the gasket in place and also is the mechanism by which the actuator retracts when pressure is released thereby returning the valve to the closed position.

5. **Mounting cup:** The mounting cup which is attached to the aerosol container serves to hold the valve in place. Because the undersigned of the mounting cup is exposed

to the formulation, it must receive the same consideration as the inner part of the container with respect to meeting criteria of compatibility. If necessary, it may be coated with an inert material to prevent an undesired interaction.

6. **Housing:** The housing located directly below the mounting cup serves as the link between the dip tube and the stem and actuator. With the stem, its orifice helps to determine the delivery rate and the form in which the product is emitted.

7. **Dip tube:** The dip tube which extends from the housing down into the product concentrate serves to bring the formulation from the container to the valve. The viscosity of the product and its intended delivery to rate dictate the inner dimensions of the dip tube and housing for a particular product.

Spray valves are used to obtain fine to coarse wet sprays. Depending on the formulation and the design of the valve and actuator, the particle size of the emitted spray can be varied. The spray is produced as an aerosol solution passes through a series of small orifices which open into chambers that allow the product concentrate to expand into the proper particle size.

Vapor tap valves are used with powder aerosols, water-based aerosols, aerosols containing suspended materials, and other agents that would tend to clog a standard valve. This valve is basically a standard valve except that a small hole has been placed into the valve housing. This allows vaporized propellant to be emitted along with the product concentrate and produces a spray with greater dispersion. These valves are used with aqueous and hydroalcoholic product concentrates and hydrocarbon propellants.

Foam valves have only one orifice that leads to a single expansion chamber. The expansion chamber also serves as the delivery nozzle or applicator. The chamber is the appropriate volume to allow the product concentrate to expand into a ball of foam. Foam valves are used for viscous product concentrates such as creams and ointments because of the large orifice and chamber. Foam valves also are used to dispense rectal and vaginal foams. If the size of the orifice and expansion chamber are appropriately reduced, a product concentrate that would produce a foam will be emitted as a solid stream. In this case, the ball of foam begins to develop where the stream impinges on a surface.

Metered dose inhaler (MDI) valves (metering values) are used to accurately deliver a dose of medication. Metered valves are used for all oral, inhalation, and nasal aerosols. The metered valves reproducibly deliver an amount of product concentrate accurately from the same package and also allow for the same accuracy between different packages.

The amount of material emitted is regulated by an auxiliary valve chamber of fixed capacity and dimensions. This metering chamber volume can be varied so that about 25 to 150 l of product concentrate is delivered per actuation. Access in and out of the metering chamber is controlled by a dual valve mechanism. When the actuator is closed, a seal blocks emission from the chamber to the atmosphere. However, the chamber is open to the contents of the container and it is filled. When the actuator is depressed, the seals reverse function; the chamber becomes open to the atmosphere and releases its contents and at the same time becomes sealed from the contents of the container. When the actuator is again closed, the system prepares for the next dose.

Two basic types of metering valves are available; one for inverted use and the other for upright use. Generally, the valves for upright use are used with solution type aerosols and contain a thin capillary dip tube. Suspension or dispersion aerosols use the valve intended for inverted use that does not contain a dip tube.

In general, valves should retain the material in the metering chamber for fairly long periods. However, it is possible for the material in the chamber to slowly return back to the container. The degree to which this occurs depends on the construction of the valve and length of time between actuations of the valves. Some valves have been fitted with a "drain tank" to overcome this problem.

Containers

Aerosol containers are generally made of glass, metals (e.g. tin-plated steel, aluminum, and stainless steel), and plastics. The selection of the container for a particular aerosol product is based on its adaptability to production methods, compatibility with the formulation, ability to sustain the pressure necessary for the product, the design and aesthetic appeal, and the cost.

Glass containers would be the preferred container for most aerosols. Glass presents fewer problems with respect to chemical compatibility with the formulation compared to metal containers and is not subject to corrosion. Glass is also more adaptive to design creativity and allows the user to view the level of contents in the container.

However, glass containers must be precisely engineered to provide the maximum pressure safety and impact resistance. Therefore, glass containers are used in products that have lower pressures and lower percentages of propellants. When the pressure is below 25 psig and less than 50% propellant is used, coated glass containers are considered safe (Table 5.5).

Table 5.5: Pressure limitations of aerosol containers

Container material	Maximum pressure (psig)	Temperature (°F)
Tin-plated steel	180	130
Uncoated glass	<18	70
Coated glass	<25	70
Aluminum	180	130
Stainless steel	180	130
Plastic	<25	70

To increase the resistance to breakage, plastic coatings are commonly applied to the outer surface of glass containers. These plastic coatings serve many purposes:

1. Prevent the glass from shattering into fragments, if broken.
2. Absorb shock from the crimping operation during production thus decreasing the danger of breakage around the neck.
3. Protect the contents from ultraviolet light.
4. Act as a means of identification since the coatings are available in various colors.

Glass containers range in sizes from 15 to 30 ml and are used primarily with solution aerosols. Glass containers are generally not used with suspension aerosols because the visibility of the suspended particles presents an esthetic problem. All commercially available containers have a 20 mm neck finish which adapts easily to metered valves.

Tin-plated steel containers are light weight and relatively inexpensive. For some products, the tin provides all the necessary protection. However, when required, special protective coatings are applied to the tin sheets prior to fabrication so that the inside of the container will be protected from corrosion and interaction between the tin and the formulation. The coating usually is an oleoresin, phenolic, vinyl, or epoxy coating. The tin-plated steel containers are used in topical aerosols.

Aluminum is used in most MDIs and many topical aerosols. This material is extremely light weight and is less reactive than other metals. Aluminum containers can coated with epoxy, vinyl, or phenolic resins to decrease the interaction between the aluminum and the formulation. The aluminum can also be anodized to form a stable coating of aluminum oxide. Most aluminum containers are manufactured by an impact extrusion process that make them seamless. Therefore, they have a greater safety against leakage, incompatibility, and corrosion.

Aluminum containers are made with a 20 mm neck finish that adapts to the metered valves. For special purposes and applications, containers are also available that have neck finishes ranging from 15 to 20 mm. The containers are available in sizes ranging from 10 ml to over 1,000 ml.

Stainless steel is used when the container must be chemically resistant to the product concentrate. The main limitation of these containers is their high cost.

Plastic containers have had limited success because of their inherent permeability problems to the vapor phase inside the container. Also, some drug–plastic interactions have limited the efficacy of the product.

Methods of Manufacturing

Two methods are used to manufacture aerosols: The cold fill process and the pressure fill process. The cold fill process takes advantage of the property that some ingredients will liquefy when cooled, and the pressure fill process uses the property that some ingredients will liquefy when placed under pressure.

In the cold fill process, both the product concentrate and the propellant must be cooled to temperatures between 30°C to 60°C where they will remain liquefied. The cooling system may be a mixture of dry ice and acetone or a elaborate refrigeration system. The chilled product concentrate is quantitatively added to the equally cold aerosol container and then the liquefied gas is added. The heavy vapors of the cold liquid propellant will generally displace the air present in the container. When filling is complete, the valve assembly is inserted into the container and crimped into place. The container is then passed through a water bath of about 55°C to check for leaks or distortion in the container.

Aqueous solutions cannot be filled by this process since the water will turn to ice in the low temperatures. For non-aqueous systems, some moisture usually appears in the final product due to the condensation of atmospheric moisture within the cold containers.

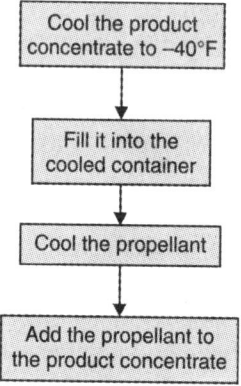

Pressure filling is carried out essentially at room temperature. The product concentrate is placed in the container, the valve assembly is inserted and crimped into place, and then the liquefied gas, under pressure, is added through the valve. The entrapped air in the package might be ignored, if it does not interfere with the stability of the product, or it may be evacuated prior to filling or during filling. After the filling operation is complete, the valve is tested for proper function. This spray testing also rids the dip tube of pure propellant prior to consumer use. Pressure filling is used for most pharmaceutical aerosols. It has the advantage that there is less danger of moisture contamination of the product and also less propellant is lost in the process.

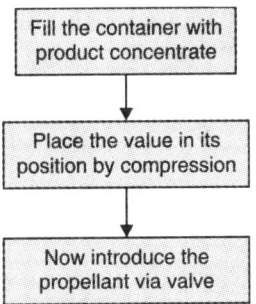

Fill the container with product concentrate

↓

Place the value in its position by compression

↓

Now introduce the propellant via valve

Aerosols are used to deliver active drugs to the pulmonary airways, the nasal passages, or the oral cavity. They are also used to administer drugs topically and into body cavities such as the vagina and rectum. Pulmonary, nasal, and oral administration is intended to achieve either local or systemic therapeutic effect, while topical, vaginal, and rectal administration is only intended for local effect. Inhalation therapy (i.e. drug delivery to the pulmonary airways and nasal passages) was once accomplished using nebulizers or atomizers that were cumbersome to use and restricted to institutional or home use. The development of the metered dose inhaler in the mid 1950s provided the convenience of portability with the accuracy of dosing. Successful inhalation therapy requires that the formulation emit droplets or particles that are the optimum size. Large particles (about 20 μm) deposit in the back of the mouth and throat and are eventually swallowed rather than inhaled. Particles in the 1 to 10 μm range will reach the bronchioles. Very small particles (0.6 μm) penetrate to the alveolar sacs but have limited retention since a large fraction of the particles are exhaled in the breath. The most therapeutically effective particle size range appears to be between 3 and 6 μm. Therefore, it is important that the aerosol system produce most of its particles between approximately 1 and 10 μm. MDIs are the most commonly used product for inhalation therapy and is also one of the most difficult dosage forms to administer properly. One of the most critical maneuvers during administration is to coordinate the actuation of the aerosol with the patient's inspiration. The mouthpiece adapter on the aerosol package has been repeatedly modified since the mid 1970s in an attempt to help patients receive the correct dosage when this coordination is not performed correctly. Larger adapters (sometimes called tube spacers) permit the propellant to completely evaporate before the aerosol reaches the patient. This results in a reduced particle size and velocity. The reduced particle size improves the depth to which the drug will penetrate into the lungs and the lower velocity decreases the amount of drug that will impact on the back of the throat. The biggest disadvantages of these larger adapters are the cost, difficulty to clean, and inconvenience to use because of their size. Nasal aerosols deliver the drug directly to the nasal mucosa. The most common nasal aerosols contain steroids used to treat nasal congestion, sneezing, and running nose associated with hay fever, allergies, and rhinitis. Such products use steroids such as beclomethasone dipropionate, triamcinolone acetonide, dexamethasone sodium phosphate, and budesonide. Aerosols used to deliver drugs to the oral cavity generally administer the product sublingually. One such product is a sublingual nitroglycerin formulation that is sprayed under the tongue and delivers 0.4 mg of nitroglycerin per actuation. Topical aerosol formulations are available for local anesthetics, antiseptics, germicides, first aid preparations, and spray on protective films. These aerosols deliver particles that are larger and more course than the inhalation aerosols. Topical aerosols deliver the active drug in the form of a powder, a wet spray, a stream of liquid, or an ointment like product. Vaginal and rectal foams are available that contain estrogens, contraceptives, and anti-inflammation agents. These products are packaged in containers that have an application device which is filled with foam when the valve is actuated and then the device is placed in the vagina or rectum and the foam is instilled with the device plunger.

Gas molecules travel in random paths and collide with one another and the walls of their container. These collisions exert a pressure per unit area and also cause the gases to occupy a volume. Both the pressure and volume are affected by temperature. The interrelationships between these three variables were formulated by Boyle, Charles, and Gay-Lussac, and can be applied to pharmaceutical aerosols.

Boyle's law states that:

$$P \propto \frac{1}{V} \text{ when temperature does not change}$$

and   PV = K

where V = the volume (ml or L)

P = the pressure (atm)

K = the proportionality constant

Charles's or Guy-Lussac's law states that:

$V \propto T$ when pressure does not change

and   V = KT

where T = the absolute temperature ($^{\circ}$K)

If two sets of conditions (i.e. P, V, and T) are being considered, equations can be combined to obtain the relationship:

$$\frac{P_2 V_2}{T_2} = \frac{P_1 V_1}{RT_1}$$

where the subscripts 1 and 2 refer to the two different conditions. Although the P, V, and T of each condition may be different, the ratio $\frac{V_1}{V_2}$ is constant and can be mathematically expressed as R, where R = the constant value of the ratio.

The above equation is derived considering only 1 mole (i.e. one gram molecular weight) of ideal gas. If n moles of gas were to be considered, it becomes:

$$PV = nRT$$

which is known as the general ideal gas law. R is the molar gas constant and is used with many different units depending on the mathematical application: 8.314 J/$^{\circ}$K/mole, 0.08205 L atm/$^{\circ}$K/mole, and 1.987 cal/$^{\circ}$K/mole.

The relevance of the gas laws to pharmaceutical aerosols can be seen in the following examples.

Example: What is the weight of nitrogen in an 8 fluid ounces aerosol container filled with 6 fluid ounces of viscous ointment?

The container is pressurized to 90 psig and the temperature is 25°C.

Determine the following values: Fluid ounce, volume, pressure, and temperature.

Fluid ounce = 29.57 ml. Volume of gas is 29.57 ml × 2 = 59.14 ml

Pressure (psia) = pressure (psig) + 14.7. Pressure of gas is 90.0 + 14.7 = 104.7 psia

Pressure (atm) = pressure (psia)/14.7 = 104.7/14.7 = 7.1 atm

Temperature (°K) = 273.2 + degrees °C = 273.2 to 25 = 298.2°K

From a rearrangement of the General Ideal Gas Law

$$n = \frac{P_2}{104.7 \text{ psia}} = \frac{n_a}{n_a + n_b} = 0.017 \text{ mole}$$

Converting the number of moles to a weight can be done using the atomic weight of nitrogen (i.e. 14) and its valence which is 2:

weight of nitrogen = (0.017 mole) (14 g/mole) (2) = 0.476 g

Example: If 3 fluid ounces of the aerosol is dispensed, what is the resulting pressure in the container?

The stated equation can be rearranged noting that $T_1 = T_2$ (i.e. temperature has not changed), setting V_1 and P_1 to the initial values for the container (i.e. 2 fluid ounces of gases), and solving for V_2 and P_2 after the container was emitted 3 fluid ounces (i.e. there is now 5 fluid ounces of gas):

$$\frac{n_b}{n_a + n_b} = P_{total}$$

$$\frac{70 \text{ g}}{137.38 \text{ g/mole}} = \frac{30 \text{ g}}{120.93 \text{ g/mole}}$$

$P_2 = 41.9 \text{ psia} = 27.2 \text{ psig}$

Example: What is the pressure remaining in the container when all of the product has been dispensed?

As in the previous example, the stated equation can be used. However, the gas now occupies 8 fluid ounces.

$$P_{11}^0 = \frac{0.5095 \text{ mole}}{0.5095 \text{ mole} + 0.2481 \text{ mole}}$$

$P_2 = 26.2 \text{ psia} = 11.5 \text{ psig}$

A liquefied gas propellant can be considered as a solution. Molecules of the solution will have escape tendencies will create a vapor pressure above the solution. According to Raoult's law, if a solute is added to a solvent, the solvent vapor pressure will be decreased proportional to the mole fraction of the solute added. If the added solute has an appreciable vapor pressure itself, its vapor pressure will also be decreased as the result of its dilution in the solvent. The total vapor pressure of a mixture of propellants can be determined as the sum of the partial pressures of each component (Dalton's law). The partial pressure of a component can be determined as the mole fraction of the component multiplied by the vapor pressure of the pure compound. If propellant a and b are mixed, the partial pressures can be calculated as:

$$pa = \frac{n_{12}}{n_{11} + n_{12}} \quad \frac{0.2481 \text{ mole}}{0.5095 \text{ mole} + 0.2481 \text{ mole}}$$

$$pb = \frac{n_b}{n_a + n_b} \, p_b^0$$

where pa and pb = partial pressure of propellants a and b

n_a and n_b = mole fraction of propellants a and b

and = vapor pressure of pure propellants a and b

The total vapor pressure of the aerosol would be the sum of the two partial pressures calculated above:

$$P_{total} = pa + pb$$

Example: What is the vapor pressure of a mixture of propellants 11 and 12 in a 70 g to 30 g ratio?

Chemical name	Chemical formula	Numerical designation	Vapor pressure 70°F (psia)	Molecular weight
Trichloromono-fluoromethane	CCl_3F	11	13.4	137.38
Dichlorodifluoro-methane	CCl_2F_2	12	84.9	120.93

Determine the mole fractions of each propellant.

$$p11 = \frac{n_{11}}{n_{11} + n_{11}} \; p_{11}^0 \; \frac{0.5095 \text{ mole}}{0.5095 \text{ mole} + 0.2481 \text{ mole}} \; 13.4 \text{ psia}$$

$$= 9.01 \text{ psia}$$

$$p12 = \frac{n_{12}}{n_{11} + n_{12}} \; p_{12}^0 \; \frac{0.2481 \text{ mole}}{0.5095 \text{ mole} + 0.2481 \text{ mole}} \; 84.9 \text{ psia}$$

$$= 27.8 \text{ psia}$$

The total vapor pressure for the propellant mixture will be:

$P_{total} = p11 + p12 = (9.01 + 27.8) \text{ psia} = 36.81 \text{ psia or } 22.11 \text{ psig.}$

ISOLATED KEY POINTS

- *A pharmaceutical aerosol* is defined as a system that depends on the power of a compressed or liquefied gas to expel the contents from the container or pressurized dosage form, containing one or more active ingredients, which upon actuation emit a fine dispersion of liquid and solid materials in gaseous medium.

- *Components of aerosol package:* (i) Propellant; (ii) Container; (iii) Valve and actuator; (iv) Product concentrate. Advantages: 1. A dose can be removed without contami-nation of remaining materials. 2. The medication can be delivered directly to the affected area in a desired form such as spray, stream, quick-breaking foam or stable form. 3. Irritation produced by mechanical application of topical medication is reduced or eliminated. 4. Ease, convenience of application of medication in a thin layer.

- *Propellants*: Propellant is responsible for developing the proper pressure within the container, and it expels the product when the valve is opened and aids in the atomization or foam production of the product. Types of propellants: i. Liquid gas propellant: A. Chlorofluoro-carbons; 1. Trichloromonofluoromethane or propellant 11. 2. Dichlorofluoromethane or propellant 12. 3. Dichlorotetra fluoroethane or propellant 114. B. Hydrocarbons: 1. Butane, 2. Isobutane, 3. Propane.

- *Compressed gas propellant:* 1. Nitrogen, 2. Oxygen. 3. Carbondioxide.
- *Containers:* They must be stand at pressure as high as 140 to 180 psig. Types of containers: 1. Tin plate containers consists of sheet of steel plate that has been electroplated on both sides with tin. 2. Aluminum containers greater resistance to corrosion, light weight, good for light sensitive drugs. 3. Stainless steel container limited for smaller size, extremely strong and resistant to most materials pressure stand. 4. Glass containers available with plastic or without plastic coating compatible with many additives no corrosion problems can have various shape because of molding not for light sensitive drugs.
- *Valves and actuator:* Valves are important for aerosols containers as they help in expelling the contents from the container. The performance of the aerosol depends on the type of formulation and valve they regulate the flow of the product and discharge the desired amount, the valve helps the loss of product when the container is not in use. With the help of actuator present on the valve, the foam product present in the container can dispensed in the form of spray or wet stream the type of product formed, i.e. foam spray or wet stream depends on the proper selection of propellant during formulation.
- Actuators to ensure that aerosol product is delivered in the proper and desired form. Different types of actuators: Spray actuators, foam actuators, solid steam actuators, mist actuators.
- *Metered dose inhalers (mdis):* Metered dose inhalers are pharmaceutical delivery systems designed for oral or nasal use, which deliver discrete doses of aerosolized medicament to the respiratory tract, e.g. salbutamol 100–200 µg, terbutaline sulfate 250–500 µg, sodium chromoglycate 5 mg. The metering valve is placed in inverted position. Depression of the valve stem allows the content of the metering chamber refill with liquid from the bulk is ready to dispense next dose.
- *Types of aerosol system:* There are four types of aerosol system: Solution system/two-phase system, water-based

system/three-phase system, suspension or dispersion system, foam system—aqueous stable foam, non-aqueous stable foam, quick breaking foam, thermal foam.

- *Manufacture of pharmaceutical aerosols:* 1. Pressure filling apparatus; 2. Cold filling apparatus; 3. Compressed gas filling apparatus.

- Pressure filling product concentrate is placed in aerosol container. Valve assembly is inserted. Liquefied gas (propellant) is metered under pressure by means of pressure burette into the container. The desired amount of propellant is allowed to flow through the aerosol valve into the container under its own vapor pressure. When the pressure is equalized between the burette and the container, the propellant stops flowing. Additional propellant is added with compressed air (N_2, CO_2, NO) to increase pressure of the propellant in the container. Trapped air inside the container was evacuated.

- *Cold filling:* The principle of cold filling method requires the chilling of all components including concentrate and propellant to a temperature of -30 to $-40°F$. This temperature is necessary to liquefy the propellant gas. The cooling system may be a mixture of dry ice and acetone or refrigeration system. First, the product concentrate is chilled and filled into already chilled container followed by the chilled liquefied propellant. The heavy vapor of the cold liquid propellant generally displaces the air in the container.

- Compressed gas filling product concentrate is placed in the container. Valve assembly is inserted. Air is evacuated from the container by a vacuum pump. Compressed gas is passed into the container. When pressure is equal to the pre-determined and regulated pressure, the gas flow stops.

- *Evaluation of pharmaceutical aerosols:* a. Flammability and combustibility: 1. Flame projection; 2. Flash point; b. Physicochemical characteristics: 1. Vapor pressure; 2. Density; 3. Moisture; 4. Identification of propellants performance; 5. Aerosol valve discharge rate; 6. Spray patterns; 7. Dosage with metered valves; 8. Net contents; 9. Foam stability; 10. Particle size determination;

11. Leakage. c. Biological testing: 1. Therapeutic activity; Toxicity

- *Spray pattern:* Spray the product on the coated (dye + talc) paper. Depending upon the nature of aerosol, water/oil soluble dye is used.

- Dosage with metered valves weigh accurately the filled container. Dispense no. of doses. Reweigh the container and calculate the weight difference. Weight diff/no. of times dose dispensed gives avg. dose. We should note the time of the each dose dispensed also. Dose is measured in gm/sec.

- *Net content:* The difference in the weight of the full container and tarred container gives the content in the container. Net wt = gross wt. – tare wt.

LONG ANSWER TYPE QUESTIONS

Q 1. Define the term aerosols. What are their advantages and disadvantages?

Q 2. What are different components of an aerosol product? Discuss in brief the significance of each product.

Q 3. What are propellants? Discuss in detail the use of various types of propellants.

Q 4. Explain how the name of trichloromonofluoromethane (CCl_3F) is derived.

Q 5. Discuss in detail the various methods used for the manufacture of aerosol.

Q 6. Write short notes on the following:
   a. Compressed gases
   b. Product concentrates
   c. Basic parts of a valve assembly
   d. Containers
   e. Metered dose inhaler

Q 7. Write down the full forms of the followings
   1. CFC
   2. HFC
   3. HCFC

OBJECTIVE TYPE QUESTIONS

1. .... are defined as the products containing therapeutically active ingredients dissolved, suspended or emulsified in a propellant or a mixture of solvent and propellant and intended for oral or topical administration into body cavities.

2. An aerosol formulation consists of two major components firstly the .... and the...................

3. MDIs stand for ....

4. .... is responsible for developing the proper pressure within the container of the aerosol and it expels the product when the valve is opened and aids in the atomization or foam production of the product.

5. .... are pharmaceutical delivery systems designed for oral or nasal use, which deliver discrete doses of aerosolized medicament to the respiratory tract. Types of aerosol system: There are four types of aerosol system: solution system/two-phase system, water-based system/three-phase system, suspension or dispersion system, foam system—aqueous stable foam, non-aqueous stable foam, quick breaking foam and thermal foam.

6. Net content is the difference in the weight of .... and .... of the container in an aerosol system.

ANSWERS

1. Aerosols
2. Product concentrate, propellant
3. Metered dose inhaler
4. Propellant
5. MDI (metered dose inhaler)
6. Gross weight, tare weight

Cosmetology and Cosmetic Preparations

INTRODUCTION

Cosmetics are substances used to enhance the appearance or odor of the human body. They are generally mixtures of chemical compounds, some being derived from natural sources, many being synthetic.

In the US, the Food and Drug Administration (FDA) which regulates cosmetics, defines cosmetics as "intended to be applied to the human body for cleansing, beautifying, promoting attractiveness, or altering the appearance without affecting the body's structure or functions." This broad definition includes, as well, any material intended for use as a component of a cosmetic product.

Before understanding cosmetic products application and composition, it is important to understand structure of skin.

STRUCTURE AND FUNCTIONS OF THE SKIN

Skin Structure (Fig. 6.1)

The skin is the largest organ of the body. It has three main layers:

1. The epidermis
2. The dermis
3. The subcutaneous layer.

Epidermis

The epidermis is an elastic layer on the outside that is continually being regenerated. It includes the following:

Keratinocytes: Keratinocytes are the main cells of the epidermis formed by cell division at its base. New cells continually move towards the surface. As they move, they gradually die and become flattened.

Corneocytes: Corneocytes are the flattened dead keratinocytes that together make up the very outer layer of the epidermis is called the stratum corneum or horny layer. This protective layer is continually worn away or shed.

Melanocytes: Melanocytes produce the pigment melanin that protects against UV radiation and gives skin its color.

Dermis

The dermis is the inner layer that includes the following:

Sweat glands: They produce sweat that travels via sweat ducts to openings in the epidermis called pores. They play a role in temperature regulation.

Hair follicles: They are pits in which hairs grow. Hairs also play a role in temperature regulation.

Sebaceous glands: They produce sebum (an oil) to keep hairs free from dust and bacteria. Sebum and sweat make up the 'surface film'.

Subcutaneous Layer

The subcutaneous layer under the dermis is made up of connective tissue and fat (a good insulator).

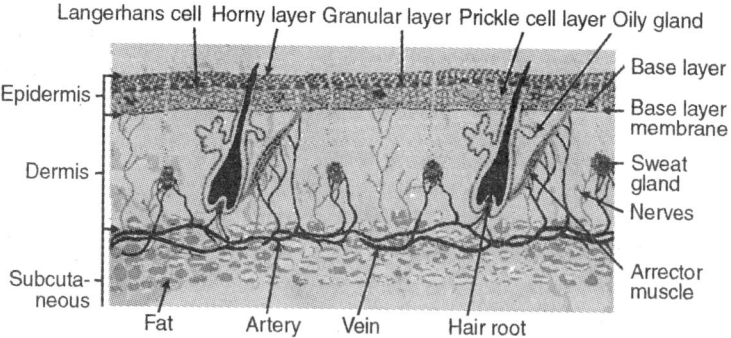

Fig. 6.1: Different layers of skin (i.e. epidermis, dermis and subcutaneous)

This skin diagram (Fig. 6.2) clearly shows all the layers of skin. We will now go over the skins layers in more detail.

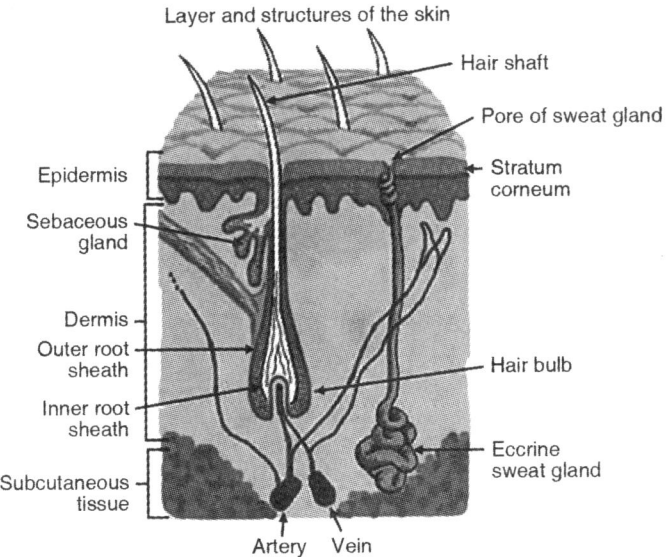

Fig. 6.2: Skin diagram

Epidermis Layer

As can be seen in the skin diagram (Fig. 6.2), the outermost layer of the skin is called the epidermis layer. There are no blood vessels in the epidermis but its deepest layer is supplied with lymph fluid. It is thickest in the palms and on the bottom of the feet.

There are various layers of cells within the epidermis, the outermost of which is called the stratum corneum (or horny layer). These can be clearly seen in the diagram of skin (Fig. 6.2). This surface layer is composed of 25 to 30 sublayers of flattened scale-like cells. These are continually being cast off by friction and replaced by the cells of the deeper epidermal layers. This surface layer is considered the real protective layer of the skin. These cells are commonly called keratinized cells because the living matter inside the cell (termed protoplasm) is changed to a protein (keratin) that helps to give the skin its protective properties.

New skin cells are formed in the deepest layer within the epidermis. This area is called the stratum germinativum. The new cells will gradually move towards the outer layers of the skin as the stratum corneum is abraded or shed. The new cells gradually change in form as they move upward to the outer layers, becoming keratinized in the process.

Dermis or Corium Layer

The dermis is a tough and elastic layer containing white fibrous tissue interlaced with yellow elastic fibers. As you can see in the skin diagram (Fig. 6.2), many structures are embedded in the dermis including:

- Lymphatic capillaries and vessels
- Blood vessels
- Sweat glands and their ducts
- Sebaceous glands
- Sensory nerve endings
- The arrectores pilorum (or arrector pilli), involuntary muscles are sometimes activated in cold weather to give 'goose bumps'
- Hair follicles, hair bulbs and hair roots.

Hypodermis or Subcutaneous Layer

This is the deepest of the layers of skin, and is located on the bottom of the skin diagram (Fig. 6.2). It connects or binds the dermis above it to the underlying organs. This layer is mainly composed of loose fibrous connective tissue and fat (adipose) cells interlaced with blood vessels. In females, the hypodermis is generally about 8% thicker than in males. The main functions of the hypodermis include insulation, storing of lipids, cushioning of the body and temperature regulation.

Functions of the Skin

1. Protects the body against physical injury.
2. Provides some protection for the body against numerous pathogenic microbes and chemical agents.
3. Helps to restrict fluid and water loss.
4. Helps to prevent excessive water absorption by imparting water resistance to the skin.

5. Is involved in temperature regulation of the body.
6. Is the body's main sensory organ for temperature, pressure, touch and pain.
7. Provides protection from UV light.
8. Plays a key role in metabolism, including vitamin D synthesis and biotransformation of some chemicals. Lack of vitamin D can lead to soft bones and many associated problems.
9. Energy storage in the form of fat.

The cosmetics are mainly external or topical preparations and are meant to be applied to external parts of the body. In other words, they may be applied to skin, hair and nails for the purposes of covering, coloring, softening, cleansing, nourishing, waving, setting, mollification, preservation, removal and protection.

Types of Skin

There are five basic skin types, including:

1. Normal Skin

This type of skin has a fine, even and smooth surface due to having an ideal balance between oil and moisture contents and is, therefore, neither greasy nor dry. People who have normal skin have small, barely-visible pores. Thus, their skin appears clear and does not develop spots and blemishes. This type of skin needs minimal and gentle treatment.

2. Dry Skin

Dry skin has a parched appearance and tends to flake easily. It is prone to wrinkles and lines due to the inability to retain moisture, as well as, the inadequate production of sebum by sebaceous glands. Dry skin often has problems in cold weather as it dries up even further. Constant protection in the form of a moisturizer by day and a moisture-rich cream by night is essential.

3. Oily Skin

As its name implies, this type of skin's surface is slightly to moderately greasy, which is caused by the over secretion of sebum. The excess oil on the surface of the skin draws dirt and dust from the environment to stick to it. Oily skin is usually prone to black heads, white heads, spots and pimples. It needs to be cleansed thoroughly every day.

4. Combination Skin

This is the most common type of skin. As the name suggests, it is a combination of both oily and dry skin where certain areas of the face are oily and the rest dry. The oily parts are usually found on a central panel, called T-zone, consisting of the forehead, nose and chin. The dry areas consist of the cheeks and the areas around the eyes and mouth. In such cases, each part of the face should be treated accordingly where the dry areas are treated as for dry skin and the central panel is treated as for oily skin. There are also skin care products made especially for those who have combination skin.

5. Sensitive Skin

Sensitive skin has a very fine texture and is excessively sensitive to changes in the climate. This skin type is easily irritated, bruised and/or scarred from bleaching, waxing, threading, perfumes, temperature extremes, soap, shaving creams, etc. People who belong to this skin type should avoid products with dyes, perfumes, or unnecessary chemical ingredients that may aggravate the skin.

General Purpose of Skin Care Products

Cleansing

Cleansing is the first essential step to any daily skin care routine. Cleansing the face at least twice a day is suitable for normal skin. If skin is oily, a more frequent cleansing or about four to five times a day is required. However, products that are water-based and gentle are ideal so as to not overdry the skin. For dry skin, it is best to avoid frequent washing and a suitable oil-based cosmetic cleanser instead of soap is preferred. There are several alternatives to soap and water cleansing. Cleansers can be in the form of creams, milks, lotions, gels and liquids. All are a mixture of oil, wax and water which have been formulated to suit different skin types. A cotton-pad dipped in fresh milk available at home, is an equally effective natural cleanser. To complete the cleansing process, the skin must be rinsed with water. Some who wear long wearing foundation may find it beneficial to pre-cleanse the face with a cleansing oil to remove any silicones left over from the foundation.

Masks

Essentially, all facemasks have some sort of a cleansing action. Various ingredients are used in the masks, depending on the skin type. Clay forms an important constituent of many face masks that helps to remove dirt, sebum, and dead skin to refresh and soften the skin surface. Fullers earth is a special type of clay often used in face packs. It contains aluminum silicate and as it dries on the skin, it absorbs the superficial dead cells and blots up any excessive oil. It is, therefore, excellent for oily skin but should not be used on dry skin. Kaolin is also a fine clay which removes grime, oils and dead cells. Again it is best for oily skin and should be avoided on dry skin. Another ingredient of some of the masks is a peeling or exfoliating agent which helps remove the top layer of dead cells from the skin, leaving behind fresh youthful skin. Oatmeal and bran are the commonly used peelers. In addition, natural ingredients such as cucumbers, curds, lemon juice and Brewer's yeast are added to many masks to restore the acid/alkali balance of the skin. There are three general forms that masks come in: Clay, Peel, and sheet. The clay formulation is one of the most common. It is usually composed of different clays to draw out the impurities in the skin. Peel masks usually have a gel-like consistency and are peeled off of the skin to help exfoliate. Sheet masks are becoming more common in America, they are very popular in Asia. Sheet masks can be used to treat different skin concerns, but one of the most popular concerns is skin brightening.

Toning

Many skin care products include skin fresheners, toners and astringents which generally contain alcohol and water. These products are used after cleansing the skin to freshen and tone up and remove any traces of dirt or impurities from the skin, as well as restore the skin's acid/alkali balance. Non-alcoholic fresheners are for dry and sensitive skin. Those with alcohol (astringent) are for oily skin. People with combination skin should use both kinds for the different areas of their face.

Moisturizing

Regular use of a suitable moisturizer benefits the skin as it not only replaces water lost from the skin but also prevents the loss of water. It protects the skin against the drying influences of the environment including the harsh effects of the sun, cold and heat. Tinted moisturizers can be used under foundation cosmetics. It allows make-up to remain moist. Using a moisturizer is particularly beneficial for dry skins. Oil free moisturizers are also available for oily skins. There are two types of moisturizers: Oil-in water emulsions and water-in-oil emulsions. For normal and combination skin, a water-based moisturizer containing mineral oil is suitable. Sensitive and dry types of skin need moisturizers containing a high content of oil.

Protecting

The sun is the most damaging environmental factor to the health and appearance of skin. Ultraviolet radiation from sunlight can cause permanent damage to the skin causing it to sag, lose elasticity and form wrinkles. Severe sunburn can even cause skin cancer. Therefore, sunscreen and SPF-foundations protect the skin against these damaging effects. They also shield the skin from direct contact with dirt or pollutants in the air and help the skin retain necessary moisture. Sunscreen's come in lotions and creams. A sunscreen with the sun protection factor (SPF) of number 15 can block most of the sun's ultraviolet radiations before it can damage the skin. The SPF number indicates the length of time that the product will protect the skin, i.e. 15 hours. Sunscreens should be applied at least 10 minutes before exposure to the sun to ensure proper absorption and effective protection.

CLASSIFICATION OF COSMETICS

1. Skin cosmetics
2. Hair cosmetics

3. Nails cosmetics
4. Oral hygiene cosmetics

All cosmetics are formulated as solids, semisolids or liquids. Their formula design is very similar to drug dosage forms.

SKIN COSMETICS

Skin cosmetics include:
1. Powder
2. Lipstick
3. Cold cream
4. Shaving preparation
5. Antiperspirant and deodorant

Powder

Face Powder (Fig. 6.3)

Face powder is basically a cosmetic product which has as its prime function, the ability to complement skin color by imparting a velvet finish to it (Table 6.1).

Desired characteristics or attributes of face powder:

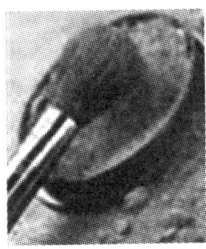

Fig. 6.3: Face powder

1. It should produce a smooth finish to the facial skin.
2. Mask visible imperfections of the face.
3. Shine due to moisture or grease from perspiration or secretion of sebaceous and sweat glands or from preparations used on the skin.
4. The powder must produce a lasting effect, so that frequent application is unnecessary.
5. The preparation should make the face pleasant to look and touch. The degree of opacity can vary from opaque, in case of clown make-up, to almost transparent.

6. It must adhered to the skin and be reasonably resistant to the mixed secretion of the skin.

Table 6.1: Formulae of face powders

Ingredients	% w/w
Talc	50–70
Kaolin	15–25
Calcium carbonate (light)	5–7
Zinc oxide	5–9
Zinc stearate	2–8
Magnesium carbonates	0.5–1.5
Color	0.1–0.9
Perfume	0.1–0.9

Note: The said range and composition stated in this example and examples there of, can vary on the discretion of formulation scientist and product requirement.

Manufacturing process: The preparation of powders is simple as it is simply a matter of dry mixing of finely powdered materials. Add the perfume with part of the absorbent materials like calcium carbonate or with magnesium carbonate and keep it aside for some time. Mix the color with part of the talc properly and add the other powders and then the perfume mixture. Mix and sieve the powder mixture using a silk mesh or an old washed nylon cloth (Flow chart 6.1).

Flow chart 6.1: Manufacturing process of face powder

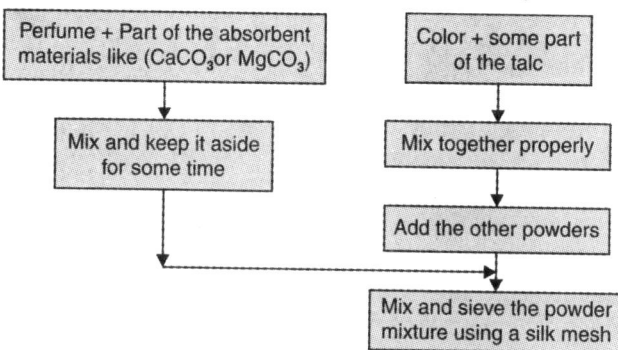

Body Powder

Amongst the various cosmetics, body powder is one of the widely consumed cosmetic preparations. Body powders are also known as talcum powders or dusting powders.

Purpose of using body powder: The main use of body powders or talcum powders is to absorb moisture or perspiration specifically after bathing particularly in warmer countries. These also provide good slip, a cooling effect and efficient lubrication, and prevent irritation of skin due to chafing. The very fine particle size of these covers a large surface area per unit weight and can cover a large body area which results in strong light dispersion and, therefore, visual covering of the skin underneath.

The surface covered by the powders is much more than the surface uncovered which leads to a cooling effect, if the ingredients of the powder have good heat conductivity. These fine powder particles with light weight adhere to the skin by the stickiness of the fat film.

Composition of body powder

Normally, they contain covering material, adhesives, absorbency material, slip, antiseptics and perfumes.

Body powders consist mainly of talc, with small proportions of a metallic stearate like zinc stearate, aluminium stearate, etc., and precipitated calcium carbonate (chalk) or magnesium carbonate (light). For antiseptic action, boric acid, chloro-hexidine diacetate, bithional, etc. are used to suppress proliferation of microorganism responsible for development of perspiration odor. Talcum powders containing antiseptic substances are also used for prickly heat and fungus infections (Table 6.2).

Table 6.2: Formulae of body powder

Ingredients	% w/w
Talc	60–80
Colloidal kaolin	10–20
Colloidal silica	5–7
Magnesium carbonates	2–6
Aluminum stearate	2–6
Boric acid	0.2–0.6
Perfume	0.4–0.8

Manufacturing process

Mix the perfume oil with magnesium carbonate properly and keep it aside for some time. Mix other ingredients together properly and add the perfumed magnesium carbonate to this mixture. Mix properly, then sieve and pack it in containers (Flow chart 6.2).

Flow chart 6.2: Manufacturing process of body powder

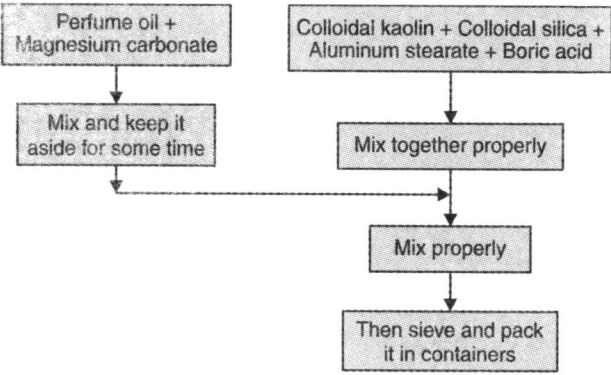

Lipsticks (Fig. 6.4)

Lipsticks also termed lip cosmetics are widely used by women. Lipsticks are basically dispersions of coloring matter in a base consisting of a suitable blend of oils, fats, and waxes suitably perfumed and flavored, molded in the form of a stick and enclosed in a case.

A lipstick should have the following characteristics:

1. It should cover the lips adequately with some gloss and last for long time.
2. It should make the lips soft.

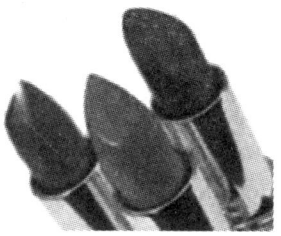

Fig. 6.4: Lipsticks

3. The film must adhere firmly to the lips without being brittle and tacky.
4. It should have high retention of color intensity without any change in shade.
5. It should be completely free from grittiness and be non-drying.
6. It should be non-irritating to the skin of lips.

Table 6.3: Formulae of lipstick

Ingredients	% w/w
Carnauba wax	3–4
Candelilla wax	4–6
Ozokerite wax	3–4
Beeswax	4–6
Lanolin	6–8
Castor oil	40–60
Isopropyl myristate	4–6
Halogenated fluorosceins	1–3
Lake colors	15–19
Propyl-p-hydroxy benzoate	0.1–0.5
Perfume	0.6–0.8

Manufacturing Process (Flow chart 6.3)

1. The lake colors are first dispersed by mixing with suitable quantity (as 25% w/w) of castor oil.
2. The color paste obtained is passed through a triple roll mill until it is smooth and free from agglomerates and gritty particles. If titanium dioxide is used in the formula, the same is also made into a paste similarly and mixed with the color mix.
3. The color mixture is then mixed with the bromo-acid mixture.
4. All the ingredients of the base are identified and arranged in order of increasing melting point. The lower melting point fats and waxes are next melted together and mixed with colors and bromo mixtures at the same temperature. This mixture is re-milled until perfectly smooth.
5. The preservative and antioxidant are dissolved in any remaining oil and added to the mixture.
6. The high melting point waxes are now melted and added to the bulk at the same temperature.

Flow chart 6.3: Manufacturing process of lipsticks

```
┌─────────────────────┐
│  Lake colors +      │
│ castor oil (25% w/w)│
└─────────────────────┘
          │
          ▼
┌─────────────────────┐
│  Mix them properly  │
└─────────────────────┘
          │
          ▼
┌─────────────────────┐
│    Color paste      │
└─────────────────────┘
          │
          ▼
┌─────────────────────┐         ┌─────────────────────┐
│  Passed through     │         │ Lower melting point │
│  a triple roll mill │         │   fats and waxes    │
└─────────────────────┘         └─────────────────────┘
          │                               │
          ▼                               ▼
┌─────────────────────┐         ┌─────────────────────┐
│    Mixed with       │         │   Melted together   │
│ bromo-acid mixture  │         └─────────────────────┘
└─────────────────────┘
          │                               │
          └───────────────┬───────────────┘
                          ▼
          ┌─────────────────────────┐      ┌──────────────────────────────┐
          │ Mix them properly at    │◄─────│ Add preservative and antioxidant│
          │ same temperature.       │      │ (dissolved in any remaining oil)│
          │ Mixture is re-milled    │      └──────────────────────────────┘
          └─────────────────────────┘
                          │
                          ▼
          ┌─────────────────────┐      ┌──────────────────────────┐
          │  Mix them properly  │◄─────│ Add melted high melting  │
          └─────────────────────┘      │       point wax's        │
                          │            └──────────────────────────┘
                          ▼
          ┌─────────────────────┐
          │ Apply gentle stirring│
          └─────────────────────┘
                          │
                          ▼
          ┌─────────────────────┐
          │    Pour it in       │
          │ lubricated molds    │
          └─────────────────────┘
```

7. The perfume is finally added and the mass stirred thoroughly but gently to avoid entrapment of air.

8. The mass should not be melted after the high melting point waxes have been added.

9. Gentle stirring is continued until the mass is homogeneous and it is then poured in lubricated molds.

Cold Cream (Fig. 6.5)

Cold cream is water-in-oil type of emulsion. Cold cream is called cold cream because breaking up of emulsion on application to skin leads to evaporation of water giving cooling effect. Cold cream is primarily used to prevent excessive drying of skin. It has emollient action and prevents dehydration of skin. The key chemical constituent of cold cream is beeswax.

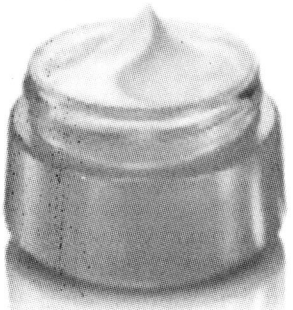

Fig. 6.5: Cold cream

Emulsifier usually prepared inside by reaction between borax and beeswax stabilizes cold cream emulsion. Beeswax, spermacitin, paraffin wax are used as thickening agent and also provide fatty acid soap formation during the preparation of cold cream. Non-ionic and ionic emulsifiers are also used to supplement borax beeswax emulsion adding increase flexibility and stability to emulsion.

Example of emulsifiers that can be used alone or in combination are sorbitol fatty acid esters and other co-emulsifier that can be used are glyceryl stearate, cetyl alcohol, stearyl alcohol, phosphate fatty alcohols and fatty alcohol sulfate.

Since this preparation contains both oil and water. It is susceptible to microbial attack. Hence a cold cream preparation should also be preserved by adding preservatives.

Marketed Cold Cream Products

- Pond's cold cream
- Charmis cold cream
- Nivea cold cream

Steps to make cold cream as per Formula 5 (Table 6.4 and Flow chart 6.4)

Step 1: Triethanol amine was weighed according to formula and dissolved in given quantity of water and heated to 70°C

Table 6.4: Five examples of cold cream formulae

Ingredients	Cold cream formula 1 Qty in gm	Cold cream formula 2 Qty in gm	Cold cream formula 3 Qty in gm	Cold cream formula 4 Qty in gm	Cold cream formula 5 Qty in gm
Beeswax	14	–	4	18	30
Cetyl alcohol	2	4	–	–	–
Stearyl alcohol	2	2	–	–	–
Mineral oil	53	53	18.5	60.5	46
Lecithin	2	–	–	–	–
Borax	1	–	0.25	1	1
Water	26	20	37	–	6
Olive oil	–	8	20	–	–
Lanolin	–	4	37.5	–	6
Glyceryl monostearate	–	1	–	–	–
Sodium lauryl sulfate	–	1	–	–	–
Spermacitin	–	–	1	–	–
Oleic acid	–	–	–	–	1
Triethanolamine	–	–	–	–	1
Stearic acid	–	–	–	–	6.5
Glycerin	–	–	–	10	1
Perfume	Quantity sufficient	Quantity sufficient	Quantity sufficient	Quantity sufficient	Quantity sufficient
Methylparaben	0.18	0.18	0.18	0.18	0.18
Propylparaben	0.02	0.02	0.02	0.02	0.02

in a suitable pharmaceutical grade container. This would make the aqueous phase of the cold cream.

Step 2: Beeswax, lanolin, spermacitin wax, oleic acid, paraffin wax are next weighed as per formula and then dissolved in mineral oil and heated to 70°C. This makes the oily phase of cold cream water-in-oil emulsion.

Step 3: Now this is the most important step and requires experience and skill to execute. At 70°C, both the phases are mixed and stirred to form water-in-oil type of emulsion. It is important to stir continuously while adding aqueous phase to the oily phase to get stable water in oil emulsion. Keep stirring till the temperature comes down to room temperature.

Step 4: Sufficient quantity of perfume is added before packing the finished product to suitable wide mouth labeled containers.

Flow chart 6.4: Manufacturing process of cold cream

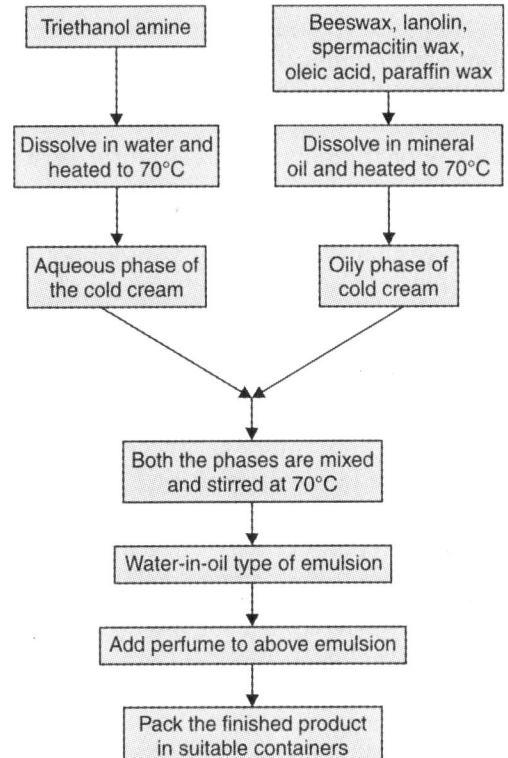

The label should display the following information:
1. Name of the product
2. *Contents:* Name and percentage of any active ingredient, if added to preparation.
3. *Net weight:* As present in the final container.
4. *Manufacturing license number:* As obtained by regulatory authority of your country.

5. *Manufacturing batch number:* As applicable.
6. *Manufacturing date:* Month and year of manufacturing.
7. *Expiry date:* Month and year of expected expiry.
8. *Maximum retail price:* As applicable.
9. *Place of manufacturing:* The plant where it is manufactured.

Vanishing Cream

As name indicates, vanishing creams, these creams are disappeared after applied and rubbed on to the skin. Vanishing cream is oil-in-water emulsion, oily phase is composed of stearic acid which gives a shiny and pearly appearance to vanishing cream. Emulsion is formed *in situ* by reaction of stearic acid with either alkali or triethanol amine to form stearate soap.

If alkali soap is formed, mixture of sodium hydroxide (NaOH) and potassium hydroxide (KOH) is used because they give hard and soft soap, respectively, if used alone. Vanishing cream differs from cold cream in having smaller quantity of oily phase; hence it is easy to rub on skin and leaves non-greasy film on skin with glow. This combined with evaporation of water, gives cooling effect.

Since creams contain large proportion of water, it tends to dry near the top of container. To prevent drying near the rim, large quantity of humectants about 15% w/w is added to vanishing cream.

Many marketed preparation now integrate sunscreen agents, natural agents to market the product as fairness creams.

Marketed preparations based on vanishing cream formula (Table 6.5):

- Fair ever
- Naturally fair
- Fair and lovely

Procedure for making vanishing cream (Flow chart 6.5)

Step 1: The oil-soluble ingredients such as stearic acid, lanolin, propylene glycol and propylparaben are mixed and heated to 70°C in a suitable container generally borosilicate glass apparatus is used when making on lab scale. For large-scale production, stainless steel containers are used. This makes the oily phase of vanishing cream.

Table 6.5: Vanishing cream formulae

S. no.	Ingredients	Formula 1 % w/w	Formula 2
1	Stearic acid	20%	25 %
2	Triethanolamine	–	1.35%
3	Lanolin	–	4%
4	Propylene glycol	–	5%
5	Potassium hydroxide	1%	–
6	Sodium hydroxide	0.133%	–
7	Glycerin	5%	–
8	Methylparaben	0.18%	0.18%
9	Propylparaben	0.02%	0.02%
10	Perfume quantity sufficient to make it pleasing		
11	Water	100% qs	

Flow chart 6.5: Manufacturing process of vanishing cream

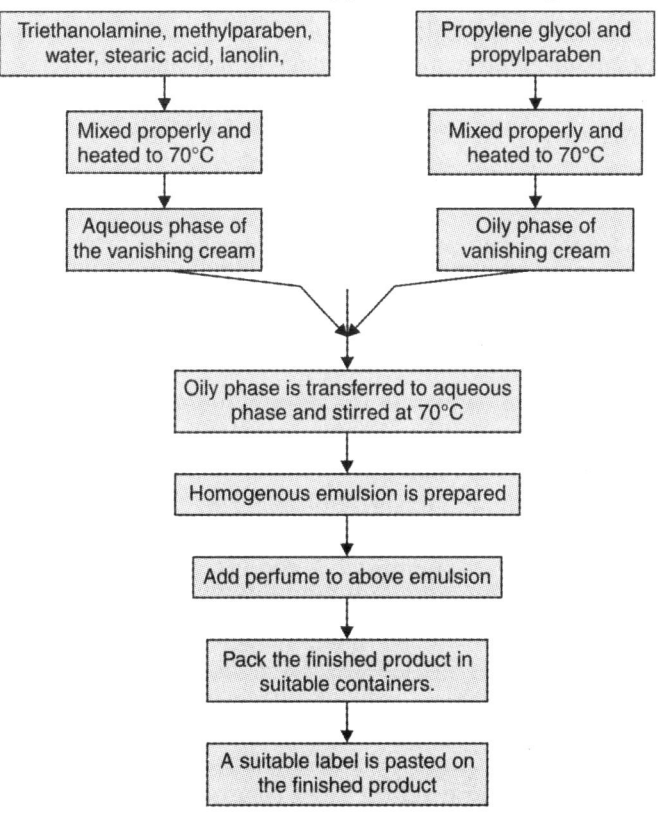

Step 2: The water-soluble ingredients such as triethanol-amine, methylparaben and water are mixed and heated to 70°C simultaneously in another suitable container. This makes the aqueous phase of the vanishing cream.

Step 3: When both phases are at 70°C, oily phase is transferred to aqueous phase in small portions with continuous stirring in manner that a homogenous emulsion is formed. Now, once the transfer is complete, it is allowed to come at room temperature all the while being stirred.

Step 4: Perfume is added just before the finished product is transferred to suitable container for the consumers.

Step 5: A suitable label is pasted on the finished product. As per Drug and Cosmetic Act, the label should contain following information:

1. Name of the product
2. *Contents:* Name and percentage of any active ingredient, if added to preparation.
3. *Net weight:* As present in the final container.
4. *Manufacturing license number:* As obtained by regulatory authority of your country.
5. *Manufacturing batch number:* As applicable
6. *Manufacturing date:* Month and year of manufacturing.
7. *Expiry date:* Month and year of expected expiry.
8. *Maximum retail price:* As applicable.
9. *Place of manufacturing:* The plant where it is manufactured.

Cleansing Cream (Table 6.6)

Cleansing cream or lotion is required for removal of facial make-up, surface dirt, oil, and water and oil-soluble soil efficiently, mainly from the face and throat. A good and properly formulated cleansing cream should be able to remove, quickly and efficiently, applied cosmetics as face powder, rouge, foundation bases, cake make-up, and lipstick. The excessive increase in eye make-up also necessitates use of cleansing products specially formulated to remove such make-up.

Although adequate washing with soap and water will perform the cleaning action but a cleansing cream has certain advantages. Washing with soap-water makes the skin look dry. The cleansing cream can readily remove the chemical substances of the facial make-up by dissolving or lifting away the greasy binding materials holding pigments or grime on the skin.

Ease of application is an important feature of the cleansing cream and so most of these creams are liquids so that excess cream and soil are then easily removable with tissue. The resultant layer left on the skin must not be occlusive but should be sufficiently emollient to prevent drying.

Table 6.6: Formulae of cleansing cream	
Ingredients	% w/w
Beeswax	10–14
Mineral oil	45–51
Paraffin wax	2–4
Spermacitin	1–3
Water	34–35
Borax	0.4–0.6
Preservative	q.s
Perfume	q.s

Manufacturing Process (Flow chart 6.6)

These preparations are emulsion type; the total ingredients can be classified into oil phase and aqueous phase. Ingredients of oil phase should be taken in increasing melting point. The materials of least melting point should be taken and melt it. Add the other oil or wax gradually in increasing melting point and melt them with continuous stirring. Take separately the ingredients of aqueous phase and mix them and heat to same temperature as oil phase. Emulsifying agents should be added to specific phase. Mix the two phases with continuous stirring until a smooth cream is formed. Finally, the product can be milled by triple roller mill. Preservative should be dissolved in the water before making cream. Perfume should be added after the primary cream is formed and cooled but before final milling.

All Purpose Cream

They are somewhat oily but non-greasy type and can spread easily on the skin to give a protective film. They can also function,

Flow chart 6.6: Manufacturing process of cleansing cream

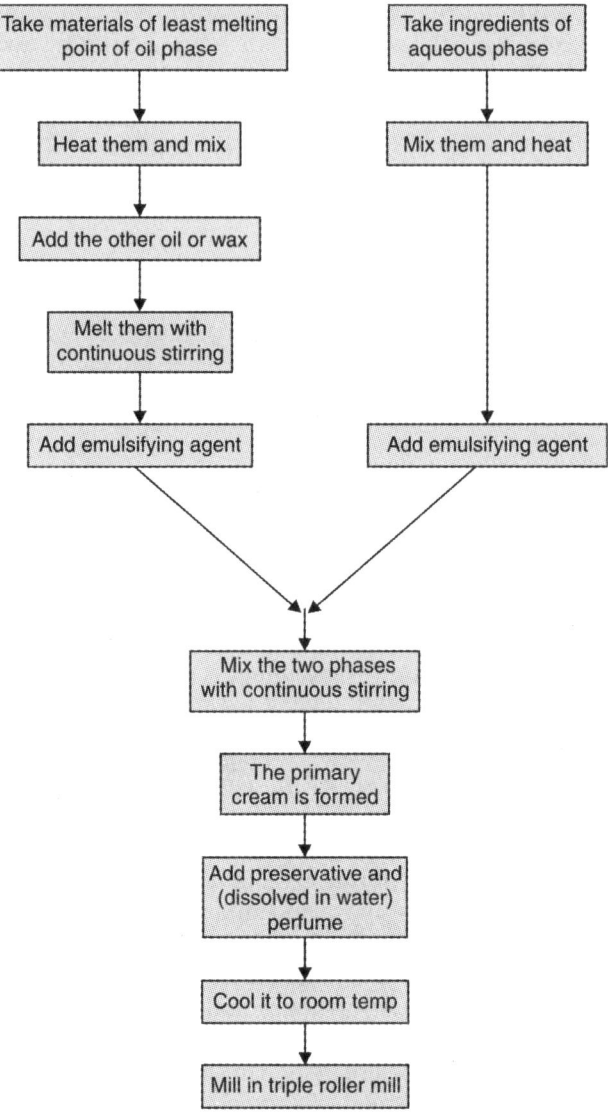

when applied excessively as a skinfood or nourishing cream or night cream or protective cream for prevention or alleviation of sunburn, or for the treatment of roughened skin area. Also when applied sparingly, they function as hand creams or foundation creams. Thus they are called as all purpose creams.

So, the composition of these creams is such that it can act:

1. As a foundation cream to provide a foundation base for make up.
2. As a cleansing cream and liquefy easily.
3. As a hand cream and should have emollient character.
4. As a protective cream and should form a continuous non-occlusive film.
5. As a cream to smooth the rough surface of the skin.

Table 6.7: Formulae of all purpose cream

Ingredients	% w/w
Stearic acid	10–14
Lanolin	2–4
Beeswax	2–4
Mineral oil	20–24
Myrj 52	5–7
Sorbitol solution	10–14
Water	37–45
Perfume	q.s
Preservative	q.s
Antioxidant	q.s

Manufacturing Process (Flow chart 6.7)

Heat and mix oil phase components such as stearic acid, lanolin, beeswax, mineral oil and myrj 52 at above 75°C. Add preservative to water and mixed with sorbital solution to get aqueous phase then heat to 75°C. Mix both the phases with continuous stirring. Finally, cool and add perfume while stirring.

Shaving Preparations

Shaving preparations are used for softening the beard for wet shaving and also to produce rich foam to facilitate shaving by razor, safety blade or electric shaving. These preparations can further be classified into two as follows:

1. Preparations used for shaving with razor blade.
2. Preparations used for electric shaving.

Flow chart 6.7: Manufacturing process of all purpose cream

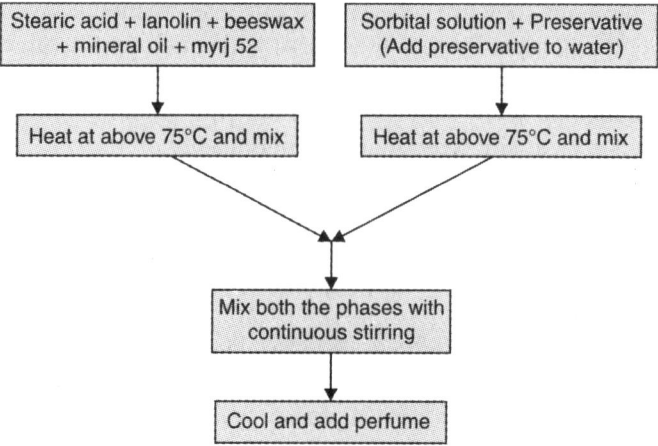

1. Preparations Used for Shaving with Razor Blade

Water can soften the hair. But, normally, water gets evaporated before sufficient wetting of the hair as it takes some time to soften hair. These drawbacks can be overcome by use of shaving preparations like shaving soaps, and creams and others, though water is main component for such softening.

These preparations can be classified into three groups:
1. Shaving soaps
2. Shaving creams
3. Aerosol preparations

Shaving Soap (Table 6.8)

Soaps are marketed in three forms such as cake and solid stick. Earlier, solid soaps or cakes or sticks were used widely.

Table 6.8: Formulae of shaving soap	
Ingredients	*% w/w*
Stearic acid	45–54
Coconut oil	10–16
Caustic potash	20–24
Caustic soda	10–14
Water	1–1.5
Sodium dioxystearate (50%)	0.5–1

(Contd...)

Table 6.8: Formulae of shaving soap *(Contd.)*

Ingredients	% w/w
Sorbitol liquid	1–1.5
Glycerol	0.5–1
Perfume	q.s
Preservative	q.s

Shaving Creams (Table 6.9)

Presently shaving creams have largely replaced the solid soaps. The creams have replaced the solid products because of ease of application.

Table 6.9: Formulae of shaving cream

Ingredients	gm/batch
Glycerol monostearate	15.0
Stearic acid	7.0
Glycerin	4.0
Mineral oil	5.0
Water	69.0
Perfume	q.s
Preservative	q.s

Aerosol Preparations

These preparations are more popular than shaving soap and cream in the present scenario because of easy in application on skin. Pressurized bottle should be shaken well before use to get good lather when discharge from the pressurized bottle. Formulation of aerosol for making shaving preparation should be carefully design to get good foam and its stability.

2. Preparations used for Electric Shaving

Generally, powder is used before electric shaving to get dry and lubricated skin which helps smooth electric shaving (Table 6.10).

Table 6.10: Formulae of shaving powder

Ingredients	% w/w
Magnesium stearate	6–10
Kaolin	4–8
Talc	84–88
Perfume	q.s

Aftershave Lotion

The aftershave preparations are basically applied to cool and refresh the skin, to overcome irritation on the skin, to neutralize the soreness, to disinfect or heal the skin damage or cut. They are used in the form of lotions, creams or powders (Tables 6.11 and 6.12).

Most of the lotions are used as aftershave preparations. Powders are also used to some extent but use of creams is comparatively less.

The lotions are clear solutions containing 25 to 50% alcohol. Additionally, they may also contain antiseptic, emollient substances. Also they may contain extract of menthol, glycerin, boric acid, alum, potassium oxyquinoline sulfate and chloroform.

If alcohol content is less, the perfume should be water-soluble or soluble in less concentrations of alcohol. Alternatively, solubilizing agents may be used.

Table 6.11: Formulae of aftershave lotion

Ingredients	*% w/w*
Glycerine	1–3
Chlorhexidine diacetate	0.1–0.5
Menthol	0.5–1.5
Alcohol	35–45
Water	56–60
Perfume	q.s

Table 6.12: Formulae of aftershave powder

Ingredients	*% w/w*
Boric acid	1–5
Magnesium stearate	2–6
Talc	91–95
Perfume	q.s

Antiperspirant and Deodorant (Figs 6.6 and 6.7)

Most people think that antiperspirants and deodorants are the same thing, but they aren't.

The fundamental differences lie in the way these products work, and potentially affect health. Essentially they use different chemical processes for minimizing body odor. Certain ingredients in either product may be unhealthy, but deodorant is frequently cited as a better alternative than many anti-perspirants.

Antiperspirants contain fragrance, but they also contain chemical compounds that block the pores to stop the discharge of perspiration. No sweat, no odor. Antiperspirants contains things like wax and aluminum in one form or another.

- Aluminum chloride
- Aluminum chlorohydrate
- Aluminum zirconium tricholorohydrex glycine
- Aluminum hydroxybromide

The way it works is that the aluminum ions go into the cells that line the ducts of the eccrine glands, these can be found on the epidermal layer, that is the top layer of skin.

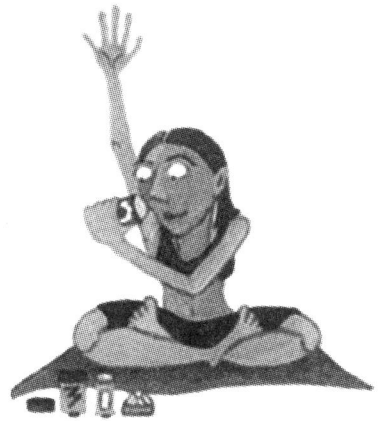

Fig. 6.6: Women using antiperspirant stick

Deodorant allows the release of perspiration, but prevents odor by combating it with antiseptic agents, which kill odor-causing bacteria.

Many consumers do not realize how deodorant works, assuming it is simply a fragrance that covers up body odor. Some choose antiperspirant, because rather than cover the odor, they prefer to eliminate it.

Consumer advocacy groups continue to voice concerns over questions regarding common health and beauty products, including deodorant and antiperspirant. Certain studies indicate potential health risks associated with aluminum compounds found in many antiperspirants. Similar studies find like risks with parabens found in some deodorants. Both have been tenuously linked to serious illnesses, including breast cancer.

Manufacturers and various health agencies claim such studies are flawed, stating concerns are unfounded.

Despite assurances, many healthcare professionals recommend deodorant over antiperspirant, believing that obstructing pores and preventing perspiration may not be the healthiest choice. Consumers are left to make their own judgements.

Those who would rather forgo a typical antiperspirant or deodorant are beginning to look for more natural alternatives. There are several brands of natural deodorant that are currently available. However, these products do not always contain purely organic ingredients, so check labels carefully before purchasing. For the true maverick, a homespun deodorant consists of equal parts cornstarch and baking soda, applied with a damp washcloth.

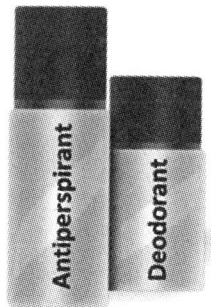

Fig. 6.7: Antiperspirant and deodorant spray

Hair Cosmetics

Hair cosmetics are:

1. Shampoo
2. Conditioner.

To study and design hair preparations, it is very much essential to have knowledge of hair. Hair is one of the vital parts of the body. Hairs are also known as epidermal derivatives as they originate from the epidermis during embryological development.

Hair production is a process of mutual involvement of both dermis and epidermis and originates from hair follicles. Hair follicles extend deep into the dermis, typically projecting into the underlyings subcutaneous layer. The base of the hair follicle, called hair papilla, is a peg of connective tissue containing capillaries and nerves.

The hair follicle is composed of multiple layers with the outermost continuous with the epidermis and the innermost being the cortex surrounded by its cuticle, which gives rise to the shaft that extends above the cutaneous surface (Fig. 6.8). The hair follicle is positioned at an angle with its base in the subcutaneous fat. A muscle is attached to the side of the follicle and runs to the upper dermis, forming an obtuse angle. When the muscle contracts, the hair rises, resulting in goose bumps. The sebaceous gland, located above the attachment of the muscle, connects to the pilar canal through a duct.

The hair shaft is a very porous structure and softens rapidly with wetting. The hair is most brittle when dry, a time when it is most susceptible to mechanical injury. Fibrous proteins fill the cortical cells and are surrounded by a matrix protein, and these are locked together by disulfide bonds. The hair shafts can be damaged by sunlight, especially lightly colored hair, and by chemicals used to bleach or color the hair. Reduction of disulfide bonds is commonly done to straighten or permanently curl hair. This results in cumulative injury and must be done with care to avoid breakage.

Functions of Hair

1. Hairs on the head protect the scalp from ultraviolet light, cushion round the head and insulate the skull.

2. Eyebrows protect the eye from small foreign particles and insects. Also it diverts sweat from the eyes.

3. The hairs, guarding the entrances to nostrils and external ear canals filter the air and help prevent the entry of foreign particles.

4. Body hairs help in evaporation of perspiration and draining of external water from the body.

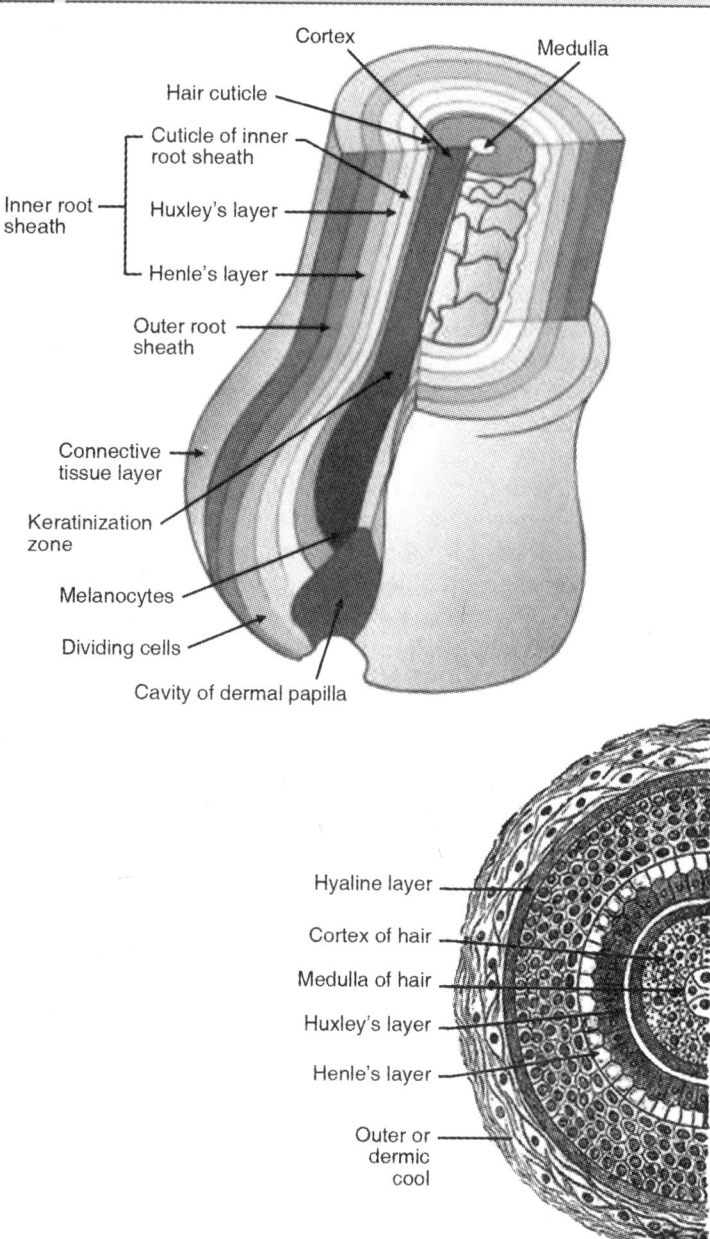

Cortex

Medulla

Hair cuticle

Cuticle of inner root sheath

Inner root sheath

Huxley's layer

Henle's layer

Outer root sheath

Connective tissue layer

Keratinization zone

Melanocytes

Dividing cells

Cavity of dermal papilla

Hyaline layer

Cortex of hair

Medulla of hair

Huxley's layer

Henle's layer

Outer or dermic cool

Fig. 6.8: Schematic structure of hair

Shampoo

The functions of a shampoo are expected to be various. A good and acceptable shampoo should have the following characteristics:

- It should effectively and completely remove dust or soil, excessive sebum or other fatty substances from the hair and other residual substances of hair dressings or settings or other materials.
- It should effectively wash the hair.
- The shampoo should be easily removed by rinsing with water.
- It should leave the hair non-dry, soft, lustrous with good manageability and less fly away.
- It should impart a pleasant fragrance to the hair.
- It should not have any side effects or causes irritation to skin or eye.

Types of Shampoo

1. Powder shampoos
2. Clear liquid shampoos
3. Liquid cream or lotion shampoos
4. Solid cream/gel shampoos
5. Oil shampoos
6. Miscellaneous including anti-dandruff medicated shampoos

1. Powder Shampoos (Table 6.13)

Table 6.13: Formulae of powder shampoos

Ingredients	% w/w
Sodium bicarbonate	40–60
Disodium phosphate	10–30
Soap powder	20–40
Perfume	q.s

Manufacturing Process (Flow chart 6.8)

They are prepared by simple mixing process. In powder shampoos, the ingredients are simply mixed and the perfume is added last.

Flow chart 6.8: Manufacturing process of powder shampoos

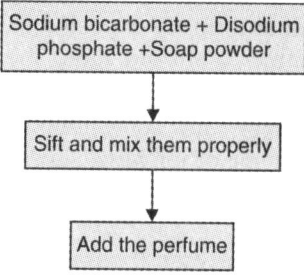

2. Clear Liquid Shampoos (Table 6.14)

Table 6.14: Formulae of clear liquid shampoos

Ingredients	% w/w
Triethanolamine lauryl sulfate	40–50
Coconut monoethanolamide	1–3
Water	50–56
Perfume	q.s
Color	q.s
Preservative	q.s

Manufacturing Process (Flow chart 6.9)

In case of clear liquid shampoos, the detergents are first dissolved in half of the water with little heat, if necessary. Other

Flow chart 6.9: Manufacturing process of clear liquid shampoos

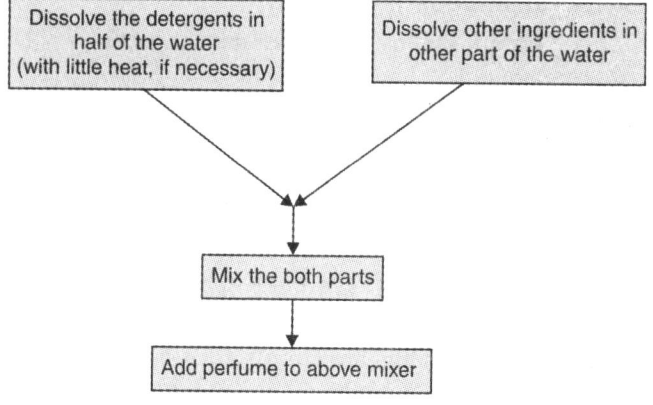

ingredients are added to other part of the water and then mixed with the first part. The perfume is added at last.

3. Liquid Cream or Lotion Shampoos (Table 6.15)

Table 6.15: Formulae of liquid cream or lotion shampoos

Ingredients	% w/w
Monoethanolamine lauryl sulfate (25% active)	30–50
Ethylene glycol monostearate	3–7
Water	50–60
Perfume	q.s
Preservative	q.s

Manufacturing Process (Flow chart 6.10)

Heat and mix the ethylene glycol monostearate with a small quantity of the detergent to form a homogeneous mixture. Add more detergent slowly and then water, mix thoroughly before addition of next. Perfume is added last after cooling to 35°C.

Flow chart 6.10: Manufacturing process of lotion shampoos

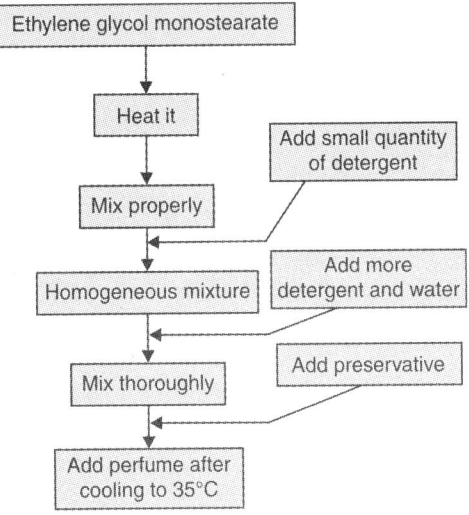

4. Solid Cream/Gel Shampoos (Table 6.16)

Table 6.16: Formulae of solid cream/gel shampoos

Ingredients	gm/batch
Sodium lauryl sulfate	15–25
Coconut monoethanolamide	0.5–1.5
Propylene glycol monostearate	1–3
Stearic acid	3–7
Sodium hydroxide	0.5–1
Water	65–75
Perfume	q.s

Manufacturing Process (Flow chart 6.11)

Mix water, oleic acid and sodium lauryl sulfate paste and heat to 60°C. Slowly add triethanolamine with continuous stirring. Add perfume after cooling to 35°C.

Flow chart 6.11: Manufacturing process of gel shampoos

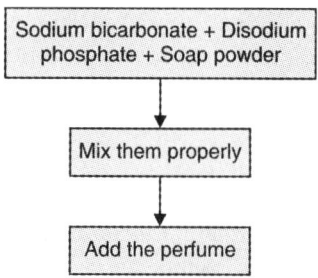

5. Oil Shampoos (Table 6.17)

Table 6.17: Formulae of oil shampoos

Ingredients	% w/w
Sulfonated olive oil	12–20
Sulfonated castor oil	12–20
Water	62–72
Perfume	q.s
Preservative	q.s
Color	q.s

Manufacturing Process (Flow chart 6.12)

Mix all the ingredients together. Color and preservatives should be dissolved in a small quantity of water. Perfume can be added at last.

6. Antiseptic/Antidandruff Shampoos (Table 6.18)

Table 6.18: Formulae of antiseptic/antidandruff shampoos

Ingredients	% w/w
Sodium lauryl sulfate	20–30
Stearic acid	5–9
Sodium hydroxide	0.5–1.5
Biosulfur powder	1–3
Water	60–70
Perfume	q.s
Preservative	q.s

Flow chart 6.12: Manufacturing process of oil shampoos

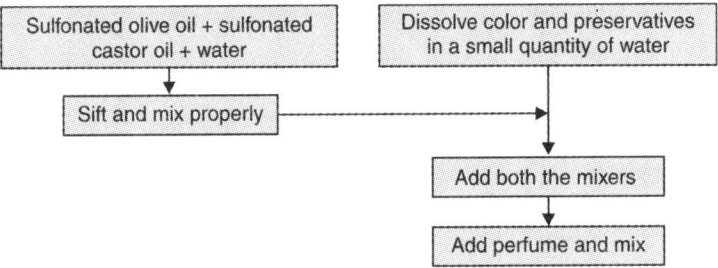

Manufacturing Process (Flow chart 6.13)

Dissolve the sodium hydroxide in a small quantity of water with heating at 75°C. Add biosulfur to the sodium hydroxide solution. Take sodium lauryl sulfate and stearic acid together and mix with heating at about 60°C and then add to the aqueous solution. Stir and cool and add perfume and preservative.

Flow chart 6.13: Manufacturing process of antiseptic and antidandruff shampoos

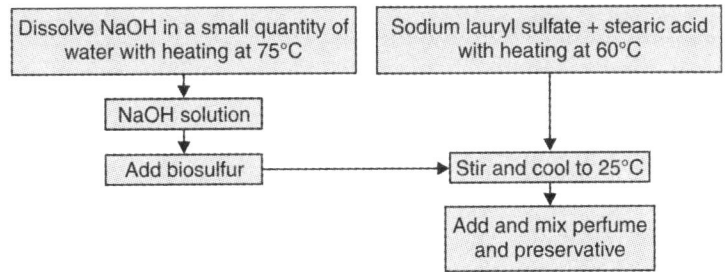

Conditioner (Table 6.19)

Conditioners are used after shampooing the hair, to render the hair more lustrous, easy to comb, and free from static electricity when dry. They are also used to improve damaged hair. Hair may be damaged by excessive use of bleaches and permanent waves. Conditioners are usually based on cationic detergents and fatty materials like lanolin or mineral oil.

Table 6.19: Formulae of conditioner

Ingredients	% w/w
Stearyl alcohol	0.25–0.75
Glyceryl monostearate	2–6
Sodium chloride	0.1–0.3
Benzalkonium chloride	1–2
Water	95–99
Color	q.s
Perfume	q.s

Manufacturing Process (Flow chart 6.14)

Dissolve the sodium chloride in a small quantity of water with heating at 75°C. Add color to the sodium chloride solution. Take glyceryl monostearate and stearic acid together and mix with heating at about 60°C and then add to the aqueous solution. Stir and cool and add perfume and preservative.

Flow chart 6.14: Manufacturing process of conditioner

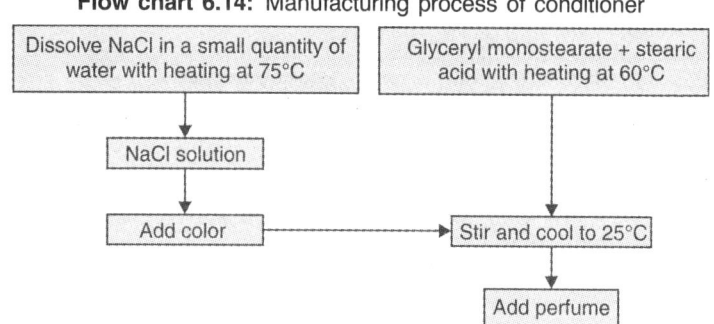

Nails Cosmetics

The body of the nail basically consists of tightly compressed dead cells packed with keratin. The protein structure contains a high proportion of sulfur-rich amino acid cystine with small proportion of methionine, tyrosine, lysine, and histidine. The nail is composed of three layers, a soft lower layer called central nail, with hard keratin forming the intermediate layer, and the outer layer called dorsal nail. The nail also contains 12 to 14% of water and fatty materials mainly of cholesterol.

The knowledge of composition suggests that the manicure preparations should possibly avoid use of materials that remove natural fat or water-soluble substances as these could damage the lattice-like structure of nail and may hasten the splitting or breaking. Sometimes fatty materials are incorporated in manicure preparations to supplement them.

Nail cosmetics are:

1. Nail lacquer
2. Lacquer removers

Nail Lacquer (Fig. 6.9)

The nail lacquers are the largest and most important group of manicure preparations (Table 6.20).

The application of nail lacquers covers the nail with a water and air impermeable membrane which remains for days and normally can be removed only by suitable solvent. So there is demand for removers as much as that of lacquers, as users change the color or shade frequently to suit their choice and necessity.

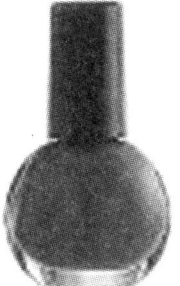

Fig. 6.9: Nail lacquer

Table 6.20: Formulae of nail lacquer

Ingredients	% w/w
Nitrocellulose	6–10
Dibutyl phthalate	4–8
Polyvinyl acetate	5–9
Methylene chloride	25–30
Ethylene glycol monomethyl ether	25–29
Diethyl glycol monomethyl ether	2–5
Ethyl alcohol	10–20
Perfume oil	3–7
Color	0.25–0.75

Manufacturing Process (Flow chart 6.15)

The base is prepared separately or diluted from the mother lacquer available in the market. Nitrocellulose or film former is dissolved in the solvent. Resin, plasticizer can be dissolved directly or may be dissolved in a small amount of solvent and then may be mixed with nitrocellulose solution. Dispersed pigments are also available readily in the market. The pigments are first dispersed by milling in a suitable vehicle and then incorporated in the base. Alternatively, the milled dispersion

Flow chart 6.15: Manufacturing process of nail lacquer

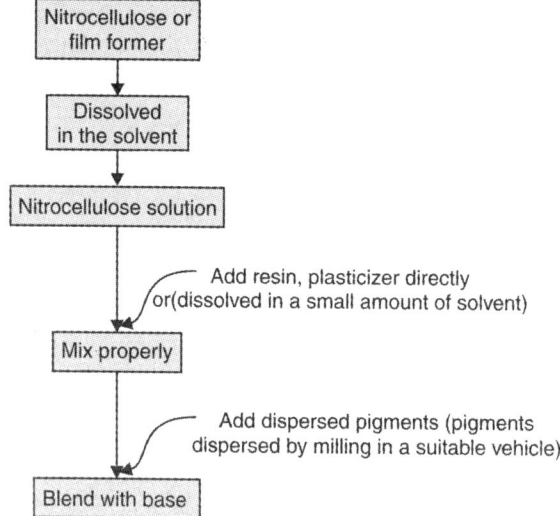

is converted into colored chips. The colored chips are dissolved in the lacquer base and blended to prepare suitable shades. Also concentrated colors are available, which can be suitably diluted and blended with base.

Lacquer Removers (Table 6.21)

These products are also called nail cleansers. They are totally different from other cleansers, such as hair, skin and teeth cleansers, as nail cleansers are required to remove only nail lacquers, whereas others are used to remove greasy materials, dirt, dust, etc. As nail cleansers are required to be applied on a smooth and highly resistant surface, composition can be different. These preparations rarely come in contact with the surrounding skin, which is not so in the case of other cleansers. So, the chance of damage is much less than shampoos or other cleansers.

Table 6.21: Formulae of lacquer removers	
Ingredients	% w/w
Castor oil	2–6
Diethylene glycol monoethyl ether	12–20
Acetone	70–90
Perfume	q.s

Prepare by simple solution.

Oral Hygiene Cosmetics

Maintenance of health of the teeth and gums well is very important for having good general health. Health of teeth and gum of a person is an indication of his/her general health. So, it is necessary to take care of health of teeth and gums. Various preparations are used for cleansing and maintenance of good health of teeth, gum and oral cavity. The products, termed as dentifrices, are used to keep the teeth clean, shiny and to inhibit the formation of unpleasant odor in mouth and freshen the breath.

Oral hygiene cosmetics are:

1. Dentifrices
2. Toothpaste
3. Tooth powder
4. Mouthwash

Dentifrices (Fig. 6.10)

Maintenance of teeth clean and in good health is essential and also important for everyone. This can be achieved by using various dental care preparations or dentifrices. Dentifrices are the preparations used for cleaning the surfaces of teeth and keep them shiny and to preserve the health of the teeth and gums. These preparations may also expected to help inhibit the formation of unpleasant odors and freshen the breath. Regular use of dentifrices helps to prevent occurrence of tooth decay. A good dental health increases the possibility of a good general health.

Dentifrices can be either simple cleansing dentifrices or also be therapeutic dentifrices. Therapeutic dentifrices are basically cleansing preparations containing additionally, some drugs or chemicals which decrease the occurrence of dental caries or help in control of periodontal disease. These are achieved by the bactericidal, bacteriostatic, enzyme-inhibiting or acid-neutralizing qualities of the drugs or chemicals used. Therapeutic dentifrices containing stannous fluoride are widely used products.

Dentifrices are prepared in paste, powder and to a lesser extent in liquid and block forms.

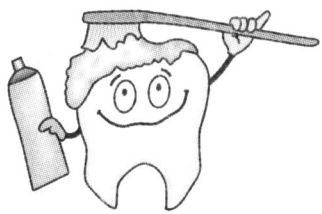

Fig. 6.10: Dentifrices

Functions of Dentifrices

Though the primary function of a dentifrice is the cleaning of the accessible surfaces of the teeth, but it can have some other functions also. The expected functions of a dentifrice are as follows:

- Cleansing of tooth
- Prevention of formation or removal of dental plaque
- Prevention of formation of calculus

- Polishing of tooth
- Reduction of the occurrence of tooth decay
- Reduction of periodontal disease
- Prevention or reduction of mouth odors and freshening of breath

Some commercial dentifrices may be performing all of the above functions and some may be fulfilling partial functions.

Toothpaste (Table 6.22)

Toothpastes are most popular, valuable and widely used preparations for cleansing the teeth. They have largest share of dental cleansing and care preparations. Though they are expensive than tooth powders but still they are more preferred.

Toothpastes are preferred because of the following reasons:

1. Easy to take measured quantity and spread on the tooth brush.
2. No spillage or wastage.
3. Attractive consistency.
4. Proper distribution in mouth.

Table 6.22: Formulae of toothpaste	
Ingredients	*% w/w*
Calcium carbonate	50–60
Sodium lauryl sulfate	0.5–1.5
Glycerin	20–26
Gum tragacanth	1–2
Water	17–20
Saccharine	0.1–0.3
Flavor	q.s
Preservative	q.s

Manufacturing Process (Flow chart 6.16)

These preparations are preferably made in stainless steel mixer container. It can be done in a planetary mixer or similar mixer used for semisolid preparations. Small scale batch can be made in a glass container.

The gum is mixed with a suitable quantity of humectant, without any water for proper dispersion. Chloroform or alcohol can also be used for dispersion of binding agents. Other colloids may be dispersed in water. Preservative can be dissolved in glycerine or water. Methylcellulose should be mixed with cold water, but ethylcellulose should be dispersed in warm water. Other powder ingredients are sifted together and added gradually to mucilaginous mixture with continuous gentle stirring. Then aqueous media are mixed and stirred further to get the product flavor and detergent should be added at the last.

In an alternative method, the binder is premixed with solid abrasives and other powders and then poured in a suitable mixer (dough-type mixer) along with aqueous solution of the humectant, preservative, sweetening agent and mixing is done. After obtaining a homogeneous paste, flavor and detergent are added.

Flow chart 6.16: Manufacturing process of toothpaste

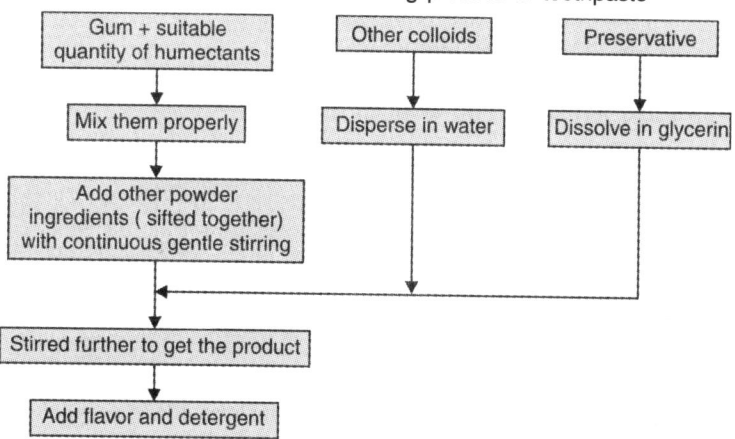

Tooth Powder (Table 6.23)

Tooth powders are, structurally, the oldest and simplest preparations and they are also the cheapest. Over the years, their market share has been reduced by popularity and advantages of pastes, but still they have a considerable share of the market and population. The main problems encountered with tooth powders are floating of powders in air during manufacturing, formation of cake on storage, and uneven distribution in mouth. The oldest tooth powder is reported to be camphorated chalk. More or less every dental care manufacturer also markets tooth powders along with tooth paste products.

Table 6.23: Formulae of tooth powder

Ingredients	% w/w
Calcium carbonate	80–85
Tricalcium phosphate	5–15
Sodium lauryl sulfate	1–5
Sodium perborate	1–5
Saccharine sodium	1–2
Flavor	q.s
Color	q.s

Manufacturing Process (Flow chart 6.17)

This is done by simple mixing. First ingredients of small quantity are premixed and then mixed with other ingredients in ribbon-type or agitator type of mixer. Flavor can be sprayed on to the bulk or can be premixed with part of some abrasive and polishing agent and then mixed with the bulk.

Flow chart 6.17: Manufacturing process of tooth powder

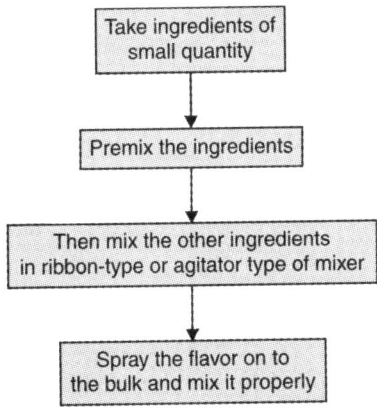

Mouthwash (Table 6.24)

Mouthwashes are basically deodorants and antiseptics. Mouthwashes, apart from their main function of deodorants and antiseptics, can also help in cleansing by removing water-soluble substances or loose debris from the surfaces or between the teeth or from oral cavity.

Mouthwashes are mainly alcoholic or hydroalcoholic solution as they are used in oral cavity (Fig. 6.11), which need to be suitably diluted, if required.

Mouthwash should have the following characters:
- Good and quick antiseptic action at the dilution it is used
- Attractive flavor to impart a odor to the mouth.
- Sweet taste
- Not much expensive
- Non-irritant and non-toxic to mouth and mucous membrane

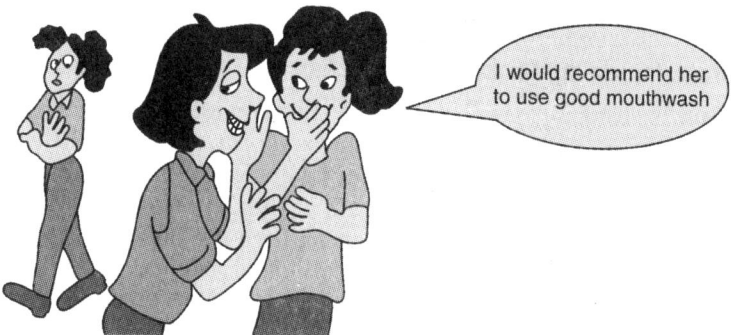

Fig. 6.11: Mouthwash is used to enhance oral hygiene

Table 6.24: Formulae of mouthwash	
Ingredients	*% w/w*
Anethol	0.5–1
Methyl salicylate	05–1.5
Menthol	0.1–0.5
Propylene glycol	20–30
Glycerin	20–30
Tween 80	15–25
Saccharin sodium	1–3
Ethyl alcohol	22–30
Color	q.s

Application of Mouthwash

The preparation is to be diluted with water in definite proportion, as suggested on the label, before use.

Dilution with water may have another advantage as dilution with water just before use, may lead to the precipitation of flavors and disinfectants. This will lead to better adherence of the above substances on the oral cavity and membrane and thus longer action.

No dilution with water for the above formulation is required but with other formulation dilution may need as per the direction on the label.

ISOLATED KEY POINTS

- Cosmetics arise from a Greek word *kosmeticos* which means adorn. If any material used for beautification or improvement of appearance is known as cosmetics. In other words, they may be applied to skin, hair and nails for the purpose of covering coloring, softening, cleansing, nourishing, setting and protection.

- *Classification of cosmetics:* Cosmetics for skin, hair, nail: Hygienic powder, compact, creams, lotion, colorants, hair remover, hair conditioner, shampoos, hair dyes, lotion, eyelash (mascaras), eye brow pencils, eyelid inside (Kohls), face powder, compact powder, body powder, prickly heat powder, cold cream, vanishing cream, all purpose cream, cleansing cream, foundation cream, emollient cream, astringent lotion, lipsticks rouges, nail lacquers, lacquer removers, nail polish, cuticle removers, Dental powders, paste, dentifrices, lotion, mouthwash, bath soap.

- *Skin introduction:* Skin is the heaviest single organ of the body combine with the mucosal lining of the respiratory, digestive and urogenital tract. A square centimeter of skin covers 10 hair follicles, 12 nerves, 15 sebaceous glan, 100 sweat glands. pH of the skin varies from 4–5.6.

- *Function of the skin:* Protection from external stimuli like chemicals, light, heat and cold, radiation. It regulates the body temperature, controls blood pressure, acts as a barrier for invasion of various microorganisms, has bactericidal fungicidal activities due to presence of sebum secretion and has important role in the synthesing of vitamin D_3–calcitriol.

- The human skin consist of mainly three types: Epidermis, dermis, subcutaneous.

- *Epidermis:* It is multilayered. It varies in thickness depends on cell size and area—soles, palm-0.8 mm; eye lid-0.06 mm. The epidermis comprises 5 distinct layers—stratum corneum (horny layer), stratum lucidum, stratum granulosum (granular layer), stratum spinosum (prickly cell layer), stratum germinativum (basal layer).

- *Stratum corneum:* It consists of epidermal cells of lipophilic nature. The membrane provides about 10–15 layers of flattened keratinized dead cells. It is 10 µm when it is dry. But it can take up moisture up to 15–20 % when occlusive dressing/cream applied over the skin prevent the evaporation of water. It plays a role in controlling the percutaneous absorption of chemical substance.

- *Stratum lucidum:* It is thin translucent layer. *Stratum granulosum:* It consists of keratin protein. *Stratum spinosum:* It consists of flattened polygonal cells. *Stratum germinativum:* It consists of melanocytes.

- *Dermis/corium:* It consists of dense network of structural protein fibres–collagen, mucopolysaccharide, ground substance. It is about 0.2–0.3 mm thick. It contains blood vessels, lymphatic vessels, nerve ending.

- *Subcutaneous:* It consists of fat rich areolar tissue. It is otherwise called superficial fascia. It is quite elastic. Large arteries and veins are present.

- Skin appendages, sebaceous gland, hair follicle/pile, pilosebaceous unit, sweat gland : Eccrine gland/salty sweat gland–present overall body surface. Apocrine gland–axillae, anogenital region, around nipple. Sebaceous gland–secretes sebum (waxes, sterols, f. acid).

- *Skin powders:* Powders are widely used for face and body care not only for woman but also for men. Powders are differ from liquid skin care ppn, e.g. body powder/ talcum powder/dusting powder. Very fine powder can cover large surface area of the body.

- *Ideal characters of powder:* Should be good covering power and hide skin blemishes. Should adhere to the skin and not blow of easily. Should not completely dissipated in a few minutes to avoid repowdering. The finish given to the skin must be preferably peach like character. Shine on around the nose must be completely eliminated. Must be absorbent. Must be slip enable the powder to spread on the skin by the puff.

- *Ideal characters for raw materials:* The material should not be too hard. If the materials are crystals in nature, they must not have any sharp edges. Otherwise, they can damage the skin. It should be non-irritating, non-toxic. It should be chemically neutral. It should be compatible with other ingredients and should not be soluble in water and fat

- *Face powder:* Face powder is basically a cosmetic product which imparts velvet like finish to it. A good face powder should produce smooth finish to facial skin masking visible imperfection of the face and shine due to moisture or grease or oily secretion. The preparation should make the face pleasant look and touch. It must adhere to the skin and mixed secretion of skin.

- *Types of face powder: Light type:* Suitable for dry skin. (no oil, and little moisture), contains large quantity of talc. Medium type: Suitable for normal or moderate oily skin. High covering power compare to light type contains less talc balanced by ZnO. *Heavy type:* Suitable for extreme oily skin, contains lower quantity of talc and high quality of zinc oxide.

- *Body powder:* It is called talcum powder/dusting powder. It is used as multi-purpose. It is used to absorb moisture or perspiration specific after bath. It also acts as cooling effect and prevent irritation of skin due to chafing. It contains covering material, adhesive, absorbancy material, slip antiseptic and perfumes. It consists of small portion of metallic stearate and talc, ppt chalk. Aseptic material used to proliferation of microbes.

- *Face primer:* Come in various formulas to suit individual skin concerns. Most are meant to reduce the appearance of pore size, prolong the wear of makeup, and allow for a smoother application of makeup. Applied before foundation.

- *Eye primer:* Used to prolong the wear of eyeshadows on the eye as well as intensify color payoff from shadows.

- *Lipgloss* is a sheer form of lipstick that is in a liquid form.

- *Lipstick*, lip gloss, lip liner, lip plumper, lip balm, lip conditioner, lip primer, and lip boosters. Lip stains have a water or gel base and may contain alcohol to help the product stay on the lips. The idea behind lip stains is to temporarily saturate the lips with a dye, rather than covering them with a colored wax. Usually, designed to be waterproof, the product may come with an applicator brush or be applied with a finger.

- *Concealer*, makeup used to cover any imperfection of the skin. Concealer is often used for any extra coverage needed to cover blemishes, or any other marks. Concealer is often thicker and more solid than foundation, and provides longer lasting, and more detailed coverage. Some formulations are meant only for the eye or only for the face.

- *Foundation*, used to smooth out the face and cover spots or uneven skin coloration. Usually, a liquid, cream, or powder, as well as most recently, a light and fluffy mousse, which provides excellent coverage as well. Foundation primer can be applied before or after to get a smoother finish. Some primers come in powder or liquid form to be applied before foundation as a base, while other primers come as a spray to be applied after you are finished to help make-up last longer.

- *Face powder*, used to set the foundation, giving a matte finish, and also to conceal small flaws or blemishes.

- *Rouge, blush or blusher, cheek coloring* used to bring out the color in the cheeks and make the cheek bones appear more defined. This comes in powder, cream, and liquid forms.

- *Contour powder/creams*, used to define the face. It can be used to give the illusion of a slimmer face or to even modify a person's face shape as desired. Usually, a few shades darker than ones own skin tone and matte in finish to create the illusion of depth. A darker toned foundation/ concealer can be used instead to contour to create a more natural look.

- *Highlight*, used to draw attention to the high points of the face as well as to add glow to the face. It comes in liquid, cream, and powder form. Often contains shimmer, but sometimes does not. A lighter toned foundation/concealer can be used instead to highlight create a more natural look.

- *Bronzer*, used to give skin a bit of color by adding a golden or bronze glow. Can come in either matte, semi-matte/ satin, or shimmer finishes.
- *Mascara* is used to darken, lengthen, and thicken the eyelashes. It is available in natural colors such as brown and black, but also comes in bolder colors such as blue, pink, or purple. There are many different formulas, including waterproof for those prone to allergies or sudden tears. Often used after an eyelash curler and mascara primer. There are now also many mascaras with certain components to help lashes to grow longer and thicker. There are specific minerals and proteins that are combined with the mascara that can benefit, as well as beautify.

LONG ANSWER TYPE QUESTIONS

Q 1. What do you understand by the term cosmetics? Elaborate in detail about the applications of cosmetics in the healthcare systems.

Q 2. Define the face powder. Write in detail about the manufacturing process evolved in the face powder manufacturing.

Q 3. How face powder can enhance the appearance of the skin? Comments.

Q 4. Differentiate between the face powder and body powder.

Q 5. What do you mean by the word "lipsticks"? How will you prepare it? Write in detail about the precautions taken while manufacturing lipsticks.

Q 6. Write the ideal formula to prepare the lipsticks.

Q 7. What do you mean by the term "cold creams"? Discuss its role in cosmetology.

Q 8. Define cold creams. Discuss its manufacturing process with the help of suitable flow charts.

Q 9. Cold cream is o/w or w/o type emulsion? Explain with the formula.

Q 10. How vanishing creams are different from cold creams?

Q 11. What do you mean by all purpose creams? Explain the manufacturing process and applications of all purpose creams.

Q 12. Define shaving cream. Discuss in detail the role of key ingredients of the shaving cream.

Q 13. How the deodorants are different from the antiperspirants? Explain by using suitable example.

Q 14. How deodorants are useful in the management of the bad odor? Explain their mechanism.

Q 15. Write the advantage and disadvantage of deodorants usage.

Q 16. Define shampoo. Explain its manufacturing process.

Q 17. Discuss in brief:
   a. Clear liquid shampoo
   b. Gel shampoos
   c. Oil shampoos
   d. Antiseptic/antidandruff shampoo

Q 18. What do you mean by the word "conditioner"? How it is different from shampoo, explain with the formula?

Q 19. Write in detail about the role of dentifrices.

Q 20. Write note on skin (with diagram).

SHORT ANSWER TYPE QUESTIONS

1. Substances which are intended to be applied to the human body for cleansing, beautifying, promoting attractiveness, or altering the appearance without affecting the body's structure or functions are called as ....

2. There are various layers of cells within the epidermis, the outermost layer of skin is called as ....

3. Vanishing creams are .... type emulsion, as name indicates, these creams get.................... after applied and rubbed on to the skin.

4. ....contain fragrance, but they also block the pores to stop the discharge of perspiration while ....allows the release of perspiration, but prevents odor by combating it with antiseptic agents, which kill odor-causing bacteria.

5. Hair .... are used after shampooing the hair, to render the hair more lustrous, easy to comb, and free from static electricity when dry.

6. Which of the following is false in context to function of skin?
    1. Protects the body against physical injury and microbes
    2. Homeostasis
    3. Provides protection from UV light.
    4. Vitamin E synthesis and biotransformation of some chemicals.
7. Cold cream is:
    1. w/o emulsion
    2. w/o/w emulsion
    3. Provides protection from UV light.
    4. Forms a dry layer on skin.
8. To remove the make up and foundation bases, cream used is:
    1. Vanishing cream
    2. Cleansing cream
    3. Moisturiser
    4. Cold cream
9. Which of the following is not the function of hair?
    1. Hairs on the head protect the scalp from ultraviolet light, cushion round the head and insulate the skull.
    2. Eyebrows protect the eye from small foreign particles and insects.
    3. Body hair helps in biochemical synthesis of vitamins.
    4. The hairs, guarding the entrances to nostrils and external ear canals filter the air and help prevent the entry of foreign particles.
10. Which of the following is not an oral hygiene cosmetic?
    1. Dentifrices
    2. Toothpaste
    3. Gargle
    4. Mouthwash

ANSWERS

1. Cosmetics	6. 4
2. Stratum corneum (or horny layer)	7. 1
3. o/w, disappeared	8. 2
4. Antiperspirants, deodorant	9. 3
5. Conditioners	10. 3

7

Laboratory Manners

1. Always enter a laboratory with permission.

2. Keep your belongings and other materials properly in safe area.

3. Enter the laboratory wearing a clean apron and carrying other essential required materials.

4. Before starting experiment clean your work place and keep minimum things with you to avoid congestion.

5. Light burners only with matchstick or lighter and never light with adjacent burner or by any other means.

6. Put off burner by closing gas connection knob and not by blowing by mouth.

7. Keep important belongings in rack or pocket of apron for maximum utilization of workplace.

8. Maintain silence in laboratory and ask your teacher in case of any query.

9. Use dustbin for throwing waste material and not on floors or platform or in sink.

10. Put off electrical fans when gas burners are in use.

11. In case of gas leakage, immediately report to lab-assistant or teacher.

12. During any injury report immediately to your teacher for first-aid help.

13. Clean your working place after completion of experiment.

14. Always wash your hands with detergent or disinfectant and with fresh water after every experiment.

15. Do not carry costly things in laboratory which may be lost or damaged.

16. Before leaving your table—check gas connection, water supply and electricity plug and ensure they are off.

GLASSWARE HANDLING

Different types and makes of glassware are used in laboratory for performing experiments. Mostly glassware of borosilicate glass are preferred because of its clarity and heat and chemical resistance. Silica, boric acid and sodium and aluminum oxide are the components of borosilicate glass.

Washing

1. Before use of any glassware wash them under tap water.

2. Use detergent and scrubber to clean and remove adhesive material.

3. Rinse glassware, before use with materials for which it is to be used.

4. If glassware is new, before use soak it in 1% hydrochloric acid for some time because such glassware are alkaline and may affect the results.

5. If glassware contains unwanted sticky material that is difficult to remove, then treat it with nitric acid or chromic acid solution.

Drying

1. After washing keep glassware's on stand for stand for draining. Carry out drying at room temperature.

2. Glassware for volumetric procedures should be dried in hot air oven. For faster drying of glassware, it is advisable to dry them by hot air using a hair dryer.

3. Dried glassware are kept covered to protect from dust and any other contaminants from the atmosphere.

Heating

1. While heating any glassware do not leave it unattended because overheating may cause serious problem.
2. Keep hot glasswares in right place and handle it carefully to avoid burns.
3. Do not keep hot glassware on damp or wet surface.
4. Use pair of tong or napkin to hold hot glassware.

Glassware Care

1. Do not leave any sticky material in glassware for long periods.
2. Glassware for reuse must be emptied immediately after use.
3. Label all glassware that contains corrosive or any other chemicals to avoid confusion and accidents.
4. Always clean glassware before and after use.

MATERIALS REQUIRED FOR PRACTICAL

Make a separate small bag for practical which should contain the following:

1. Clean apron
2. Practical note book
3. Journal
4. Graph paper sheets
5. Pencil, eraser, ruler, sharpener
6. Permanent marker pen
7. Butter paper
8. Dusting and cleaning cloth
9. Calibrated small and big weight boxes
10. Match box/lighter
11. Self-adhesive labels of different sizes
12. Colored sketch pens
13. Scientific calculator

JOURNAL WRITING

The practical journal should be of 150 to 200 pages for 20–25 experiments. It should be covered with waterproof brown paper. On the cover of the journal, stick label containing information as given below.

Name:	Semester/Year
Subject:	Roll No.
Name of Institute:	

Writing in Index

While writing in the index write experiment number, complete aim or title, page number and date on which experiment performed. To have an attractive index, leave one line between two titles and draw over it with a black marker to look attractive.

Writing Experiment

Leaving one page blank after index start writing experiment with fresh page. Journal contains three types of pages, namely blank on left side, ruled on right side and graph page in between. Use these pages as mentioned in the following table.

Details of Journal Writing

If page numbers are not printed, write page number on all pages on both sides in a sequence. While writing headings, use official shortforms only as given in table below and avoid using your own shortcuts for different words. Also do not use the word like sol^n(solution), temp (temperature), etc. in the text.

Ruled page	Blank page	Graph page
Experiment number	Diagram (if any)	Title of the experiment
Date	Observations	Graph number
Title	Observation table	Scale
Aim	Formula	Graph
Requirements	Calculations	
References		
Theory or principle		
Procedure		
Precaution		
Result		
Conclusion (if any)		

Do not copy from seniors or other journals. Try to write journal on your own by taking help of reference books or your laboratory book, use the term properly mentioned below:

S. no.	Words	Proper	Improper
1.	Date	Date	Dt.
	1 Jan 2007	Jan 1, 2007	J. 1, 2007
		01.01.2007	01, J. 2007
			1st Jan 2007
2.	Page numbers	01, 02, 03	‹1›, (1), [1], 1
3.	Experiment	Experiment no.	Ex. No.
	Number	Experiment no.	Expt. No.
			Ex. No
4.	Requirements	Requirements	Req.
5.	Procedure	Procedure	Proc., Proce., Pro.
6.	Serial number	S. No., Serial no.	s. no., no.
7.	Observation table	Observation table	Ob. Table
			Obser^n. Table
8.	References	References	Ref.
9.	Calculations	Calculations	Cal^n., Cals.
10.	Conclusion	Conclusion	Concl., Concl^n.
11.	Observations	Observations	Obs., obs^n.

Aim: Keeping in mind the objective of experiment—write completely the aim of experiment beginning with word 'To'.

Requirement: Divide requirements of the experiment into two parts, namely chemicals and apparatus. All the solid and liquid chemicals including water must be written under chemicals. Apparatus includes glassware, instruments, equipment and accessories.

References: At least one reference should be written for every experiment. While writing references, refer journals such as Indian Drugs, Indian Journal of Pharmaceutical Sciences or any other journal of your choice and see how references are written. Once the style of writing (sequence) a reference is selected, continue it for all other experiments.

Theory: Under theory part of experiment write definition, classification, principle, formula, method, applications and other related information that can be helpful while studying for viva-voce.

Procedure: The first important point is to write procedure in past tense because you are narrating the way you have worked for experiments. Avoid style of writing in passage form. It is always better to follow stepwise procedure for better understanding of sequence of work and for representation. Procedure should be brief to understand the way of performing each step.

Observations: Under observations you need to write conditions that were observed while performing a particular experiment.

Observation table: Draw complete observation table giving sufficient column width and row space. If keywords are used in table, meaning of keywords should be mentioned immediately after table. Remember to specify units.

Calculations: You may have to calculate number of parameters. While doing this, give heading for calculation of each parameter. For highlighting the answer, underline it or put it in a square box or brackets. Specify appropriate unit to each value obtained.

Result: Conclude the result in compact and truthful manner. Do not forget to specify the unit for observed or calculated values.

Journal checking: Always get your journal checked at next practical. Avoid presenting journal for checking at the end of term. Before submission, check your journal for different entries and see that it is completed in all respect.

EXAMINATION

In most universities throughout India, annual pattern of examination is followed. However, recently a shift over from annual pattern semester pattern is observed. For an examination of 100 marks (practical), either 70:30 or 80:20 marking scheme is in existence for university and internal examinations, respectively.

No fixed criterion is laid down for marks distribution but generally it has been observed that the distribution of subject matter in relation with marks is as follows:

1. Synopsis (based on theory and practical) —15–20 per cent
2. Experiment —55–60 per cent
3. Viva-voce —10–15 per cent

VIVA-VOCE QUESTIONS

It is observed that as such there are no specific guidelines for asking questions at the time of examination during viva-voce session. Any question related to the subject, either from theory or practical or general knowledge, can be asked. Following are a few examples of questions and expected answers.

1. Why are you performing a particular experiment?
   - You should explain the objective of that experiment.
2. How to perform the experiment?
   - Explain stepwise detailed procedure or method of the experiment.
3. What is principle of experiment?
   - Explain principle on which experiment is based.
4. Name other methods of doing same experiment (if any).
   - Give list of other methods.
5. What is the significance or application of the experiment?
   - Explain the application with examples.
6. Different definitions related with experiment.
   - Definition must cover all points so that it can have meaning.
7. Name instrument or equipment used with its parts in the experiment.
   - Answer correct name of instrument or equipment with its parts.
8. Various standard values of properties or parameters can be asked.
   - When standard values are asked, your answer should be with the unit of the same.
9. Any questions from other subjects of pharmacy related with experiment performed may be asked.
   - To answer such type of questions, you have to attend all theory lectures and practicals. Listen to your teachers when they explain. Also make habit of reading reference books and subject related journals.

LIST OF EXPERIMENTS

Experiment Number 1

Object: To prepare 20.5 g of ORS powder (I.P), label it and dispense it in a suitable container.

Principle: A pharmaceutical powder is a mixture of finely divided drug and/or chemicals in dry form. These are solid dosage form of medicament, which are meant for internal and external use. They are available in crystalline or amorphous form. The particle size of powder plays an important role in physical, chemical and biological properties of the dosage forms. There is a relationship between particle size of powder and dissolution, absorption and therapeutic efficacy of drugs.

Powders are classified as:

1. Bulk powder for external use
2. Bulk powders for internal use
3. Simple and compound powders
4. Effervescent granules
5. Cachets.

Observation Table

S. no.	Ingredients	Quantity given	Quantity taken
1.	Sodium chloride	12.638 g	2.6 g
2.	Potassium chloride	7.317 g	1.5 g
3.	Sodium bicarbonate	14.14 g	2.9 g
4.	Dextrose	65.86 g	13.5 g

Procedure

1. Weigh the required amount of sodium chloride, potassium chloride, sodium bicarbonate, and dextrose.
2. Mix them in mortar and pestle and pass through the sieve no. 80
3. Dispense the powder and label it.

Category: As an electrolyte replenisher.

Storage: Stored in a well-closed airtight container, keep it in a cool and dry place.

Uses

1. Used in dehydration, dysentery and diarrhoea.
2. As a electrolyte replenisher.
3. To be diluted with 1 litre of sterile water.

Experiment Number 2

Object: To prepare 100 g of absorbable dusting powder (USP/NF), label it and dispense it in a suitable container.

Principle: Dusting powder is the powder in a fine state of subdivision of such substance for external application. They are usually mixture of substance zinc oxide, starch and boric acid or natural mineral substance such as kaolin or talc, the later may be contaminated with pathogenic organism and should therefore be sterilized by heat. Dusting powders are not intended for oral use. Dusting powder should be passed through sieve number 80 (#80) before dusting to avoid partial loss. It is better to weigh for some extra quantity, dusting powders are of two types:

1. Medical
2. Surgical

Observation Table

S. no.	Ingredients	Quantity given	Quantity taken
1.	Purified talc	500 g	50 g
2.	Starch	250 g	25 g
3.	Zinc oxide	50 g	5 g
4.	Salicylic acid	200 g	20 g

Procedure

1. Weigh the required quantity of starch, talc, zinc oxide and salicylic acid.
2. Mix them in ascending order of their weight.
3. Pass the mix powder through a sieve number 80.
4. After sieving, again mix the contents.
5. Dispense dusting powder in six sub-divided glass, label and dispense it.

Category: As medical and surgical.

Storage: *"Store in a cool and dry place".*

Uses: As an antiperspirant.

Experiment Number 3

Object: To prepare and submit 20 ml of cresol with soap solution I.P (lysol solution)

Principle: Solutions are liquid preparations that contain one or more soluble chemical substances dissolved in liquid solvents. Solutions are generally prepared by four methods:

a. By simple solution.
b. By chemical reactions.
c. By simple solution with sterilization.
d. By extraction.

Solution is a mixture of two compounds, namely solute and solvent. Solute is the smaller component present in the solution and is usually non-volatile in nature. Solvent is the larger component present and is also known as vehicle. Most of the drugs are non-polar or semi-polar. Hence they cannot be easily solubilized in water. Therefore special methods are used to prepare solutions. Solubility can be enhanced by using co-solvents (examples are glycerin, ethyl alcohol, propylene glycol) or complexation (example is a combination of iodine and potassium iodide) or surfactants (example is cresol with soap solution). Solutions are usually used for their specific therapeutic effect of solute either internally or externally. To increase the shelf life and aesthetic value of solutions, various additives are also added such as stabilizers, preservatives, coloring agents, flavoring agents, and sweetening agents. Solutions form most of the dosage forms like mixtures, enemas, mouthwashes, gargles, eardrops, eye drops, etc.

Cresol is a mixture of O, m and p-cresol. It acts as disinfectant. The solubility of cresol in water is only about 3%, whereas the quantity of cresol present in this preparation is 50%. To dissolve this much quantity of cresol, a solubilising agent is required. Vegetable oil contains free fatty acids, which react with potassium hydroxide and form soap. This soap acts as solubilising agent. The vegetable oil may be cottonseed, linseed, soybean or similar oils, which have a saponification value not greater than 205 and an iodine value, not less than 100. Solubilization is a process which allows a poorly water-soluble solute to go into solution and hence increases the solubility of the materials. It requires the presence of surface-active agents, which form colloidal aggregates when added in higher concentrations. The concentration of the surfactant at which the micelle formation takes place called the critical micelle concentration or CMC. The poorly soluble material either dissolves or gets absorbed onto the micelle at CMC, which ultimately increases the solubility of the material.

Observation Table

S. no.	Ingredients	Quantity given	Quantity taken
1.	Cresol	500 ml	10 ml
2.	Vegetable oil	180 g	3.6 g
3.	Potassium hydroxide	42 g	0.84 g
4.	Purified water (q.s)	1000 ml	20 ml

Procedure: Dissolve the potassium hydroxide in 250 ml of purified water, add the vegetable oil and heat on a water bath, mixing thoroughly, continue to heat until a small portion dissolves in water without separation of oily drops. Add the cresol, mix thoroughly and add sufficient purified water to produce the required volume.

Category: Disinfectant.

Storage: Store in cool and dry place, keep away from the children.

Direction : For external use only as a general disinfectant. It is unsuitable for use on human beings.

Uses: Lysol (cresol with soap) solution is a phenolic compound used as a disinfectant for domestic or hospital use like disinfection of floors, bathrooms, washbasins, organic waste such as sputum, faeces, urine, etc.

Precautions

1. Not to be used in the vicinity of infants such as nursery, children wards, etc.
2. Not to be used in places where food is prepared and served.

Experiment Number 4

Object: To prepare and submit 20 ml of aqueous iodine solution I.P. (Lugol's solution)

Principle: Practically the iodine is insoluble in water; its solubility is 1:2950. Iodine in presence of potassium iodide is soluble in water due to the formation of poly iodides. Iodine reacts with potassium iodide to form compounds called polyiodides.

$$KI + I_2 \rightarrow KI. I_2 \text{ or } K$$

The higher polyiodides are more soluble than the lower ones. Hence a rapid solution of the iodine is affected by using the potassium iodide in concerned solution. Iodine is an essential element of our body and its deficiency leads to development of goiter. The minimum daily requirement of an adult is about 100 µg. This preparation is used in the treatment or perpetrated treatment of thyro toxicosis. It can also be used as an antiseptic. Iodine slowly volatilizes at room temperature, therefore, the preparation should be stored in a well-closed container.

Observation Table

S. no.	Ingredients	Quantity given	Quantity taken
1.	Iodine	50 g	1 g
2.	Potassium iodide	100 g	2 g
3.	Purified water (q.s)	1000 ml	20 ml

Procedure: First dissolve the potassium iodide in a little volume of water. Dissolve the iodine in the above solution; add sufficient purified water to produce the required volume.

Category: Internally as a source of iodine, externally as an antiseptic.

Storage: Store in a well-closed container, the container materials of which are resistant to iodine.

Uses: It is used as an antiseptic and disinfectant, for emergency disinfection of drinking water and as a reagent for starch detection in medical tests. It is a source of iodine. It is used as a local anti-infective.

Experiment Number 5

Object: To prepare and submit 20 ml of strong iodine solution I.P.

Principle: Strong iodine solution contains 10% w/v of iodine (limits 9.5 to 10.5) and 6.0% w/v of potassium iodide KI (limits 5.7 to 6.3). Iodine with potassium iodide forms compounds called polyiodides. The higher polyiodides are more soluble than lower ones. Hence a rapid solution of the iodine is affected by using the potassium iodide in concentrated solution. Alcohol in the preparation is used as a menstruum. Another advantage of alcohol is that it quickly evaporates when the solution is applied over the skin leaving behind the iodine in very fine particle size. Due to this a larger surface area of iodine comes in contact with the body, which results in quicker absorption. It also dissolves cutaneous fat and hastens penetration and absorption and provides some additional antibacterial effect. The preparation is used as a topical antiseptic agent. The preparation cannot be applied to wounds and abrasions because the alcohol in the tincture is very irritating to open tissues. The preparation is stored in a well-closed container because alcohol and iodine are volatile in nature. The iodine stains the skin, clothes and vessels made from porcelain and metal, therefore, it should be stored only in glass containers. The iodine stain can be removed by sodium thiosulphate solution.

Observation Table

S. no.	Ingredients	Quantity given	Quantity taken
1.	Iodine	100 g	2 g
2.	Potassium iodide	60 g	1.2 g
3.	Purified water	100 ml	2 ml
4.	Alcohol (90%) sufficient to produce	1000 ml	20 ml

Procedure: First dissolve the potassium iodide in little volume of water. Dissolve the iodine in above solution; add sufficient alcohol 90% to produce the required volume.

Category: Antiseptic

Storage: Store in a well-closed container, the materials of which are resistant to iodine.

Direction: 'For external use only'.

Uses: Strong iodine is used to treat overactive thyroid, iodine deficiency, and to protect the thyroid gland from the effects of radiation from radioactive forms of iodine.

Experiment Number 6

Object: To prepare and submit 20 ml of weak iodine solution I.P. (tincture iodine)

Principle: Weak iodine solution is used internally in hypothyroidism and externally as antiseptic to treat wounds. In this preparation the concentration of iodine required is 20 mg/ml. As this preparation is used internally as well as externally, alcohol 50% (absolute alcohol 50 ml + water 50 ml) is used as a vehicle. Iodine is very slightly soluble in water. Its solubility can be increased using potassium iodide. Potassium iodide reacts with iodine to form polyiodides that are more soluble in alcohol 50%

$$Kl + nl_2 \rightarrow Kl\, l_2 + Kl\, 2l_2 + Kl\, 3l_2 + \ldots + Kl\, nl_2$$
Polyiodides

Polyiodides are more soluble in water by ion-induced dipolar interaction. Alcohol is used in this preparation because of two reasons: (a) when this preparation is applied to the wounds, alcohol precipitates the proteins and forms a protective layer, (b) alcohol absorbs heat from the body and gets evaporated, thereby causing cooling effect. Since iodine (present in iodine solution) reacts with some ingredients of ordinary glass container, iodine resistant container like amber colored container is used to store iodine solutions.

Observation Table

S. no.	Ingredients	Quantity given	Quantity taken
1.	Iodine	20 g	0.4 g
2.	Potassium iodide	25 g	0.5 g
3.	Alcohol (50%) (q.s)	1000 ml	20 ml

Procedure: Dissolve the potassium iodide and iodine in sufficient alcohol 50% to produce the required volume.

Category: Antiseptic, iodine supplement in hypothyroidism.

Storage: Store in a well-closed container, the materials of which are resistant to iodine.

Direction: 'For external use only'

Uses: As a disinfectant.

Experiment Number 7

Object: To prepare and submit 20 ml of strong ammonium acetate solution I.P.

Principle: This preparation contains 57.5 % w/v of ammonium acetate and it is prepared by reacting glacial acetic acid with ammonium bicarbonate and strong solution of ammonia.

$$NH_4HCO_3 + CH_3COOH \rightarrow CH_3COONH_4 + H_2O + CO_2$$
$$CH_3COOH + NH_4HCO_3 \rightarrow CH_3COONH_4 + H_2O + CO_2$$

A large open vessel is used to allow easy escape of the carbon dioxide and avoid spillage due to frothing. It is not possible to prepare the solution by reacting glacial acetic acid with ammonium bicarbonate alone, because the reaction between these substances ceases before the formation of required amount of ammonium acetate. As more and more ammonium acetate is going to form, concentration of acetate ions is going to increase and ionization of CH_3COOH is going to decrease and will stop ultimately. Ammonium hydroxide is used to neutralize the unreacted acid and to make the preparation alkaline with pH range of 7.6 to 8.1. The pH is adjusted by using two indicators, i.e. bromothymol blue and thymol blue. They give different colorations at different pH. Blue and yellow colors are obtained only in pH range of 7.6 to 8.1. Bromothymol blue checks the lower limit, i.e. pH 7.6 and thymol blue checks the upper limit, i.e. pH 8.1. Bromothymol blue changes color as follows:

Yellow → pH 6.0 green → pH 7.6 blue → pH 14

Thymol blue changes color as follows:

Red → pH 2.1 — yellow → pH 8.1 — green — pH 9.2 — violet → pH 14

The preparation is stored in lead free glass containers because ammonium acetate dissolves lead salts readily and due to extraction of lead from the glass, the preparation will become toxic and can cause lead poisoning. Diaphoretic mixture is used to lower the raised body temperature by increasing the excretions of body fluids in the form of sweat and urine.

Observation Table

S. no.	Ingredients	Quantity given	Quantity taken
1.	Glacial acetic acid	453 g	9.06 g
2.	Ammonium bicarbonate	470 g	9.4 g
3.	Ammonium solution strong	100 ml	2 ml
4.	Purified water (q.s)	1000 ml	20 ml

Note: Glacial acetic acid Wt/ml 1.047–1.052 g

Procedure: Mix the glacial acetic acid with about 350 ml purified water, add the ammonium bicarbonate in small quantities at a time and stir until it is completely dissolved. Add sufficient quantity of ammonia solution until one drop of the resulting solution, diluted with 10 drops of water, gives a full blue color with 1 drop of bromothymol blue, and a full yellow with thymol blue. Add sufficient purified water to produce the required volume.

Category: Bactericidal.

Storage: Store in a well-closed lead-free glass container.

Direction: For external use only

Uses: As a bactericide.

Experiment Number 8

Object: To prepare and submit 100 ml of aluminum hydroxide antacid suspension.

Principle: Suspensions are disperse systems in which finely divided insoluble solid drug particles are dispersed in a suitable liquid vehicle. The solid particles are known as dispersed phase, whereas liquid vehicle is known as continuous phase. A good suspension should have the following characteristics.

1. Finely divided solid particles should not settle rapidly and should be readily re-dispersed on gentle shaking of the container, if particles settle.

2. The suspension should be easily removed from the container.

3. The suspended particles should not form hard cake.

4. The suspension should have optimum viscosity, which facilitates the easy removal from the container and easily spread on the body surface.

5. The suspension should be free from gritty particles.

Suspension should be packed in suitable containers. For less viscous preparations, use narrow mouthed bottles and wide mouth bottles for thick preparations.

Based on the nature of the solids, present suspensions can be classified as follows:

a. Flocculated suspensions, e.g. Tetanus toxoid suspension

b. Deflocculated suspensions, e.g. procaine penicillin G suspension.

Aluminum hydroxide gel is an antacid suspension. It is also known as aluminum hydroxide suspension or Aluminum hydroxide mixture. It is colloidal suspension, hence does not require the use of suspending agent because of the strong affinity that exists between the dispersed phase of aluminum hydroxide and water. As a result there is increase in viscosity and aluminum hydroxide gel gets easily dispersed in water.

Aqueous aluminum hydroxide antacid suspension tends to thicken as gel during shelf life. This gelling accelerated during storage under warm conditions (30–40°C). This problem can be circumvented by the addition of sorbitol in concentration from 0.5–7% depending on the concentration of aluminum hydroxide in suspension. Aluminum hydroxide has constipating effect; therefore, it is normally combined with magnesium hydroxide, which provides laxative effect in commercial antacid formulations.

The taste of an antacid must be considered for consumers' acceptance. Sorbitol imparts a cool sweet pleasant taste. The parabens are used as preservatives. Peppermint oil is used as flavoring agent. Alcohol serves as vehicle. Amaranth solution is added to impart color to the preparation.

Observation Table

S. no.	Ingredients	Quantity for 1000 ml	Quantity for 100 ml
1.	Aluminum hydroxide gel dried	360 g	36 g
2.	Sorbitol	70 ml	7 ml
3.	Sodium saccharine	0.5 g	0.05 g
4.	Methyl paraben	2 g	0.2 g
5.	Propyl paraben	0.2 g	0.02 g
6.	Peppermint oil	0.05 ml	0.005 ml
7.	Alcohol	10 ml	1 ml
8.	Amaranth solution	q.s	q.s
9.	Purified water	q.s to 1000 ml	q.s to 100 ml

Procedure: Dissolve methyl paraben, propyle paraben, sodium saccharine, and peppermint oil in alcohol in clean dry vessel. In another beaker take nearly one-half of volume of purified water and add sorbital solution. Mix well. To this solution add the alcoholic solution and stir well. Add aluminum hydroxide in small proportions with continuous stirring. Add amaranth solution and mix. The entire product may be passed through a colloidal mill or homogeniser. Transfer to a measuring cylinder, add sufficient purified water to produce required volume. Mix well. Transfer to suitable bottle.

Category: Antacid suspension

Storage: Store in a cool and dry place, away from sunlight.

Direction: "Shake well before use".

Use: As antacid in peptic ulcers and hyperchlorhydria.

Experiment Number 9

Object: To prepare and submit 20 ml of liquid paraffin emulsion I.P

Principle: Emulsions are defined as disperse systems consisting of two immiscible liquids, one of which is distributed through the other in the form of minute globules, the system being stabilized by adding the third substance, the emulsifying agent. Emulsions are of two types.

1. Oil in water (O/W), in which the oil is dispersed in the water continuous phase. These emulsions are preferred for internal use. In these emulsions gum acacia, tragacanth and soaps of monovaslent bases like Na^+, NH_4^+, K^+ are used as emulsifying agents.

2. Water in oil (W/O), in which the water is dispersed in the oil, the continuous phase. In these emulsions wool fat, resins, bees wax and soaps of divalent bases like Ca^{++}, Mg^{++}, Zn^{++} are used as emulsifying agents.

Emulsions are prepared by different methods. They are dry gum method, wet gum method and bottle method.

While preparing the acacia emulsions for extemporaneous use, primary emulsion formula must be used. Based on the nature of the oil different formulas are there.

Nature of oil	Examples	Ratios of ingredients		
		Oil	Water	Acacia gum
Fixed oil	Castor oil	4	2	1
Mineral oil	Liquid paraffin	3	2	1
Volatile oil	Turpentine oil	2	2	1
Oleo gum resin	Male fern extract	1	2	1

Liquid paraffin emulsion is oil in water emulsion, made by the dry gum method, containing 50% v/v of liquid paraffin (limits 45.0–55.0). Liquid paraffin constitutes oil phase and purified water constitutes water phase.

Acacia is used as an emulsifying agent, which forms oil in water type of emulsion. Tragacanth is used as an emulsifying agent as well as viscosity-increasing agent, which stabilize the o/w acacia emulsion. Sodium benzoate is used as the preservative, especially for the oil phase. It prevents the surface growth of the microorganisms when emulsion is packed. High vapour pressure of chloroform allows it to concentrate on the surface of the emulsion and also fill the empty area of the bottle, which will not allow any growth of microorganisms on the surface of the mixture.

Observation Table

S. no.	Ingredients	Official quantity	Quantity taken
1.	Liquid paraffin	500 ml	10 ml
2.	Indian gum, in powder form	125 g	2.5 g
3.	Tragacanth, in powder form	5 g	0.1 g
4.	Sodium benzoate	5 g	0.1 g
5.	Vanillin	0.5 g	0.01 g
6.	Chloroform	2.5 ml	0.05 ml
7.	Glycerin	125 ml	2.5 ml
8.	Purified water, sufficient to produce	1000 ml	20 ml

Procedure: Triturate liquid paraffin and the chloroform with the Indian gum, the tragacanth and vanillin. Add in one quantity 250 ml of purified water and triturate until a creamy emulsion formed. Add the glycerin and the sodium benzoate dissolved in 2.5 ml of purified water. Add sufficient purified water to produce 20 ml. Mix.

Category: Laxative.

Storage: Store in a well-closed container; protected from light.

Direction: 'Shake well before use'

Uses: It is used as laxative in chronic constipation and also used during pregnancy for the emptying of faecal material in body before surgery.

Experiment Number 10

Object: To prepare and submit 20 ml of castor oil emulsion.

Principle: Castor oil is a fixed oil and is not miscible with water. To make it miscible, a third substance known as emulsifying agent in the ratio of 4:2:1, i.e. oil: water: gum will be used for the preparation of primary emulsion. Gum acacia will be used as emulsifying agent because emulsions prepared with gum acacia remain stable for sufficient long time.

Observation Table

S. no.	Ingredients	Official quantity	Quantity taken
1.	Castor oil	8 ml	5.33 ml
2.	Water	30 ml	20 ml

Procedure: By *wet gum method:* Thoroughly clean and dry a pestle and mortar. Weigh out 2 gm gum acacia and transfer it to the mortar. Measure 4 ml water and triturate it with gum so as to form mucilage. To this add 8 ml castor oil in small quantities at a time with thorough trituration after each addition. Triturate briskly without ceasing until a clicking sound is produced and the product becomes white or nearly white. At this stage the emulsion is known as primary emulsion. Add about 10 ml more of vehicle in small quantities at a time with constant trituration so as to get a homogeneous product.

Transfer the emulsion to a measure, add more of vehicle to produce the final volume 30 ml, stir thoroughly so as to form a uniform emulsion. Transfer the preparation to a bottle, cork, polish the bottle to remove fingerprints, label and dispense. "Shake well before use".

Category: Purgative.

Storage: Store in a well-closed container; protected from light.

Direction: 'Shake well before use'

Uses: As a purgative for the free evacuation of especially causing evacuation of the bowels.

Precautions: Because of its prompt action, castor oil should not be administered at bedtime, preferably it should be given early in the morning.

Experiment Number 11

Object: To prepare and submit 20 ml of cod liver oil emulsion IP.

Principle: Cod liver oil is fixed oil obtained from the fresh liver of the cod fish. This emulsion is given in case of the deficiency of vitamins A and D as an anti-rachitic. The emulsion should be protected from light to prevent the degradation of vitamin A.

The emulsion is prepared by the dry gum method. Acacia is the emulsifying agent and tragacanth is the emulsion stabilizer. Saccharin sodium is used as the sweetening agent. Benzaldehyde spirit is used as the flavoring agent and chloroform is used as the preservative.

Observation Table

S. no.	Ingredients	Official quantity	Quantity taken
1.	Cod liver oil	500 ml	10 ml
2.	Acacia, in powder form	125 g	2.5 g
3.	Tragacanth, in powder form	7.5 g	0.15 g
4.	Benzaldehyde spirit	2.5 ml	0.05 ml
5.	Saccharin sodium	1 gm	0.02 g
6.	Chloroform	2.5 ml	0.05 ml
7.	Purified water (q.s)	1000 ml	20 ml

Procedure: Take the cod liver oil in dry mortar and disperse acacia powder and tragacanth powder in it. Add the required volume of water, as for the primary emulsion formula, all at once to the mortar and triturate in one direction only until primary emulsion is formed. Dilute carefully, transfer to a measure, add the saccharin sodium solution, benzaldehyde spirit and chloroform with constant stirring and make up the volume with purified water.

Category: Source of vitamins A and D (anti-rachitic)

Storage: Store in a well-closed container in a cool place.

Direction: 'Shake well before use'

Uses: As a nutritional supplement. Since it is obtained from fish oils, it has high levels of the omega-3 fatty acids, EPA and DHA.

Also as a source of vitamins A and D.

Experiment Number 12

Object: To prepare and submit 5 boric acid suppositories.

Principle: Suppositories are conical or ovoid, solid preparations for insertion into the rectum where they melt dissolve or disperse and exert a local or less often, a systemic effect. Their basis is fat, a wax or a glycerol-gelatin jelly. They weigh 1, 2 or occasionally 4 g. Earlier, small suppositories known as cones were prescribed for ear infections and long, very narrow forms, called bougies, were used for nasal and urethral infections. There are virtually absolute today. Medicaments are prescribed in suppositories for these reasons.

1. To exert a direct action on the rectum.
2. To promote evacuation of the bowel.
3. To provide a systemic effect.

Systemic treatment by the rectal route is of particular value for,

a. Treating patients who are unconscious, mentally disturbed or unable to tolerate oral medication because of vomiting or pathological conditions of the alimentary tract.

b. Administering drugs, that cause gastric irritation, such as aminophylline.

c. To produce mechanical action on the lower bowel and facilitate evacuation in the treatment of hemorrhoids, anal irritation, constipation, etc.

d. Treating infants.

Suppositories are usually prepared by melting a suitable base, incorporating the prescribed amounts of finely powdered medicament(s) and pouring the mixture into molds.

Displacement value: The volume of suppository that occupy in a given mold remains same. The weight of a medicated suppository varies when compared to a plain suppository. It is due to the variation of the densities of the medicament and the base. It means the weight of the medicament may not displace the same weight of the base for the same volume. Therefore, an allowance is made for the alteration in the density of the total mass, due to the added medicament. It is calculated by applying displacement value.

Calculation is done for extra quantity to manipulate the loss during preparation. Boric acid is insoluble in cocoa butter. Therefore, mixed with a portion of melted cocoa butter on a warm tile. The warm tile prevents the cooling and solidification of the base during mixing only 2/3 of the base is melted, as this prevents overheating of the base and the formation of unsatisfactory suppositories. When cocoa butter is heated above its melting temperature (about 36°C) and chilled to its solidification point (below 15°C), immediately after returning to room temperature this cocoa butter attains a melting point of about 24°C, therefore cocoa butter must not be heated at higher temperature. Cooling the mold dissipates the contain heat and hastens settling of the base. Overfilling of the mold is done to prevent hollows and depressions forming at top of the suppository due to contraction of the base.

Observation Table

S. no.	Ingredients	Quantity given	Quantity taken
1.	Boric acid	120 mg	600 mg
2.	Cocoa butter (q.s)	1 g	5 g

Note: Displacement value of boric acid is 1.5

Procedure: Clean the suppository mold with hot water and detergent. Lubricate the mold with the lubricant fluid and invert the mold in ice. Weigh the cocoa butter and transfer to a china dish. Melt 2/3 of it on a water bath, remove from the water bath and stir well until all that has melted.

Warm a small tile on a water bath. Place the boric acid on the warmed tile. Pour half of the melted base on the boric acid powder on the tile and mix well to get a smooth dispersion. Transfer the dispersion to the porcelain dish and stir well to form a homogeneous mixture.

Fill 6 cavities of the mold to overflow. Allow the mass to set. Trim of the excess with a sharp blade. Keep the mold for half an hour on ice. Open the mold and remove the suppositories. Blot off the excess lubricant.

Select the 5 best suppositories. Wrap and dispense in a neatly labeled box.

Category: Local anti-infective.

Storage: Store in a cool place.

Direction: 'For rectal use only'

Uses: As an antifungal and antibacterial.

Experiment Number 13

Object: To prepare and submit 5 zinc oxide suppositories.

Principle: Same as of boric acid suppositories.

Observation Table

S. no.	Ingredients	Quantity given	Quantity taken
1.	Zinc oxide	600 mg	3 g
2.	Cocoa butter (q.s)	2 g	10 g

Note: Displacement value of zinc oxide is 5

Procedure

1. Calculate the quantities required, taking displacement values into account if relevant. Excess must be made because of unavoidable wastage during preparation.

2. Select a dry, clean mold and place it on a clean tile.

3. Shred the fat with a fine food grater. Weigh the required amount, avoiding lumps that will be slow to melt, and place in the smallest evaporating basin that will hold it. The shreds can be poled high because the volume contracts considerably on melting. A porcelain dish is preferable because it is easier to overheat the contents in a metal type.

4. Finely powder the medicaments and pass each through a separate no. 180 sieve. Weigh the required quantities.

5. Heat a small tile until it is comfortably warm to the hand. If this is done over a water bath, dry the tile thoroughly afterwards.

6. Mix the powders on the tile with a flexible spatula.

7. Place the base on the water bath until about two-thirds of the contents has melted and then remove from the heat the rest will melt with stirring, particularly if the dish is tightly cupped in the palm of one hand. Stir with a small, non-tapering spatula; not a glass rod, because base tends to solidify on the stirrer and is more easily removed from a spatula on to the edge of the dish. Overheating may occur if the base is left over the heat until completely melted.

8. Pour about half of the melted base onto the mixed medicaments and work into a smooth dispersion as quickly as possible by levigating with the spatula. Avoid loss over the edge of the tile. To prevent excessive cooling through spreading over a large area, use as small a tile as is consistent with avoidance of spillage. If the base solidifies, it can be softened by holding the tile over the water bath for a few seconds.

9. Transfer the disoperation to the dish, leaving virtually none on the tile, and air to form a homogeneous mixture.

10. Continue stirring until the mixture begins to thicken. Then fill each cavity of the mold to overflowing. Meanwhile stir the mass continuously; this precaution (easily forgotten

due to anxiety that setting will take place before the mold is filled), and delay in pouring until the mass is about to sedimentation of insoluble solids. If necessary, use the spatula to help the viscous base from the dish. Solidification should occur during pouring, apply the minimum of heat to start the mass moving again. The cavities are overfilled to prevent depressions in the tops of the suppositories due to contraction of the base during cooling.

11. Leave for two or three minutes until the mass has just not and then remove the excess from the mold with a sharp knife, razor blade or a slightly warm spatula.

12. Leave in a cool place for 10 to 15 min. Then open the mold and remove the suppositories. If they are difficult to separate, reclose the mold loosely and tap the base squarely and firmly on the protected bench, a procedure that generally force suppositories of the synthetic for type.

Note

- The large amount of powder in this preparation cannot be incorporated satisfactorily in a 1 g suppository; hence the official product is made in a 2 g mold.

- Preferably, these suppositories should be made with a synthetics fatty base but it is interesting to prepare them with theobroma oil for experience in the problems presented with this base.

- To obtain a homogeneous suppository of uniform composition and color, it is advisable to levigate the powders with a little water before mixing with the base. About 0.4 ml per suppository is suitable but this must be taken into account when calculating the amount of base required.

Category: Local anti-infective.

Storage: Store in a cool place.

Direction: 'For rectal use only'

Uses: As an antifungal and antibacterial.

Experiment Number 14

Object: To prepare and submit 25 g of cold cream.

Principle: Cold creams are typically beeswax-borax emulsions. They are so called because on application to skin the evaporation of water leads to cooling effect. When a solution of borax is added to molten beeswax, emulsifying agent is formed because of wax acid and borax, i.e. wax acid is saponified by borax forming Na-soap (i.e. Na-soap of wax acid). This agent is formed at the interface between oil and water, which emulsifies the mineral oil in water. It is because of beeswax, cream is able to contain appreciable amount of water. These are typically white creams of higher-class free form greasiness, which has firm consistency and on application they liquefy and spread easily.

This cream can be either o/w type (or) w/o type depending upon the ratio of water phase. 45% is considered to be the critical level of water phase, cream-containing water less than 45% is of w/o type and cream with water phase more than 45% is of o/w type of emulsion. Percentage of beeswax used ranges 5–15% and borax 5–6% of wt of beeswax. Lesser amount of beeswax gives softer cream and higher amount gives stiffer cream. Cold cream has got a neutral pH.

Both w/o and o/w emulsion can be obtained by beeswax-borax which depends upon

- Ratio of oil to water phase.
- Temperature of preparation.
- Amount of beeswax saponified.
- Other ingredient present.

Observation Table

S. no.	Ingredients	Quantity given	Quantity taken
1.	Bees wax	80 g	2 g
2.	Mineral oil	490 ml	12.25 ml
3.	Soft paraffin	70 g	1.75 g
4.	Cetyl alcohol	10 g	0.25 g
5.	Borax	4 g	0.1 g
6.	Water	346 ml	8.65 ml
7.	Perfume	q.s.	q.s

Procedure: Take 2.16 g beeswax, 1.89 g of soft paraffin, 0.27 g of cetylalcohol and 13.2 ml mineral oil in a clean dry vessel and heat on water bath to 80°C. Dissolve borax in water in another vessel and heat simultaneously with the oil phase to 70°C. Add the aqueous phase to oil phase slowly with rapid stirring. Continue stirring slowly after the additions of aqueous phase until the cream has cooled to about 50°C. Add the perfume, mix well. Weigh out 25 g of cream and fill into jar. At the time of filling the cream, it should have cooled to 40–42°C.

Category: Humectants.

Storage: Store in a cool and dry place.

Direction: "For external use only"

Uses: To prevent loss of water for dry skin, especially during winter and skin smoothener.

Experiment Number 15

Object: To prepare and submit 25 g of vanishing cream.

Principle: A cream, which spread easily and seems to disappear rapidly when applied on the skin, are termed vanishing cream. These creams are composed of emollient esters, which have a little apparent film on the skin. Low percentage of oil phase is chosen for the abovementioned reasons. Traditional formula of vanishing cream is based on the stearic acid. The acids melt above the body temperature and crystallize in suitable form so as to be immiscible providing a non-greasy film stearic acid to impart attractive appearance to cream.

Stearic acid makes the cream very white and because of this, vanishing cream contains partially saponified stearic acid, free stearic acid and water. Cream made with sodium hydroxide is harder than made with potassium hydroxide. Borax also can be used and these creams are white in color, but the product has the tendency to become greasy. Glycerin is used as humectant that attracts moisture and hydrates the stratum corneum. Glycerin also prevents the cream from drying up. Lanoline is used in modern formula as emollient. Triethanolamine stearate is used as emulsifier, which is obtained by reaction between triethanolamine and stearic acid.

Observation Table

S. no.	Ingredients	Quantity given	Quantity taken
1.	Stearic acid	200 g	5 g
2.	Glycerin	60 ml	1.5 ml
3.	Potassium hydroxide	4 g	0.1 g
4.	Triethanolamine	12 ml	0.30 ml
5.	Water (q.s)	1000 ml	25 ml
6.	Preservative	0.2 g	0.005
7.	Perfume	Adequate	Adequate

Procedure: Melt 5.4 g of stearic acid by heating along with glycerin to about 70°C on a water bath. Dissolve 0.108 g of KOH in water. Add triethanolamine, preservative and warm the aqueous solution to 70°C on water bath.

Add the aqueous phase to the oil phase and stir continuously all the time until the cream has formed. When it has cooled to 50°C add the perfume, mix well. Transfer to a clean mortar and triturate well until a cream of pearslescent luster is obtained. Weigh out 25 g of cream and fill into suitable container.

Category: Cosmetic.

Storage: Store in a cool and dry place

Direction: "For external use only"

Uses

1. Used as base for free powder and other makeup.

2. Used as emollient.

3. It gives better complexion to skin and also used for oily skin.

Experiment Number 16

Object: To prepare and submit 5 g of tooth powder.

Principle: Tooth powder is the simplest and cheapest form of dentifrices compare to toothpaste. Tooth powder has less solubility problem in formulation because interaction between components is less in absence of water. Oxidizing agent and fluorides retain their effective concentration longer in tooth powder than in toothpaste. It contains abrasive such as precipitated chalk, i.e. calcium carbonate. It is used in small proportion and mixed with larger quantities of other abrasive. It contains dry calcium phosphate which usually provides the toothpaste the pH ranging from 6 to 8.

It also contains detergent like sodium lauryl sulphate which is necessary to reduce interfacial tension between adherent matter and surface of teeth, thereby during cleaning, it helps in penetration and removed matter in the foam produced. It also contains sodium per borate that acts as bleaching agent, which is added to improve the whitening action of tooth powder. They are basically oxidizing agents. Artificial sweeteners such as sodium saccharin is used to an extent of 0.05–0.25%. Flavor such as peppermint oil is used which improves the characteristic taste and sensation of freshness in mouth.

Observation Table

S. no.	Ingredients	Quantity given	Quantity taken
1.	Precipitated chalk	810 g	4.05
2.	Tricalcium phosphate	100 g	0.5
3.	Sodium lauryl sulphate	50 g	0.25
4.	Sodium per borate	20 g	0.1
5.	Sodium saccharin	20 g	0.1
6.	Peppermint oil	q.s	q.s

Procedure

All solid ingredients are requiring being in fine powder.

1. Mix the weighed quantity of sodium saccharine and peppermint oil together with small amount of precipitated chalk in mortar until uniform mix is obtained.

2. In another clean mortar mix sodium lauryl sulphate with sodium per borate lightly by trituration.

3. Add flavor solution to this mix and mix by light trituration.

4. Add tricalcium phosphate.

5. Mix lightly and then gradually incorporate the precipitated chalk. Mix by light trituration until uniform mass is produced.

6. Weigh about 5 g of tooth powder and fill in container with perforated top.

Category: Dentifrice

Storage: Store in a cool and dry place, away from moisture.

Direction: To be rubbed on teeth

Use: To prevent tooth decay and maintenance of healthy gum.

Experiment Number 17

Object: To prepare and submit 20 g of toothpaste.

Principle: Toothpaste is a dentifrice and its primary function is to remove adherent matter from the tooth surface with minimal damage to it. It is a common domestic cleaning preparation, which is normally prepared by using mild abrasive agent to which surfactants are added. Surfactant aids in the penetration and removal of adherent film and to suspend removed soil matter. The foam produced has physiological effect in making tooth cleansing more pleasurable. Cleaning function is achieved in short time and at body temperature.

The basic processes in the manufacturing of toothpaste are

- Hydration gelling.
- Dispersion of the abrasive in the gel.

Hydration of the gel is normally done by adding a solid gelling agent to glycerin and part of the water under condition of vigorous agitation. The powder addition may be done in variety of steps. It is usual practice to add active ingredient late in the mixing cycle and to add surfactant and flavor last. This is done to avoid excessive foaming and to reduce loss of flavor.

Glycerin and propylene glycol are added as humectant to prevent the toothpaste drying at the tube nozzle. In order to maintain high solid suspension in stable viscous form, adding gum tragacanth increases the viscosity of liquid phase. Sodium saccharin used as sweetener, sodium lauryl sulphate as surfactant, peppermint oil as flavoring agent, precipitated calcium carbonate as abrasive.

Observation Table

S. no.	Ingredients	Quantity given	Quantity taken
1.	Precipitated chalk	400 g	8 g
2.	Sodium lauryl sulphate	12 g	0.24 g
3.	Glycerin	250 ml	5 ml
4.	Propylene glycol	60 ml	1.2 ml
5.	Sodium saccharin	0.5 g	0.01 g
6.	Sodium carboxy methyl cellulose	10 g	0.2 g
7.	Chloroform	5 ml	0.1 ml
8.	Propyl paraben	0.2 g	0.004 g
9.	Peppermint oil	Adequate	Adequate
10.	Water (q.s)	1000 g	20 g

Procedure: Dissolve sodium saccharin and propyl paraben in half the quantity of water. Mix glycerin and propylene glycol and add this to sodium saccharin solution. Weigh out required quantity of sodium CMC and place in a clean dry mortar. Add aqueous solution to the gum and triturate rapidly until a uniform dispersion is obtained. Keep aside for 20 minutes to allow binding agent to swell. To the gel produced, add precipitated chalk in small amount and triturate thoroughly after each addition to obtain smooth paste. Add chloroform, peppermint oil and mix well. Dissolve sodium lauryl sulphate in required remaining quantity of water taken in beaker. Add this solution into the mortar and triturate slowly, then fill into the container.

Category: Dentifrice

Storage: Store in a cool and dry place, away from moisture.

Direction: To be rubbed on teeth with the help of tooth brush.

Use: To clean the teeth and deodorize the oral cavity.

Experiment Number 18

Object: To prepare and submit 10 ml of shampoo.

Principle: Shampoo may be defined as a preparation containing surface-active agents, which are used to remove dirt, oil and debris from the hair, scalp without affecting the natural gloss of hair. It also helps to keep the hair fragrant, lustrous, soft and manageable. Shampoo is prepared by dissolving detergents in suitable liquid along with other ingredients like cleansing, flavoring agent and preservatives. An ideal shampoo should have the following properties.

1. It should remove dirt, grease (oil) debris from the hair and scalp.
2. It should be non-toxic.
3. It should be non-irritant.
4. It should provide sufficient fragrance to the hair after its use.
5. It should be effective in small amount.
6. It should be easily removed by washing with water.
7. It should make the hair soft and shining.

All the fatty acids oil content, which reacts with potassium hydroxide and form soap. In this preparation glycerol is used as solubilising agent and methyl paraben is used as preservative.

Observation Table

S. no.	Ingredients	Quantity given	Quantity taken
1.	Coconut oil	140 g	1.4 g
2.	Olive oil	30 ml	0.3 g
3.	Castor oil	30 ml	0.3 g
4.	Potassium hydroxide	47 g	0.47 g
5.	Glycerol	20 ml	0.2 g
6.	Methyl paraben	1.8 g	0.018 g
7.	Perfume	0.2 g	0.002 g
8.	Water (q.s)	1000 ml	10 ml

Procedure: In a beaker heat coconut oil, olive oil and castor oil with potassium hydroxide and a little quantity of water on a water bath at 70°C. Take remaining quantity of water in another beaker, add glycerol, preservative and perfume, dissolve them thoroughly. Mix both the liquids to form a clear solution.

Category: Cleaning agent.

Storage: Store in a narrow mouthed, well-closed plastic container.

Direction: To be applied on wet hair

Uses: To rinse out the dirt and give gloss to hair.

Experiment Number 19

Object: To prepare and submit 10 g of lipstick.

Principle: Lipstick is defined as a preparation, which is applied on lips to impart color and make them more attractive. It is a dispersion of colored material in base, which is a blend of oil, fat and waxes. Lipstick is generally prepared in 3 steps:

1. Preparation of component blends
2. Mix of various blends to give the lipstick mass
3. Molding of the mass and flaming.

In the first step all the color present are grounded using mills and mixed with oil or solvent to give uniform dispersion. Simultaneously other mix of the entire wax base is heated and the wax base is prepared. Oil blend and wax blend are mixed to give lipstick mass. During mixing temperature of oil blend and wax blend should be almost same in order to prevent thickening of wax in oil. The mass obtained is then poured into lipstick mold in the step 3. Before pouring, the mass is warmed to about 40°C. This is done to avoid flow of mass during setting of lipstick. Mass is overflown to prevent dispersion in the centre of stick. When mass has just cooled, the excess is cripped off. Molds are then cooled until the lipstick has completely settled. Mold is then opened and lipstick is then subjected to immediate flaming. Flaming is done after the placing of lipstick into its container. This helps to give the lipstick a smooth and glossy look. An ideal lipstick should have the following properties.

i. It should be non-irritant and non-toxic.

ii. It should not dry on storage.

iii. It should maintain the lip color long period after its application.

iv. It should be free from gritty particles.

v. It should be easily applicable and removable after its application.

vi. It should not break during use.

Observation Table

S. no.	Ingredients	Quantity given	Quantity taken
1.	Bees wax	150 g	1.5 gm
2.	Paraffin wax	100 g	1 gm
3.	Cetyl alcohol	50 g	0.5 gm
4.	Perfume	Adequate	Adequate
5.	Castor oil (q.s)	700 ml	7 ml
6.	Coloring agent	Adequate	Adequate

Procedure: Take paraffin wax and bees wax in a China dish and heat it up to 70°C on a water bath. In a beaker take caster oil and heat up to 70°C and mix into melted mixture and add perfume and coloring agent. Immediately pour the molten mass into the lubricated mold, allow it to cool by placing molds on ice cubes. And then cut the surface using sharp knife. Remove the sticks from the mold and place it in the lipstick case and label it.

Category: Cosmetic

Storage: Store in a cool and dry place.

Direction: To be applied on lips.

Uses: As a cosmetic for attractive lips.

Experiment Number 20

Object: To prepare and submit 20 ml of potassium chlorate gargles.

Principle: Generally, gargles are used to relieve soreness in mid-throat infections and most have a deodorant effect. A bactericide, e.g. phenol or thymol is usually present but not in high enough concentration for significant antibacterial activity; however, it may exert a mild anesthetic effect. Potassium chlorate is included in gargles for its weak astringent effect on superficial cells, which helps to remove the tone of a relaxed throat; it also stimulates the flow of saliva, which relieves dryness. The best-known gargles are phenol garlic, potassium chlorate and phenol garlic and thymol glycerin compound.

Observation Table

S. no.	Ingredients	Quantity given	Quantity taken
1.	Potassium chlorate	30 g	0.6 g
2.	Liquid phenol	15 ml	0.3 g
3.	Water (q.s)	1000 ml	20 ml

Procedure: Dissolve the weighed amount of potassium chlorate is about 15 ml of water. To this add liquefied phenol and add sufficient water to produce the required volume. Transfer to a container, label and dispense. The secondary label "for external use only" must be attached.

Category: Antibacterial.

Storage: Store in a cool and dry place, away from children.

Direction: These gargles should be diluted with ten times its volume of warm water before use.

Uses: These gargles are used at sialogogue and astringent. Potassium chlorate is a sialogogue (which increases the flow of saliva) and astringent (which precipitate the proteins).

Experiment Number 21

Object: To prepare and submit 20 ml of antiseptic mouthwash.

Principle: Mouthwashes are aqueous solutions with pleasant taste and odor used to clean deodorize the buccal cavity. They are very refreshing, particularly to bed-ridden patients. Generally they contain antibacterial agents, alcohol, glycerin, sweetening agents and flavoring agents. In this preparation thymol and borax used as antibacterial agents, alcohol as solvent, glycerin as sweetening agent, sodium bicarbonate can dissolve mucous.

Observation Table

S. no	Ingredients	Prescription quantity	Quantity taken
1.	Thymol	0.3 g	0.006 g
2.	Alcohol	35 ml	0.7 ml
3.	Borax	20 g	0.4 g
4.	Sodium bicarbonate	10 g	0.2 g
5.	Glycerin	80 ml	1.6 ml
6.	Flavor	Adequate	Adequate
7.	Water (q.s)	1000 ml	20 ml

Procedure: Dissolve the required quantity of thymol in alcohol. In another beaker dissolve borax and sodium bicarbonate in water and mix the both solutions. Add glycerin and sufficient quantity of flavor mix well. Add the water to produce required volume.

Category: Antibacterial.

Storage: Store in a cool and dry place, away from children.

Direction: 'Dilute with an equal volume of warm water before use'. 'Not to be swallowed in large quantities'.

Uses: To enhance oral hygiene.

Mouthwash has antiseptic and anti-plaque effect, it also kills the bacterial which causes plague, gingivitis and bad breath.

Experiment Number 22

Object: To prepare and submit 20 g of non-staining iodine ointment BPC.

Principle: Non-staining iodine ointment BPC is used as a counterirritant. The fixed oils and many fats obtained from vegetable and animal sources contain unsaturated constituents. The iodine combines with double bonds of the unsaturated constituents. Hence free iodine is not available.

$$CH_3 (CH_2)_7 CH = CH - (CH_2)_7 COOH + I_2 \rightarrow CH_3 (CH_2)_7$$

Oleic acid $CHI = CHI (CH_2)_7 COOH$

Di-iodo stearic acid

If complete iodine is not combined, then the free iodine gives brown color to the product and leaves a stain when applied. In other words, if complete iodine is combined with unsaturated oils and fats, then the final ointment attains greenish black color. It leaves no stain when rubbed onto the skin. Hence they are known as non-staining iodine ointments. Iodine is easily soluble in unsaturated oils like arachis oil. To enhance the rate of solubilization, powdered form of iodine is preferred. Iodine solution is heated to complete the reaction between iodine and arachis oil. Heating must be done at not more than 50°C, because at high temperature iodine sublimes.

Methyl salicylate is volatile in nature. To avoid evaporation of methyl salicylate, it is added when the preparation is at lower temperature. Stirring should be done slowly to prevent air entrapment when the preparation starts thickening. Iodine acts as a counterirritant. Methyl salicylate also serves as a counterirritant and a flavoring agent. Yellow soft paraffin is used as a base. This is a semisolid preparation. Some quantity of preparation will go waste during manufacture of semisolids. 2 g extra is calculated to nullify loss during manufacture of 20 g non-staining iodine ointment, i.e. quantities of ingredients are calculated for 22 g.

Observation Table

S. no.	Ingredients	Quantity given	Quantity taken
1.	Methyl salicylate	50 ml	1 ml
2.	Iodine	50 g	1 g
3.	Arachis oil	150 g	3 g
4.	Yellow soft paraffin (q.s)	1000 g	20 g

Procedure: Depending on the quantity of preparation to be submitted, the working formula is calculated.

1. Iodine is dissolved in arachis oil at room temperature by simple stirring in a beaker.
2. Heat the above solution on water bath at 50°C with occasional stirring until the brown color disappears (or greenish black color appears).
3. Sufficient quantity of yellow soft paraffin is added (previously heated to 40°C), stirred slowly, cooled to solidify.
4. When the above preparation is at semi-liquid consistency, methyl salicylate is added, stirred slowly, allowed for complete solidification.
5. The ointment is transferred to a tightly-closed wide-mouthed container.
6. The container is capped, polished, labeled, and submitted.

Composition: Each g contains 47.5 to 52.5 mg of iodine.

Category: Counterirritant

Storage: Store in a cool place

Directions: For external use only. Do not apply on broken skin.

Uses: The deeply penetrating action of ointment provides long-lasting relief from backaches, waist pains, muscle strains, and sprains.

Experiment Number 23

Object: To prepare and submit 20 g of diclofenac sodium gel.

Principle: Diclofenac sodium is a non-steroidal anti-inflammatory agent. It possesses analgesic and antipyretic actions also. It is an inhibitor of prostaglandin synthesis. It is supplied in the gel form for topical use. It is prepared in the concentration of 1% w/w. In this preparation sodium alginate gel is used as a base. Glycerin used in this preparation acts as humectant. Methyl hydroxybenzoate acts as a preservative. Calcium gluconate in small quantity is used to improve the viscosity of sodium alginate gel by cross-linking.

Observation Table

S. no.	Ingredients	Quantity given	Quantity taken
1	Diclofenac sodium	10 g	0.2 g
2	Sodium alginate	70 g	1.4 g
3	Glycerin	70 g	1.4 g
4	Methyl hydroxy benzoate	2 g	0.04 g
5	Calcium gluconate	0.5 g	0.01 g
6	Purified water (q.s.)	1000 g	20 g

Procedure: Depending on the quantity of preparation to be submitted, the working formula is calculated.

1. Sodium alginate is wet with glycerin in a mortar.
2. Methyl hydroxybenzoate and calcium gluconate are dissolved in about 3/4th of the purified water with the aid of heat in beaker. This solution is cooled to about 60°C and stirred well.
3. Add sodium alginate–glycerin mixture to the above aqueous solution in small quantities and stirred vigorously.
4. Weighed quantity of diclofenac sodium is added and stirred well.
5. The gel is packed in a well-closed, wide-mouthed container.
6. The container is capped, polished, labeled, and submitted.

Composition: Each g contains 10 mg of diclofenac sodium.

Category: Analgesic, anti-inflammatory.

Storage: Store in a cool place, do not freeze.

Direction: For external use only.

Uses: As an analgesic and antipyretic.

Evaluation of Diclofenac Sodium Gel

Principle: Diclofenac sodium is soluble in water. Therefore, drug is extracted with water. The extracted drug after necessary dilutions is measured at 279 nm in uv-vis spectrophotometer.

Procedure: Construction of a standard graph and preparation of diclofenac sodium stock solution:

1. Accurately weighed 100 mg of diclofenac sodium is transferred into a 100 ml standard volumetric flask.
2. Diclofenac sodium placed in volumetric flask is dissolved by adding 50 ml of distilled water with shaking. Then the volume is made up to 100 ml with distilled water.
3. From this, 10 ml of the drug solution is transferred into another 100 ml standard volumetric flask.
4. The solution is diluted to 100 ml accurately with distilled water.
5. The resulting solution contains 100 mg/ml. This solution is used to prepare diluted solutions for standard plot.

Preparation of Solutions for Standard Plot

1. From the stock solution, 0.5, 1, 2, 3, 4, 5, and 6 ml solutions are transferred into 10 ml test tubes (or volumetric flasks).
2. All the solutions are diluted to 10 ml using distilled water.
3. The resulting solutions contain 5, 10, 20, 30, 40, 50, and 60 mg/ml of drug.
4. The solutions are mixed to distribute the drug uniformly.
5. The absorbances of the solutions are measured at 277 nm (care should be taken to see that air bubbles are absent in the solutions while measuring absorbance).
6. Standard graph is constructed as shown in Fig. 7.1. By taking concentration (mg/ml) on x-axis and y-axis.

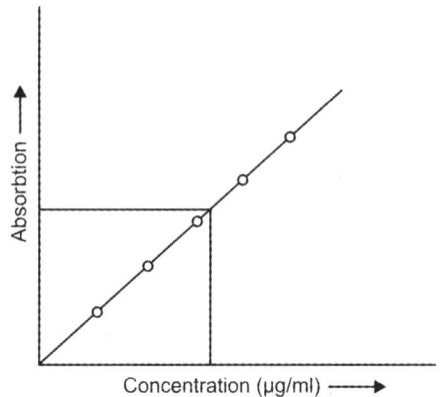

Fig. 7.1: Standard graph of diclofenac sodium

Estimation of Diclofenac Sodium in the Gel

1. Accurately weighed 1 g of the gel is placed in 100 ml volumetric flask.
2. 25 ml of distilled water is added into the volumetric flask.
3. The contents are shaken well to extract the drug.
4. The solution is filtered and the filtrate is collected.
5. Again steps 2 to 4 are repeated.
6. From this, 1 ml is pipetted into test tube.
7. The volume is made up to 10 ml with water.
8. The absorbance of the diluted solution is measured at 277 nm.
9. From the absorbance the amount of drug is estimated.

Result (Table 7.1)

Table 7.1: Standard plot data for diclofenac sodium

S. no.	Drug conc., Mg/ml	Stock solution of diclofenac sodium, ml	Distilled water, ml	Absorbance
1.	0	0	10	
2.	5	0.5	9.5	
3.	10	1	9.0	
4.	20	2	8.0	
5.	30	3	7.0	
6.	40	4	6.0	
7.	50	5	5.0	
8.	60	6	4.0	

Experiment Number 24

Object: To prepare and submit 20 g of pain balm.

Principle: Ointments are semisolid preparations for application to skin or mucous membrane, which have the ability to cling to the surface of application for a required time before it is washed or warm out. This adhesion is due to their plastic rheological behavior, which allows the semisolid to retain their shape and cling as film until acted upon by an outside force. Ointments are used for their emollient effect on the skin for the protection of lesions and for topical medication .The ointments is generally anhydrous and contains one or more medicaments in suspension or in solution form.

Pain balm is prepared by fusion method containing liquid miscible with bases. It is used to relieve pain backache, myalgia, and fibrositis. It is applied with rubbing to relieve pain and have deep penetrative action. They contain drugs having counterirritant action like methyl salicylate and camphor. In this preparation menthol, cassia oil, peppermint oil is used to impart aromatic odor. Peppermint oil also possesses antiseptic activity. Methyl salicylate is used for analgesic activity, camphor and cajuput oil for counterirritant activity. Bees wax and petrolatum are absorption type of ointment base.

Observation Table

S. no.	Ingredients	Quantity given	Quantity taken
1.	Menthol	100 ml	2 ml
2.	Camphor	250 g	5 g
3.	Methyl salicylate	50 ml	1 ml
4.	Cassia oil	50 g	1 g
5.	Peppermint oil	60 ml	1.2 ml
6.	Cajuput oil	70 ml	1.4 ml
7.	Bees wax	300 g	6 g
8.	Petrolatum	120 g	2.4 g

Procedure: Melt 6 g of beeswax and 2.4 g of petrolatum in a dry china dish. Dissolve 2 ml of menthol, 5 g of camphor in 1 ml of methyl salicylate and to this add 1.1 ml of cassia oil, 1.2 ml of peppermint oil, and 1.4 ml of cajuput oil. Add the mix to cooled base just as it starts to solidify. Stir quickly until cool. Weigh out 20 g of ointment and transfer to an ointment jar with a screw cap.

Category: Anti-inflammatory and analgesic.

Storage: Keep container tightly closed after use. Store in a cool place.

Direction: For external use only. Not to be applied on broken skin. Apply to affected area with rubbing.

Uses: As an analgesic

Experiment Number 25

Object: To prepare and submit 25 g of non-staining iodine ointment BPC.

Principle: Ointments are semisolid preparations for application to the skin or mucosa. The common property of semisolid preparation is the ability to cling to the surface of application for reasonable duration before they are washed. This adhesion is due to their plastic rheological behavior, which allows the semisolid pharmaceutical preparations are pastes, creams, gel, etc. Ointments are semisolid greasy preparations for application to the skin, rectum and nasal mucosa. The base is usually anhydrous and contains the medicament in solution or suspension form. They are used for their emollient effect on skin, for the protection of lesion and for topical medication.

Ointment bases: Apart from drug, ointment consists of ointment base. Various types of bases are used depending upon characteristic of drug and product required. The bases are classified as:

1. Oleaginous bases. Ex: Soft paraffin, hard paraffin, etc.
2. Absorption bases. Ex: Non-emulsified w/o, etc.
3. Water removable (miscible).
4. Water soluble.

Ointment base used in non-staining iodine ointment is yellow soft paraffin, which is an example of oleaginous base. Yellow soft paraffin is preferred for darker constituent.

Non-staining iodine ointment which is used as analgesic, anti-inflammatory contains iodine which is complex with fixed oil containing fatty acid at 60°C which results in color change from brown to green black. This is done because free iodine has staining property and is irritant to skin and is used for veterinary use only. Here paraffin, i.e. ointment base is only used as a carrier of drug. Paraffin can absorb only 2% of iodine but fixed oil can bind with iodine equivalent to its weight.

Equation:

$$CH_3 (CH_2)_7 CH = CH (CH_2)_7 COOH + I_2 \rightarrow$$

Oleic acid $\quad CH_3 (CH_2)_7 CHI - CHI(CH_2)_7 COOH$

di-iodo-stearic acid

Observation Table

S. no.	Ingredients	Quantity given	Quantity taken
1.	Iodine	50 g	1.25 g
2.	Arachise oil	150 ml	3.75 ml
3.	Methyl salicylate	50 g	1.25 g
4.	Yellow soft paraffin (q.s)	1000 g	25 g

Procedure: Finely powder the iodine in a glass mortar and add required amount to the oil taken in a glass stoppered conical flask and stir well. Heat at 50°C and stir occasionally until the brown color has changed to greenish black. Take the required quantity of yellow soft paraffin in a China dish and warm soft paraffin and mix well. Measure the required volume of methyl salicylate and mix with base containing the iodized oil. Then pour into a warm wide mouth light resistance glass container and allow cooling without further stirring.

Category: Counterirritant, rubifacient, and anti-inflammatory and analgesic.

Storage: Store in a cool place and protect from light. Keep container tightly closed after use.

Direction: For external use only. Not to be applied on broken skin. Apply to affected area with rubbing.

Uses: Used as an anti-inflammatory and analgesic.

Experiment Number 26

Object: To prepare and dispense 10 g of face powder.

Principle: Face powder is a cosmetic powder applied to the face to set a foundation after application. It can also be reapplied throughout the day to minimize shininess caused by oily skin. There is translucent sheer powder, and there is pigmented powder. Certain types of pigmented facial powders are meant be worn alone with no base foundation. Powder tones the face and gives an even appearance. Besides toning the face, some powders with sunscreen can also reduce skin damage from sunlight and environmental stress. It comes packaged either as a compact or as loose powder. It can be applied with a sponge, brush, or powder puff. Uniform distribution over the face is achieved easier when a loose powder is applied.

Because of the wide variation among human skin tones, there is a corresponding variety of colors of face powder. There are also several types of powder. A common powder used in beauty products is talc (or baby powder), which is absorbent and provides toning to the skin. A good face powder should produce a smooth finish to the facial skin.

Observation Table

S. no.	Ingredients	Quantity given	Quantity taken
1.	Talc	630 g	6.3 g
2.	Kaolin	200 g	2 g
3.	Calcium carbonate (light)	50 g	0.5 g
4.	Zinc oxide	50 g	0.5 g
5.	Zinc stearate	50 g	0.5 g
6.	Magnesium carbonate	10 g	0.1 g
7.	Color	5 g	0.05 g
8.	Perfume	5 g	0.05 g

Procedure

1. Take talcum powder, kaolin and zinc oxide in ascending order and mix well in mortar vessel.
2. Add calcium carbonate, zinc citrate and magnesium carbonate in mortal and mix well.
3. Finally add one drop of perfume, mix all the constituents well, label it and dispense it in a suitable container.

Category: Cosmetic

Storage: Store in well-closed air tight container.

Direction: For external use only.

Use:

1. For beautification purpose.
2. For reducing perspiration.

Experiment Number 27

Object: To prepare and submit 20 g of cleansing cream.

Principle: One popular type of face wash is cleansing cream, which washes and moisturizes the skin, getting rid of dirt, sweat, makeup and bacteria. It is usually made from a combination of mineral oil, petrolatum, water and waxes. These cleansers may come in many different kinds of creams with their own methods of application. Some kinds might need to be applied to wet skin, massaged in until it forms a rich lather and then rinsed off. Others, such as cold cream, simply might require being applied to the skin and allowed to sit for a period of time before being either wiped off or removed with water. Most cleansing creams are oil and water emulsions, or moisturizers. The oil (usually mineral oil) is gentler than fat in removing excess oil from the skin. Because there is always the risk of removing too much oil from the skin and losing the natural moisture barrier, cleansing creams generally leave behind a protective layer of moisture to prevent skin from getting too dry.

Skin cream are those emulsion which are either o/w or w/o type. It is the texture and color of these emulsion that they are also named so keeping the body cleans, most important to the skin and primitive need.

1. It should liquefy at body temp.
2. It should be an emulsion type with a small % of water.

Types of Cleansing Cream

1. *Liquefying cream:* Translucent, liquefying type, anhydrous in character and consisting a mixture of hydrocarbon oil waxes which do not contain water.

2. *Emulsifying cream:* White emulsified cold cream (borax, bee wax) type contain large proportion of mineral.

Observation Table

S. no.	Ingredients	Quantity given	Quantity taken
1.	Mineral oil	280 g	5.6 g
2.	Isopropyl myristate	140 g	2.8 g
3.	Acetoglyceride	25 g	0.5 g
4.	Petroleum jelly	75 g	1.5 g
5.	Beeswax	150 g	3 g
6.	Borax	10 g	0.2 g
7.	Perfume	Adequate	Adequate
8.	Methyl paraben and propyl paraben	2 g	0.04 g
9.	Water (q.s)	1000 g	20 g

Procedure

1. Dissolved borax in hot water, separately melt waxy material like beeswax petroleum jelly and add mineral oil to it with constant stirring.
2. Heat the melted mass above 72°C and add powdered borax in the melted mass at room temp.
3. Dissolve parabens in water to form a clear solution. Add this clear solution to above mixture with constant stirring, when the temp dropped at 40–50°C, then added perfume to preparation and keep it for 15 minutes in ice cold water.

Category: Cosmetic

Storage: Store in a cool and dry place, away from sunlight.

Direction: Cream are to be applied on skin.

Use: For cleansing action.

Experiment Number 28

Object: To prepare 10 g of coal tar and salicylic acid ointment.

Principle: Ointments are semisolid preparations for application to the skin or mucosa. The common property of semisolid preparation is the ability to cling to the surface of application for reasonable duration before they are washed. This adhesion is due to their plastic rheological behavior, which allows the semisolid pharmaceutical preparations are pastes, creams, gel, etc. Ointments are semisolid greasy preparations for application to the skin, rectum and nasal mucosa. The base is usually anhydrous and contains the medicament in solution or suspension form. They are used for their emollient effect on skin, for the protection of lesion and for topical medication.

Ointment bases: Apart from drug, ointment consists of ointment base. Various types of bases are used depending upon characteristic of drug and product required. The bases are classified as

1. Oleaginous bases. Ex: Soft paraffin, hard paraffin, etc.
2. Absorption bases. Ex: Non-emulsified w/o, etc.
3. Water removable (miscible).
4. Water soluble.

Ointment base used in non-staining iodine ointment is yellow soft paraffin, which is an example of oleaginous base. Yellow soft paraffin is preferred for darker constituent.

Observation Table

S. no.	Ingredients	Quantity given	Quantity taken
1.	Coal tar	20 g	0.20 g
2.	Polysorbate 80	40 ml	0.40 ml
3.	Salicylic acid	20 g	0.20 g
4.	Emulsifying wax	114 g	1.14 g
5.	White soft paraffin	190 g	1.9 g
6.	Coconut oil	540 ml	5.40 ml
7.	Liquid paraffin	76 ml	0.76 ml

Procedure

1. Melt the white paraffin and coconut oil.
2. Add liquid paraffin previously warmed at the same temperature and mix (A).
3. Disperse the coal tar in the polysorbate 80.
4. Incorporate the salicylic acid and mix with the previously melted emulsifying wax (B).
5. Add (A) with stirring to the (B), mix thoroughly and stir until cold.

Category: Local irritant

Storage: Preserve in a well-closed container, protect from light.

Uses: Local irritant, disinfectant.

It is used for topical treatment of conditions like acne, seborrheicdermatitis, psoriasis, warts, corns, calluses and hyperkeratotic skin disorders.

Experiment Number 29

Object: To prepare 25 g of foundation cream.

Principle: Foundation creams are applied to the skin to provide a smooth emollient base or foundation before the application of face powder and other make-up preparations. They help the powder to adhere to the skin due to possession of good holding power. They should spread well, be non-greasy and should leave non-occlusive film on the face. The humectants present in the preparation helps powder retention. Lanolin also does help in retention of powder. Apart from the materials mentioned in vanishing creams, additionally mineral oil may be added to promote powder adhesion. The low surface tension of isopropyl myristate, butyl stearate, and similar esters results in closer adhesion of the film and softer feeling of the skin.

The foundation creams can be of two types:

1. Pigmented creams which are colored.
2. Unpigmented creams.

Observation Table

S. no.	Ingredients	Quantity given	Quantity taken
1.	Lanolin	20 g	0.5 g
2.	Cetyl alcohol	5 g	0.125 g
3.	Stearic acid	98 g	2.45 g
4.	Potassium hydroxide	4 g	0.1 g
5.	Propylene glycol	80 g	2 g
6.	Perfume	Adequate	Adequate
7.	Methy paraben and propyl paraben	2 g	0.05 ml
8.	Water (q.s)	1000 g	25 g

Procedure

1. Heat ingredients of oil phase like lanolin, cetyl alcohol and stearic acid separately to 75°C (A).
2. Add the perfume when the temperature is about 35°C.
3. Dissolve potassium hydroxide, propylene glycol in water and add parabens to it (B).
4. Add (A) with stirring to the (B), mix thoroughly.
5. Finally a milling will give a good product and allow it to stand in ice cold water.

Category: Cosmetic

Storage: Store in a cool and dry place.

Uses: They are applied to the skin before the make-up.

Experiment Number 30

Object: To prepare 25 g of all-purpose cream.

Principle: In recent times there has been a tremendous increase in the consumption of preparations which are normally known as all-purpose creams. These were also known as 'sports cream' as they were used by sportsmen in skiing and outdoor activities. They are somewhat oily but non-greasy type and can spread easily on the skin to give a protective film. They can also function, when applied excessively, as a skinfood or nourishing cream, or night cream or protective cream for prevention or alleviation of sunburn, or for the treatment of roughened skin areas.

These preparations are mainly based on wool alcohols, which consist of the alcoholic fraction obtained by saponification of the grease of the wool of sheep and contain not less than 28% of cholesterol. Its value as a water-in-oil emulsifier is due to the property of absorption of water. But this character can be lost due to oxidation and thus an antioxidant, like butylated hydroxyanisole, is to be used. If oxidation occurs, water can be lost from the base and can seep out. As these preparations need to spread easily, microcrystalline wax can be used. Mineral oils, paraffin are used to get protective layer. Magnesium sulfate is used to enhance the stability of the creams by the presence of magnesium ions in aqueous phase. Methyl and propyl parahydroxy benzoates can be used as preservatives to prevent microbial growth. Suitable perfumes are also to be added. The preparations are normally water-in-oil.

Observation Table

S. no.	Ingredients	Quantity given	Quantity taken
1.	Wool alcohol	58 g	1.45 g
2.	Hard paraffin	240 g	6 g
3.	White soft paraffin	100 g	2.5 g
4.	Liquid paraffin	600 g	15 g
5.	BHT and BHA	2 g	0.05 g
6.	Perfume	Adequate	Adequate

Procedure

1. Heat the ingredients wool alcohol, hard paraffin and white soft paraffin to 75°C (A).

2. In a separate beaker take liquid paraffin add BHA and BHT (B).

3. Add the perfume when the temperature is about 35°C.

4. Add (A) with stirring to the (B) mix thoroughly.

5. Finally a milling will give a good product and allow it to stand in ice cold water.

Category: Cosmetic.

Storage: Store in a cool and dry place.

Uses: They are applied on the skin.

Experiment Number 31

Object: To prepare 100 ml of hair conditioner

Principle: A substance used, often after shampooing, to detangle and improve the condition of the hair. Like shampoo, it is applied to wet hair and then rinsed out after applying. Conditioners are used after shampooing the hair, to render the hair more lustrous, easy to comb, and free from static electricity when dry. They are also used to improve damaged hair. Hair may be damaged by excessive use of bleaches and permanent waves. Conditioners are usually based on cationic detergents and fatty materials like lanolin or mineral oil.

Observation Table

S. no.	Ingredients	Quantity given	Quantity taken
1.	Stearyl alcohol	6 g	0.6 g
2.	GMS (glyceryl monostearate)	2 g	0.2 g
3.	Sodium chloride	2 g	0.2 g
4.	Benzalkonium chloride	15 g	1.5 g
5.	Color	Adequate	Adequate
6.	Perfume	Adequate	Adequate
7.	Water (q.s)	1000 ml	100 ml

Procedure

1. Heat ingredients of oil phase like GMS, stearyl alcohol in a separate beaker to 75°C. (A).
2. Add the perfume when the temperature is about 35°C.
3. Dissolve sodium chloride, benzalkonium chloride in water (B).
4. Add (A) with stirring to the (B), mix thoroughly.
5. Finally a milling will give a good product and allow it to stand in ice cold water.

Category: As hair cleansing preparation.

Storage: Store in a cool and dry place , away from sunlight.

Uses: They are used to improve damaged hair.

To recondition and revitalize the look and texture of hair.

Experiment Number 32

Object: To prepare 25 g of brushless shaving cream.

Principle: This preparation does not require brush to produce lather. After washing off the face with soap and warm water, these shaving creams are applied to keep the beard soft till the shaving is completed. Initial washing helps in making the hair soft. The creams function is to prevent the keratin from drying and hardening. As these creams are applied on wet face, they should be miscible with water for uniform spreading. They mainly consist of stearate, soaps and additionally contain oils, humectants, viscosity enhancing agent. The fatty substances should be at least 20%. Incorporation of some waxes can enhance the viscosity and it is required as consistency is important for proper application. Perfumes and preservatives are also incorporated.

Observation Table

S. no.	Ingredients	Quantity given	Quantity taken
1.	Stearic acid	160 g	4 g
2.	Mineral oil	140 g	3.5 g
3.	Spermaceti	20 g	0.5 g
4.	Glycerin	58 ml	1.45 g
5.	Dil. Ammonia sol	20 g	0.5 g
6.	Methyl paraben and propyl paraben	2 g	0.05 g
7.	Perfume	Adequate	Adequate
8.	Water (q.s)	1000 ml	25 ml

Procedure

1. Heat ingredients of oil phase like spermaceti, mineral oil and stearic acid separately to 75°C (A).
2. Add the perfume when the temperature is about 35°C.
3. Dissolve parabens, dil ammonia sol. in water. (B)
4. Add (A) with stirring to the (B) mix thoroughly.
5. Finally a milling will give a good product and allow it to stand in ice cold water.

Category: As shaving preparation.

Storage: Store in a cool and dry place.

Uses: These shaving creams are applied to keep the beard soft till the shaving is completed.

Experiment Number 33

Object: To prepare 25 g of aftershave cream.

Principle: The aftershave preparations are basically applied to cool and refresh the skin, to overcome irritation on the skin, to neutralize the soreness, to disinfect or heal the skin damage or cut. They are used in the form of lotions, creams or powders. The lotions are clear solutions containing 25 to 50% alcohol.

Additionally they may also contain antiseptic, emollient, haemostyptic substances, boric acid, alum, potassium oxyquinoline sulphate and chloroform. If alcohol content is less, the perfume should be water soluble or soluble in less concentrations of alcohol. Alternatively, solubilizing agents may be used.

Most of the lotions are used as aftershave preparations. Powders are also used to some extent but use of creams is comparatively less. The useful antibacterial or antiseptic substances are quaternary ammonium compounds, chlorhexidine diacetate. Creams are preferred for skins sensitive to alcoholic lotions. Creams can also give extra benefit to the skin like any other emollient or protective creams.

Observation Table

S. no.	Ingredients	Quantity given	Quantity taken
1.	Toilet spirit	500 g	12.5 g
2.	Glycerin	30 g	0.75 g
3.	Cetrimide	1 g	0.025 g
4.	Perfume	Adequate	Adequate
5.	Water (q.s)	1000 g	25 g

Procedure: Heat ingredients of oil phase and aqueous phase separately to 75°C and mix the latter to the former slowly with continuous stirring. Cool while stirring. Add the perfume when the temperature is about 35°C. Preservative should be added to water before mixing with oil phase. Finally a milling will give a good product.

Category: Cosmetic

Storage: Store in a cool and dry place, away from sunlight.

Uses: Applied to the shaving area of skin to provide a smooth texture.

Appendices

ABSORBENTS

Bentonite

Kaolin

Magnesium carbonate

Magnesium oxide

Magnesium silicate

Silica (cab-o-sil, syloid, aerosol)

Starch

Tricalcium phosphate

ANTIADHESIVES

Colloidal silica

Corn starch

DL-Leucine

Magnesium stearate

Metallic stearates

Sodium lauryl sulfate

Talc

ANTIFOAMING AGENTS

Ariacel C

Atlas G 1706

Ethylene glycol fatty acid ester

(Emcol EC-50)

G.M.S.

Propylene glycol monostearate

Span 65

Span 85

ANTIOXIDANTS

Acetone

Ascorbic acid

Ascorbyl palmitate

Benzoin

Beta-naphthol

Butylated hydroxytoluene

Butylated hydroxyanisole

Citric acid

Cysteine hydrochloride

Maleic acid

Monoisopropylcitrate

Nor-dihydroguaiaretic acid

Phenyl alphanapthlamine

Propyl gallate

Pyrogallol

Pyrocatechol

Sodium bisulfite

Sodium formaldehyde sulfoxylate

Contd.

APPENDIX I *Contd.*

Dilauryl thiodipropionate	Sodium metabisulfite
Distearylthiodipropionate	Sodium sulfate
Ethylgallate	Sodium thiosulfate
Gallic acid	Thioglycerol
Glycerin	Thiosolbitol
Guaiac resin	Thiourea
Hydroquinon	Thioglycollic acid
Isoascorbic acid	Alpha tocopherol
Lecithin	Trihydroxybutyrophenone

COLORING AGENTS

1. Natural

Alizarin	Hesperidin
Anattenes	Indigo
Caramel	Quercetin
Beta-carotene	Riboflavin
Carbon black	Rubia tinctorum
Carmic acid	Rutin
Chlorophyll	Saffron
Cochineal	Titanium dioxide
Curcumin	Turmeric
Ferric oxides (red and yellow)	Tyrian purple

2. Synthetic

Alizarin cyanine	Indigo carmine 73015
Amaranth I N 16785	Napthol blue black 20470
Brilliant Blue FCS 42090	Orange G 16 30
Carmoisine 14720	Ponceaux 4 16255
Eosine G 45380	Quinazarine 61565
Erythorosin 45430	Quinoline yellow SS 47000
Fast red E 16045	Resoroin brown 20170
Fast green FCF 42053	Sudan III 26100
Green S 44090	Sunset yellow FCF 15185
Freen F 61570	Tartrazine 19140

EMULSIFYING AGENTS

1. Surfactants forming monomolecular films

Alkylpolyoxyethylene sulfates   Polyoxyethylene monolaurate
(Atlas G 2127)

Contd.

APPENDIX I *Contd.*

Benzalkonium chloride	(Polyoxyethylene alkylphenol (Igepal CA 630)
Cetrimide	Polyoxyethylene sorbitan monolaurate (Tween 20)
Dioctylsodium sulfosuccinate	Polyoxyethylene sorbitan monopalmitate (Tween 40)
Lauryldimethylbenzyl-ammonium chloride	Polyoxyethylene sorbitan (Tween 80)
Lecithin	Polyoxyethylene laurylether (Brij 35)
N-cetyl N-ethyl morpholinium ethosulfate (Atlas G -263)	Monostearate (Myrj 52)
PEG 400 monostearate	Castor oil (Atlas G 1974)
Polyoxyethylene laurylether (Brij 30)	Potassium oleate
Polyoxyethylene monostearate (Myrj 45)	Sodium oleate
Propylene glycol monostearate	Sodium lauryl sulfate
Propylene glycol monostearate (Atlas G 917)	Sorbitan monopalmitate (Span 40)
Sorbitan monolaurate (Span 20)	Sorbitan monostearate (Arlacel 60)
Glyceryl monostearate (GMS)	Sodium laurate
Sorbitan sesquioleate (Alacel C)	Triethanolmine oleate
Potassium stearate	Triethanolamine stearate

2. Surfactants forming multimolecular films

Acacia	Hectorite
Agar	Magnesium hydroxide
Alginates	Pectin
Atapulgite	Silica gel
Bentonite	Tragacanth
Gelatin	Veegum

FLAVORING AGENTS

Almond	Oil of anise
Amyl acetate	Oil of bergamot
Anethol	Oil of caraway

Contd.

APPENDIX I *Contd.*

Apricot
Apple
Banana
Benzaldehyde
Black current
Blueberry
Butterscotch
Burgundy
Cherry
Chocolate
Custard
Ethyl acetate
Ethyl vanillin
Eucalyptol
Eugenol
Ginger
Hyacinth
Jasmine
Lemongrass
Liquorice
Mango
Maple
Methyl salicylate
Melon
Narcissus
Neroli
Violet

Oil of cardamom
Oil of cinnamon
Oil of clove
Oil of coriander
Oil of fennel
Oil of lemon
Oil of lavender
Oil of nutmeg
Oil of orange
Oil of narcissus
Oil of peppermint
Oil of rosemary
Oil of rose
Oil of spearmint
Oil of thyme
Orris root
Peach
Phenyl ethyl alcohol
Pineapple
Plum
Raspberry
Sandalwood
Saffron
Strawberry
Thymol
Vanillin

FLOCCULATING AGENTS

Electrolytes like KH_2PO_4, $AlCl_3$, NaCl, etc.

Ionic and non-ionic surfactants
Hydrocolloids

PRESERVATIVES

Banzalkonium chloride
Benzoic acid and benzoates
Benzylalcohol
Cetylpyridinium chloride
Chlorbutanol

Boric acid and propyl alcohol
Cetrimide
Dichlorophene
Ortho and parachlorbenzoic acid
Parahydroxybenzoates

Contd.

APPENDIX I *Contd.*

Chlorothymol
p-Chlorphenylglyceryl ether
Dichlorometasylenol
Dehydroacetic acid

Formic acid
Formaldehyde

Parachlor metacresol
Parachlor metaxylenol
p-Chlor phenylpropanediol
Phenylmercuric nitrate and other
salts of phyenylmercuric acid
Phenol
Phenol hexachlorophene

SOLUBILISING AGENTS

Atlas G 1690
Atlas G 1794
Brij 35
Igepal CA 630
Myrj 45
Myrj 49
Myrj 51
Myrj 52

PEG 400 monostearate
Sodium oleate
Triethanolamine oleate
Tween 20
Tween 40
Tween 60
Tween 80

SUSPENDING AGENTS

Acacia
Agar
Alginates
Attapulgite
Bentonite
Carboxy methyl celluloses
Carbopol
Carbomer
Cellulose powder
Chondorus
Gelatin
Guar gum

Hectorite
Hydroxyethyl cellulose
Hydroxyl propyl cellulose
Methyl celluloses
Microcrystalline cellulose
Polyvinyl alcohol
Povidone
Psyllium seed gum
Pectin
Tragacanth
Veegum

SWEETENING AGENTS

Aspartame
Cyclamates
Dextrose
Fructose
Glycerin

Maltose
Mannitol
Neohsperidin dehydrochalone
Saccharin
Sorbitol

Contd.

Glycyrrhizin	Sucrose
Honey	Xylitol
Lactose	

WETTING AGENTS

| Tween 20 | Span 20 |
| Brij 30 | Span 40 |

APPENDIX II
UNITS AND CONVERSION FACTORS

Length	1 inch	= 0.0254 m
	1 ft	= 0.3048 m
Area	1 ft^2	= 0.0929 m^2
Volume	1 ft^3	= 0.0283 m^3
	1 gal Imp	= 0.004546 m^3
	1 gal US	= 0.003785 m^3 = 3.785 litres
	1 litre	= 0.001 m^3
Mass	1 lb	= 0.4536 kg
	1 mole	molecular weight in kg
Density	1 lb/ft^3	= 16.03 kg m^{-3}
Velocity	1 ft/sec	= 0.3048 m s^{-1}
Pressure	1 lb/m^2	= 6894 Pa
	1 torr	= 133.3 Pa
	1 atm	= 1.013 × 10^5 Pa = 760 mm Hg
	1 Pa	= 1 N m^{-2} = 1 kg m^{-1} s^{-2}
Force	1 Newton1 lb ft s^{-2}	= 1 kg m s^{-2} = 1.49 kg m s^{-2}
Viscosity	1 cP	= 0.001 N s m^{-2} = 0.001 Pa s
	1 lb/ft sec	= 1.49 N s m^{-2} = 1.49 kg m^{-1} s^{-2}
Energy	1 Btu	= 1055 J
	1 cal	= 4.186 J
Power	1 kW1 W	= 1 kJ s^{-1} = 1 J s^{-1}
	1 horsepower	= 745.7 W = 745.7 J s^{-1}
		= 0.746 kW
	1 ton refrigeration	= 3.519 kW

Contd.

APPENDIX II *Contd.*

Temperature units	(°F)	$= 5/9\ (°C) = 5/9\ (K)$
Heat-transfer coefficient	1 Btu ft^{-2} h^{-1} °F^{-1}	$= 5.678\ J\ m^{-2}\ s^{-1}\ °C$
Thermal conductivity	1 Btu ft^{-1} h^{-1} °F^{-1}	$= 1.731\ J\ m^{-1}\ s^{-1}\ °C^{-1}$
Constants	π	3.1416
	e (base of natural logs)	2.7183
	R	8.314 kJ mole^{-1} K^{-1} or 0.08206 m^3 atm mole^{-1} K^{-1}

(M) Mega = 10^6, (k) kilo = 10^3, (H) Hecto = 10^2, (m) milli = 10^{-3}, (μ) micro = 10^{-6}

Index